CLINICALLY RELEVANT RESISTANCE IN CANCER CHEMOTHERAPY

Cancer Treatment and Research

Steven T. Rosen, M.D., *Series Editor*

Goldstein, L.J., Ozols, R. F. (eds.): *Anticancer Drug Resistance. Advances in Molecular and Clinical Research.* 1994. ISBN 0-7923-2836-1.
Hong, W.K., Weber, R.S. (eds.): *Head and Neck Cancer. Basic and Clinical Aspects.* 1994. ISBN 0-7923-3015-3.
Thall, P.F. (ed): *Recent Advances in Clinical Trial Design and Analysis.* 1995. ISBN 0-7923-3235-0.
Buckner, C. D. (ed): *Technical and Biological Components of Marrow Transplantation.* 1995. ISBN 0-7923-3394-2.
Winter, J.N. (ed.): *Blood Stem Cell Transplantation.* 1997. ISBN 0-7923-4260-7.
Muggia, F.M. (ed): *Concepts, Mechanisms, and New Targets for Chemotherapy.* 1995. ISBN 0-7923-3525-2.
Klastersky, J. (ed): *Infectious Complications of Cancer.* 1995. ISBN 0-7923-3598-8.
Kurzrock, R., Talpaz, M. (eds): *Cytokines: Interleukins and Their Receptors.* 1995. ISBN 0-7923-3636-4.
Sugarbaker, P. (ed): *Peritoneal Carcinomatosis: Drugs and Diseases.* 1995. ISBN 0-7923-3726-3.
Sugarbaker, P. (ed): *Peritoneal Carcinomatosis: Principles of Management.* 1995. ISBN 0-7923-3727-1.
Dickson, R.B., Lippman, M.E. (eds.): *Mammary Tumor Cell Cycle, Differentiation and Metastasis.* 1995. ISBN 0-7923-3905-3.
Freireich, E.J, Kantarjian, H. (eds.): *Molecular Genetics and Therapy of Leukemia.* 1995. ISBN 0-7923-3912-6.
Cabanillas, F., Rodriguez, M.A. (eds.): *Advances in Lymphoma Research.* 1996. ISBN 0-7923-3929-0.
Miller, A.B. (ed.): *Advances in Cancer Screening.* 1996. ISBN 0-7923-4019-1.
Hait , W.N. (ed.): *Drug Resistance.* 1996. ISBN 0-7923-4022-1.
Pienta, K.J. (ed.): *Diagnosis and Treatment of Genitourinary Malignancies.* 1996. ISBN 0-7923-4164-3.
Arnold, A.J. (ed.): *Endocrine Neoplasms.* 1997. ISBN 0-7923-4354-9.
Pollock, R.E. (ed.): *Surgical Oncology.* 1997. ISBN 0-7923-9900-5.
Verweij, J., Pinedo, H.M., Suit, H.D. (eds.): *Soft Tissue Sarcomas: Present Achievements and Future Prospects.* 1997. ISBN 0-7923-9913-7.
Walterhouse, D.O., Cohn, S. L. (eds.): *Diagnostic and Therapeutic Advances in Pediatric Oncology.* 1997. ISBN 0-7923-9978-1.
Mittal, B.B., Purdy, J.A., Ang, K.K. (eds.): *Radiation Therapy.* 1998. ISBN 0-7923-9981-1.
Foon, K.A., Muss, H.B. (eds.): *Biological and Hormonal Therapies of Cancer.* 1998. ISBN 0-7923-9997-8.
Ozols, R.F. (ed.): *Gynecologic Oncology.* 1998. ISBN 0-7923-8070-3.
Noskin, G. A. (ed.): *Management of Infectious Complications in Cancer Patients.* 1998. ISBN 0-7923-8150-5
Bennett, C. L. (ed.): *Cancer Policy.* 1998. ISBN 0-7923-8203-X
Benson, A. B. (ed.): *Gastrointestinal Oncology.* 1998. ISBN 0-7923-8205-6
Tallman, M.S. , Gordon, L.I. (eds.): *Diagnostic and Therapeutic Advances in Hematologic Malignancies.* 1998. ISBN 0-7923-8206-4
von Gunten, C.F. (ed.): *Palliative Care and Rehabilitation of Cancer Patients.* 1999. ISBN 0-7923-8525-X
Burt, R.K., Brush, M.M. (eds): *Advances in Allogeneic Hematopoietic Stem Cell Transplantation.* 1999. ISBN 0-7923-7714-1
Angelos, P. (ed): *Ethical Issues in Cancer Patient Care* 2000. ISBN 0-7923-7726-5
Gradishar, W.J., Wood, W.C. (eds): *Advances in Breast Cancer Management.* 2000. ISBN 0-7923-7890-3
Sparano, Joseph A. (ed.): *HIV & HTLV-I Associated Malignancies.* 2001. ISBN 0-7923-7220-4.
Ettinger, David S. (ed.): *Thoracic Oncology.* 2001. ISBN 0-7923-7248-4.
Bergan, Raymond C. (ed.): *Cancer Chemoprevention.* 2001. ISBN 0-7923-7259-X.
Raza, A., Mundle, S.D. (eds): *Myelodysplastic Syndromes & Secondary Acute Myelogenous Leukemia* 2001. ISBN: 0-7923-7396.
Talamonti, Mark S. (ed.): *Liver Directed Therapy for Primary and Metastatic Liver Tumors.* 2001. ISBN 0-7923-7523-8.
Stack, M.S., Fishman, D.A. (eds): *Ovarian Cancer.* 2001. ISBN 0-7923-7530-0.
Bashey, A., Ball, E.D. (eds): *Non-Myeloablative Allogeneic Transplantation.* 2002. ISBN 0-7923-7646-3
Leong, Stanley P.L. (ed.): *Atlas of Selective Sentinel Lymphadenectomy for Melanoma, Breast Cancer and Colon Cancer.* 2002. ISBN 1-4020-7013-6
Andersson , B., Murray D., (eds.): *Clinically Relevant Resistance in Cancer Chemotherapy.* 2002. ISBN 1-4020-7200-7

CLINICALLY RELEVANT RESISTANCE IN CANCER CHEMOTHERAPY

edited by

Borje Andersson, M.D., Ph.D.
MD Anderson Cancer Center
Houston, Texas, USA.

and

David Murray, Ph.D.
Cross Cancer Institute
Edmonton, Alberta, Canada.

KLUWER ACADEMIC PUBLISHERS
Boston / Dordrecht / London

Distributors for North, Central and South America:
Kluwer Academic Publishers
101 Philip Drive
Assinippi Park
Norwell, Massachusetts 02061 USA
Telephone (781) 871-6600
Fax (781) 681-9045
E-Mail: kluwer@wkap.com

Distributors for all other countries:
Kluwer Academic Publishers Group
Post Office Box 322
3300 AH Dordrecht, THE NETHERLANDS
Telephone 31 786 576 000
Fax 31 786 576 474
E-Mail: services@wkap.nl

Electronic Services <http://www.wkap.nl>

Library of Congress Cataloging-in-Publication Data

A C.I.P. Catalogue record for this book is available
from the Library of Congress.

Printed on acid-free paper.

Printed in the United States of America.

The Publisher offers discounts on this book for course use and bulk purchases. For further information, send email to laura.walsh@wkap.com.

TABLE OF CONTENTS

Chapter 7
DNA repair in resistance to bifunctional alkylating and platinating agents. David Murray

Chapter 8
Leukemic cell insensitivity to cyclophosphamide and other oxazaphosphorines mediated by aldehyde dehydrogenase(s).
Norman E. Sládek

Chapter 15

Clinical pharmacology of melphalan and its implications for clinical resistance to anticancer agents. Roy B. Jones

Chapter 16

Pharmacological considerations of primary alkylators.
Jeannine S. McCune and John T. Slattery

Chapter 17
Genomic approaches to clinical drug resistance.
Sambasivarao Damaraju, Michael Sawyer and Brent Zanke

CONTRIBUTORS

Borje S Andersson, Department of Blood and Marrow Transplantation, The University of Texas MD Anderson Cancer Center, Houston, Texas, USA.

Michael Andreeff, Section of Molecular Hematology and Therapy, Department of Blood and Marrow Transplantation, The University of Texas MD Anderson Cancer Center, Houston, Texas, USA.

Stephen A Baldwin, School of Biochemistry and Molecular Biology, University of Leeds, Leeds, United Kingdom.

Gerald Batist, The Center for Translational Research in Cancer, McGill University and Lady Davis Institute for Medical Research, Sir Mortimer B Davis-Jewish General Hospital, Montréal, Québec, Canada.

Richard A Britten, Department of Radiation Oncology, Eastern Virginia Medical School, Norfolk, Virginia, USA.

Carol E Cass, Departments of Oncology and Biochemistry, University of Alberta, and Department of Experimental Oncology, Cross Cancer Institute, Edmonton, Alberta, Canada.

Marilyn L Clarke, Department of Experimental Oncology, Cross Cancer Institute, Edmonton, Alberta, Canada.

O Michael Colvin, Department of Medicine, Duke University Comprehensive Cancer Center, Duke University Medical Center, Durham, North Carolina, USA.

Sambasivarao Damaraju, Polyomx Program and Department of Experimental Oncology, Cross Cancer Institute, Edmonton, Alberta, Canada.

Alison J Davis, Department of Medical Oncology and Hematology, Princess Margaret Hospital and University of Toronto, Toronto, Ontario, Canada.

Lei Deng, Department of Molecular Pathology, The University of Texas MD Anderson Cancer Center, Houston, Texas, USA.

Paul Dent, Department of Pharmacology and Toxicology and Department of Radiation Oncology, Medical College of Virginia, Virginia Commonwealth University, Richmond, Virginia, USA.

Paul B Fisher, Department of Pathology and Urology, Columbia University College of Physicians and Surgeons, New York, New York, USA.

Nasser Fotouhi-Ardakani, Department of Experimental Medicine, McGill University and Lady Davis Institute for Medical Research, Sir Mortimer B Davis-Jewish General Hospital, Montréal, Québec, Canada.

Henry S Friedman, Department of Neuro-Oncology, Duke University Comprehensive Cancer Center, Duke University Medical Center, Durham, North Carolina, USA.

Michael P Gamcsik, Duke Comprehensive Cancer Center and Department of Medicine, Duke University Medical Center, Durham, North Carolina, USA.

Steven Grant, Department of Pharmacology and Toxicology and Department of Hematology/Oncology, Medical College of Virginia, Virginia Commonwealth University, Richmond, Virginia, USA.

David Hamilton, Department of Pharmacology and Therapeutics, McGill University and Lady Davis Institute for Medical Research, Sir Mortimer B Davis-Jewish General Hospital, Montréal, Québec, Canada.

Toshihisa Ishikawa, Department of Biomolecular Engineering, Graduate School of Bioscience and Biotechnology, Tokyo Institute of Technology, Yokohama, Japan.

Stewart P Johnson, Departments of Neuro-Oncology and Neurosurgery, Duke University Comprehensive Cancer Center, Duke University Medical Center, Durham, North Carolina, USA.

Roy B Jones, Bone Marrow Transplant Program, University of Colorado Health Science Center, Denver, Colorado, USA.

Marina Konopleva, Section of Molecular Hematology and Therapy, Department of Blood and Marrow Transplantation, The University of Texas MD Anderson Cancer Center, Houston, Texas, USA.

M Tien Kuo, Department of Molecular Pathology, The University of Texas MD Anderson Cancer Center, Houston, Texas, USA.

Randy Legerski, Department of Molecular Genetics, The University of Texas MD Anderson Cancer Center, Houston, Texas, USA.

Yen-Chiu Lin-Lee, Department of Molecular Pathology, The University of Texas MD Anderson Cancer Center, Houston, Texas, USA.

Susan M Ludeman, Duke Comprehensive Cancer Center and Department of Medicine, Duke University Medical Center, Durham, North Carolina, USA.

John R Mackey, Departments of Medicine and Experimental Oncology, Cross Cancer Institute, and Department of Oncology, University of Alberta, Edmonton, Alberta, Canada.

Jeannine S McCune, Department of Clinical Research, Fred Hutchinson Cancer Research Center, and Department of Pharmacy, University of Washington, Seattle, Washington, USA.

David Murray, Department of Oncology, University of Alberta, and Department of Experimental Oncology, Cross Cancer Institute, Edmonton, Alberta, Canada.

Christopher Richie, Department of Molecular Genetics, The University of Texas MD Anderson Cancer Center, Houston, Texas, USA.

Michael Sawyer, Polyomx Program and Department of Medicine, Cross Cancer Institute, Edmonton, Alberta, Canada.

Zahid H Siddik, Department of Experimental Therapeutics, The University of Texas MD Anderson Cancer Center, Houston, Texas, USA.

Norman E Sladek, Department of Pharmacology, University of Minnesota, Minneapolis, Minnesota, USA.

John T Slattery, Department of Clinical Research, Fred Hutchinson Cancer Research Center, and Department of Pharmaceutics, University of Washington, Seattle, Washington, USA.

Ian F Tannock, Department of Medical Oncology and Hematology, Princess Margaret Hospital and University of Toronto, Toronto, Ontario, Canada.

Shigaru Tatebe, Department of Molecular Pathology, The University of Texas MD Anderson Cancer Center, Houston, Texas, USA.

James D Young, Department of Physiology, University of Alberta, Edmonton, Alberta, Canada.

Brent Zanke, Polyomx Program and Departments of Medicine and Experimental Oncology, Cross Cancer Institute, Edmonton, Alberta, Canada.

PREFACE

Over the last several decades, the introduction of new chemotherapeutic drugs and drug combinations has resulted in increased long-term remission rates in several important tumor types. These include childhood leukemia, adult leukemias and lymphomas, as well as testicular and trophoblastic tumors. The addition of high-dose chemotherapy with growth factor and hemopoietic stem cell support has increased clinical remission rates even further. For the majority of patients with some of the more common malignancies, however, palliation (rather than cure) is still the most realistic goal of chemotherapy for metastatic disease. The failure of chemotherapy to cure metastatic cancer is commonly referred to among clinicians as "drug resistance". This phenomenon can, however, often be viewed as the survival of malignant cells that resulted from a failure to deliver an effective drug dose to the (cellular) target because of any one of or combination of a multitude of individual factors. Clinically, this treatment failure is often viewed as the rapid occurrence of resistance at the single cell level. However, in experimental systems, stable drug resistance is usually relatively slow to emerge. Clinical "drug resistance" may be caused by some combination of: [a] resistance of individual cells to the delivered treatment; [b] unfavorable drug-host interactions: tumor cells may be exposed to a limited drug concentration because of a high rate of metabolic drug degradation and/or altered regional blood supply; in this case, individual tumor cells may still be sensitive to the used chemotherapy; and [c] unfavorable malignant cell-host interactions that result in the survival and proliferation of the neoplastic cells.

We as a scientific community have come to realize that inter-individual genetic differences are of major importance for metabolic drug handling, and that this may be of the utmost importance for clinical treatment outcome. Furthermore, as our knowledge of the molecular mechanisms that operate to confer drug resistance at the single-cell level increases, we are developing the ability to create probes that can be used to study malignant-cell drug resistance at the clinical level, in addition to studying the clinical pharmacology of anticancer drugs both at the patient level and (sometimes) at the tumor cell level. An integration of clinical and experimental investigations will improve the understanding of clinically relevant drug resistance, and ultimately it should also assist us in improving the treatment of human cancer.

Recently, rapid technological advances have enabled high-throughput studies of genetic polymorphisms and cellular proteomes. This has opened up entirely new approaches not only to the study of drug resistance in model systems but also to the individualization of chemotherapy in order to decrease clinical toxicity and optimize treatment results. This volume reviews clinically relevant aspects of both cellular/experimental resistance to commonly used anticancer agents and the importance of the pharmacokinetics of such agents, as well as some of the developments that can be expected over the next 5-10 years.

Finally, we would like to acknowledge the major contributions from all of our co-authors, without whose hard work and patience we would not have been able to complete this volume. Our administrative assistants, Sandy Deib and Muriel Giese, are to be complimented for their never-ending tolerance and for their administrative and technical support in all aspects of the preparation of these chapters.

Borje Andersson

David Murray

Chapter 1

TUMOR PHYSIOLOGY AND RESISTANCE TO CHEMOTHERAPY: REPOPULATION AND DRUG PENETRATION

Alison J. Davis and Ian F. Tannock
Department of Medical Oncology and Hematology, Princess Margaret Hospital and University of Toronto, Toronto, Ontario, Canada

1. INTRODUCTION

Advances in the treatment of cancer with chemotherapy have been extremely limited over the past few decades. For a few malignancies, such as Hodgkin's disease and other lymphomas, testicular cancer, and leukemia in children, cure is a realistic and frequently attainable goal, even in the advanced setting. However, for the majority of solid tumors the impact of chemotherapy on survival is at best modest. For tumors that have already metastasized, chemotherapy may provide palliation through transient improvement in symptoms, but has little or no impact on the duration of survival[1]. Adjuvant chemotherapy following surgery for apparently localized disease has shown a small survival benefit in several tumor types, including node-positive breast and colon cancer. However, for the majority of patients their disease will recur despite adjuvant chemotherapy, at which point it is generally incurable. The relative cell survival after a six month course of adjuvant chemotherapy for breast cancer has been estimated to be as high as 10^{-2} or even greater[2]. This failure to eradicate all tumor cells has commonly been attributed to the intrinsic resistance of tumor cells to chemotherapy, and the vast majority of articles about drug resistance have focused on causes or effects of genetically determined stable drug resistance at the cellular level.

There are several pieces of evidence to suggest that stable drug resistance at the cellular level is only one of multiple causes of effective resistance to anticancer drugs *in vivo*. Perhaps the most direct evidence is the rarity with which genetically stable drug resistance can be induced by repeated transient exposure of tumor cells in culture to drug concentrations that are achievable in patients. Generally it requires far higher concentrations and prolonged exposure to induce a genetically stable form of drug resistance. Secondly, there is evidence that some types of drug resistance are only expressed when cells are grown in contact, such as in solid tumors or in multicellular spheroids, while the same cells exposed to drug in suspension remain fully sensitive[3,4]. Thirdly, patients who relapse following prior adjuvant chemotherapy have been reported to have rates of response to the same chemotherapy in the same range as those in patients who have not received prior treatment[5–7]. This finding suggests that selection of cells with stable intrinsic resistance may not be the only or even the major reason for limited cell kill from adjuvant treatment.

In the present chapter we describe two aspects of tumor physiology that have received only minimal attention in the literature, but which are likely to be important causes of clinical resistance to chemotherapy. These are repopulation, or proliferation of surviving tumor cells between cycles of chemotherapy, and poor penetration of drugs through tumor tissue. We show that each of these effects can have a profound effect on tumor response, and that each of them is amenable to modulation that could lead to improved clinical outcome following chemotherapy.

2. REPOPULATION

2.1 Cell Kinetic Factors Affecting Response to Chemotherapy

The rate of growth of a tumor is dependent on the mean duration of the cell cycle, the proportion of proliferating cells (the growth fraction) and the cell loss factor. There is limited but consistent data to suggest that the mean time taken for a tumor cell to cycle from one mitosis to the next (T_C) is usually in the range of 2-4 days, regardless of the cell type or the rate of tumor growth[8]. The tumor doubling time (T_D), for a clinically detectable tumor, varies between histological types and between individual tumors of the same type, with a median duration for solid tumors of about 2 months[8,9]. Historical data suggest that during a limited period of observation untreated tumors either grow exponentially, with a constant T_D[8,10], or that the growth rate decreases slowly with time, as described by the Gompertzian equation[11]. The difference between the rather short T_C and the variable and longer T_D is due to the presence of non-proliferating cells in tumors, and to a high rate of cell loss through such processes as necrosis, terminal differentiation and apoptosis. The rate of cell loss is frequently a high proportion of the rate of cell production with a median value of about 80% in human tumors[8].

Cytotoxic treatment increases tumor cell loss by direct killing in 'sensitive' tumors. It is well recognized, however, that repopulation or proliferation of surviving tumor cells (and of cells in normal tissues) occurs between fractions of radiation treatment and is an important factor influencing the probability of local control. Radiation therapy is generally given in daily fractions, with an average overall treatment time of 5-7 weeks. It is likely that repopulation has an even greater influence on the outcome of chemotherapy where 'dose fractions' are typically administered at 3-weekly intervals, and a course of adjuvant chemotherapy usually lasts 6 months. Despite this, repopulation between cycles of chemotherapy has received little attention.

Norton and Simon[12,13] have analyzed the implications of human tumors shrinking along a Gompertzian growth curve following chemotherapy, and have suggested that tumor cells might increase their rate of proliferation with increasing time of treatment and with tumor shrinkage. This mathematical analysis, however, is based on an imperfect model for tumor growth and does not take into account the changes in proliferative rate that might occur after individual cycles of treatment, often without gross changes in tumor volume. They have proposed “late intensification” of treatment to overcome repopulation as tumors respond and shrink. This approach, however, is of limited utility because drugs are already given at close to toxic levels for normal cells.

In the following paragraphs we summarize the relevant radiation literature and the limited available information about repopulation of tumor cells between courses of chemotherapy. We then model the probable effects of repopulation on outcome following chemotherapy, and suggest strategies that have the potential to inhibit the proliferative process and thereby improve the therapeutic outcome.

2.2 Repopulation and Radiation Therapy

Rates of repopulation have been estimated for a variety of transplanted tumors in experimental animals by estimating the number of surviving clonogenic tumor cells as a function of time following single or fractionated doses of radiation. These experiments have, in general, shown rates of repopulation that are equal to, or more often faster than the rates of cell production in untreated tumors[14–18]. Estimates of repopulation of human tumors following radiation have been obtained by plotting the total dose to achieve a level of control of a given type and stage of cancer (e.g., T3 larynx cancer) against the time over which treatment is given in different series. An increase in the total dose to achieve local tumor control with increased duration of treatment is indirect evidence for repopulation during treatment. Retrospective data obtained from patients with head and neck cancer suggest a delay in onset of repopulation of 3-4 weeks, followed by a doubling of cell number with a doubling time of about 4 days (Figure 1)[19,20]. This estimated rate of repopulation during the latter part of a course of radiotherapy is much faster than rates of growth of untreated tumors of the same type. Bentzen *et al.*[21] have questioned the validity of using multi-institutional retrospective data, requiring normalization of treatment doses between centers, especially as no significant dose response was seen in most centers. They have expressed doubt about the presence of an initial delay in the onset of repopulation, although not about the existence of accelerated repopulation itself. Analyses of clinical data for several tumor types, including head and neck cancer, cervical cancer and lymphomas, have shown reduced local control with interruptions in the radiation schedule and are consistent with substantial rates of repopulation[22–24].

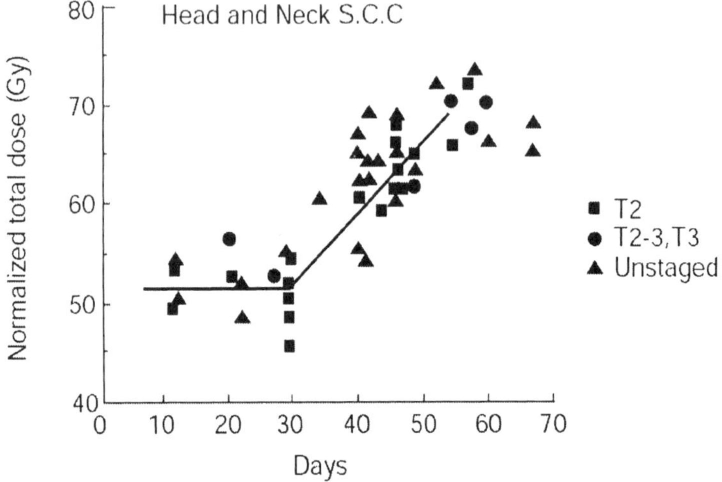

Figure 1. Relationship between total dose of radiation to control 50% of stage 3 and 4 carcinomas of the larynx plotted as a function of the total time over which the radiation was given (data reviewed by Withers *et al.*[20], figure redrawn). Note that the total dose rises rapidly (with a doubling time of about 4 days for courses of radiotherapy longer than about 4 weeks), consistent with a high rate of repopulation during the latter part of radiation treatment.

Several clinical approaches have been explored to overcome the problem of repopulation and subsequent loss of tumor control during radiotherapy. Accelerated fractionation, in which more than one fraction is given per day, or where radiation is continued during weekends, has been evaluated in randomized clinical trials. The CHART (continuous, hyperfractionated, accelerated radiotherapy) studies are large multicentre randomised controlled trials comparing CHART to conventionally fractionated radiotherapy in head and neck cancer and non-small cell lung cancer (NSCLC)[25,26]. The head and neck study showed equivalent results in terms of locoregional control and survival whilst the NSCLC study showed improvement in both local control and survival[26,27], despite lower radiation doses in the CHART schedule. These results support the importance of repopulation as a cause of radiation therapy failure. Two other recent studies in head and neck cancer, the DAHANCA study and a Polish study, have also shown improved local control; the DAHANCA study also showed improved survival with reduced overall treatment time and dose[27–29].

A second proposed strategy involves the use of concurrent biological agents to slow or inhibit cell proliferation during treatment[30]. In intriguing preliminary human studies, concurrent administration of a monoclonal antibody to the epidermal growth factor receptor (EGFR) with radiation for head and neck cancer was reported to result in a marked increase in anti-tumor effects, albeit with some increase in toxicity[31].

2.3 Repopulation and Chemotherapy

The intervals between doses of cytotoxic chemotherapy are necessarily long compared with the usual daily intervals between radiation dose fractions because of the need to allow recovery (i.e., repopulation) of normal tissues such as the bone marrow and intestinal mucosa. Most drugs are only present in cytotoxic concentrations for a few hours following administration, and although lower concentrations that inhibit cell proliferation may be present for longer, this effect is likely to be short compared with the interval between treatments. There are therefore substantial intervals following each treatment where surviving tumor cells can proliferate and repopulate the tumor.

There are very few pre-clinical studies examining the effects of anticancer drugs on tumor cell proliferation in animal or tissue culture models. The data from these studies are summarized in Table 1. Stephens and Peacock[32] treated mice bearing transplanted B16 melanomas with cyclophosphamide (CP) or 1-(2-chlorethyl)-3-cyclohexyl-1-nitrosurea (CCNU). Colony-forming-survival assays were performed at various times after treatment of the mice with doses of CP and CCNU that produced a surviving fraction of about 10^{-3}. Repopulation commenced by 5 days following injection of CP, and there was an exponential increase in number of cells with a T_D of about 1.5 days until day 15, and then the rate of increase in clonogenic cells declined. After injection of CCNU, repopulation began immediately and was very rapid, the T_D being about 0.85 days. The rate of repopulation declined after 10 days, with T_D increasing to about 3.6 days, slightly longer than the doubling time of the untreated tumors.

Rosenblum *et al.*[33,34] examined post-treatment kinetics of surviving clonogenic cells following intraperitoneal injections of 1,3-bis(2-chloroethyl)-1-nitrosourea (BCNU) to Fischer 344 rats implanted intracerebrally with 9L gliosarcoma cells. After a lag period of approximately 1-4 days, the surviving clonogenic cells proliferated with doubling times of 15, 21, and 38 hours following single doses of 0.25, 0.5, and 1 x LD_{10} (i.e., the dose leading to death of 10% of the animals), respectively; suggesting a dose-response. Post-treatment kinetics of clonogenic cells surviving two daily 0.5 x LD_{10} doses of BCNU showed that repopulation began on Day 2, with a repopulation-doubling time of 26 hours and total repopulation of the clonogenic cell pool in about 10 days.

Milas *et al.*[35] studied tumor cell repopulation in a murine sarcoma, SA-NH, treated with CP. Changes in the absolute number of clonogenic cells in tumors were determined by estimating the dose of radiation required to control 50% of tumors (TCD_{50}) under hypoxic conditions at different times after treatment with CP. These estimates were compared with those for tumors that did not receive chemotherapy. Treatment with CP depleted tumors of clonogenic cells as manifested by a reduction in the control TCD_{50} value of 64.5 Gy to 32.8 Gy at one day after CP treatment, and then remained relatively constant for two weeks. Two weeks after treatment the TCD_{50} increased rapidly, continuing until the end of the observation period of 21 days when the tumors reached the pretreatment size. The daily increase in TCD_{50} was more than twice as high in CP-treated than in control tumors: 4.5 Gy/day versus 2.1 Gy/day. This result implies that the rate of production of clonogenic cells in CP-treated tumors was twice as high as that in unperturbed tumors between 2-3 weeks after treatment.

The reason for the delay in repopulation of tumor cells following treatment, as shown in these studies, is unclear. Chemotherapy has been shown to delay cell cycle progression, and the delay lengthens with increased dose[35]. Alternatively the chemotherapy may have killed most of the cycling tumor cells and the surviving quiescent cells may have been stimulated to proliferate only when the micro-environmental conditions, such as hypoxia and poor nutrition, improved. The variability in timing of onset and the rate of repopulation following different agents might be explained by differences in the duration of activity of the drugs and their metabolites, by differential damage to the tumor matrix, or by different effects on the nutritional status of the animals and on their immunological response[32].

Multicellular spheroids have been used to model tumor cell sensitivity to multiple doses of chemotherapy. Spheroids are spherical aggregates of tumor cells that grow in culture to a diameter of about 1 mm. They resemble tumor nodules in that they have gradients of metabolites, gradients in rates of cell proliferation, and they develop central necrosis[37,38]. Chinese hamster V79 spheroids were exposed to cisplatin for 2 hours daily for 3 weeks and the total number of viable cells was counted following each treatment[39]. After an initial response, re-growth of the spheroids occurred despite continued therapy (Figure 2). The fraction of cells killed with each week of treatment did not alter significantly, suggesting that the diminishing effectiveness of the chemotherapeutic treatment was not due to selection of drug-resistant cells but to an increasing rate of repopulation between treatments. Similar results were seen when cisplatin was combined with etoposide[40].

We could find only one study of cell proliferation following the clinical use of chemotherapy for solid tumors. Bourhis *et al.*[41] assessed tumor cell proliferation in patients with oropharyngeal cancer receiving induction chemotherapy and found a statistically higher rate of cell production in treated patients as compared with patients who had no prior chemotherapy. The patients receiving chemotherapy were a select group, including only patients whose tumors had shown partial or no response to chemotherapy, as tumor was not available for study from patients who had achieved a complete remission. In addition, the mean delay between the end of chemotherapy and the time of the tumor biopsy was long (4.1 weeks). However, the results do suggest that rapid repopulation occurs in oropharyngeal cancer which had responded poorly to chemotherapy.

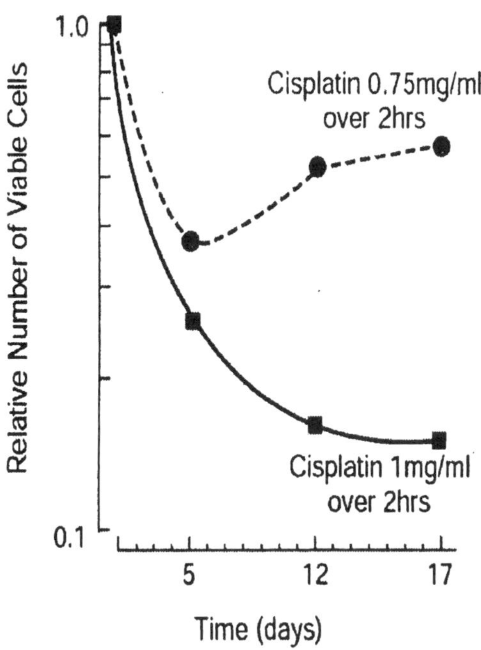

Figure 2. Survival of cells in spheroids treated daily with either 0.75 or 1.0 mg/ml of cisplatin, Monday to Friday. The data points indicate the relative number of viable cells per spheroid after the last drug exposure for each of the 3 weeks and show that after an initial response there is repopulation of the spheroid cells. (Redrawn from Durand *et al.*[39]).

2.4 Models of Repopulation Between Cycles of Chemotherapy

The simplest model for repopulation between cycles of chemotherapy assumes a constant proportion of cells killed with each cycle and a constant rate of repopulation between treatments[42]. As shown in Figure 3, the overall "response" to treatment will then depend on the ratio between cell kill induced by each treatment and the rate of repopulation. If repopulation is rapid the number of viable cells will increase despite the cells being "sensitive" to the chemotherapy. If repopulation is slow there will be a slow reduction in the number of clonogenic tumor cells. Even this simple model illustrates that rapid rates of repopulation of human tumors (with doubling times of surviving cells of a week or less) may abrogate completely the effects of substantial levels of cell kill.

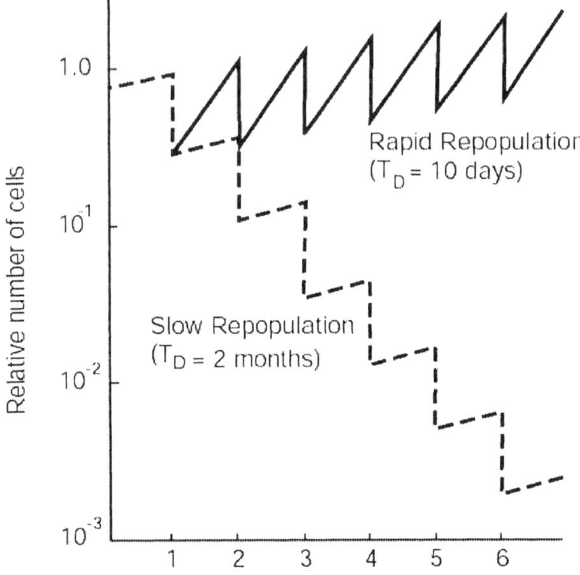

Figure 3. A model for cell killing and repopulation during a course of chemotherapy. Assuming a constant rate of cell kill of 70% with each cycle, repopulation with a doubling time of 10 days will allow tumor growth despite "sensitivity", whereas slower repopulation with a doubling time of 2 months will allow shrinkage.

Both clinical data for radiotherapy and studies of repopulation in experimental systems following chemotherapy suggest that there may be a delay in onset of repopulation, with accelerating rates of repopulation after successive treatments. In Figure 4A we assume a constant cell kill for each treatment but model the outcome if there is a halving in the doubling time for repopulation during each of the first four intervals following treatment, i.e., accelerated repopulation between cycles. Figure 4B incorporates both accelerated repopulation and a lag in onset of repopulation following each dose and allows a maximum rate of repopulation with T_D of ~4 days in the latter part of each cycle of treatment beyond the third. This value of T_D is similar to that estimated for repopulation of head and neck tumors during the latter part of fractionated radiotherapy (see Figure 1).

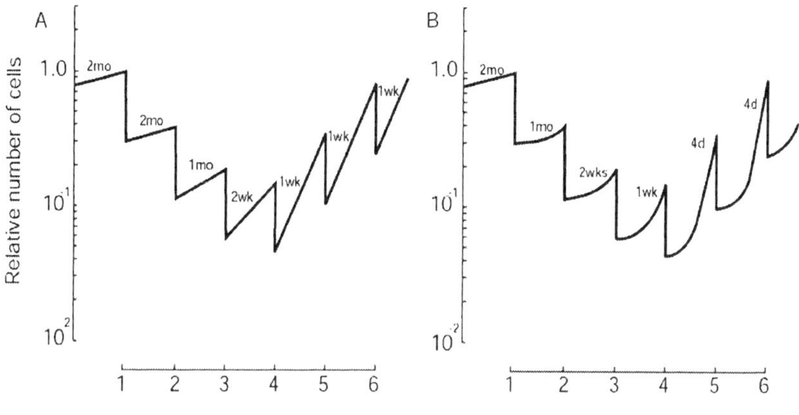

Figure 4. Model curves to illustrate the effects of accelerating repopulation during successive cycles of chemotherapy. The rate of cell kill is assumed to be constant, with 70% of cells killed with each cycle. In (A) the rate of repopulation is assumed to be constant but the doubling time halves with each of the first four cycles, from 2 months to 1 week, and remains constant thereafter. In (B) a delay to onset of repopulation is assumed followed by maximal rates of repopulation between successive cycles characterized by doubling times of 1 month, 2 weeks, 1 week, and 4 days, respectively.

The model in Figure 4B probably resembles most closely the clinical situation. It illustrates that without any selection of drug-resistant cells a tumor may shrink in response to chemotherapy and then re-grow because accelerating repopulation overcomes completely the effect of drug-induced cell kill. We are all too familiar with the frustrating clinical scenario of initial tumor shrinkage followed by re-growth despite ongoing treatment. This has usually been assumed to reflect the development of tumor cell resistance, but an alternative or additional explanation is the induction of accelerated repopulation of surviving tumor cells.

2.5 Potential Methods for Inhibition of Repopulation Following Chemotherapy

Despite the paucity of data concerning repopulation following chemotherapy, there is good reason to expect that repopulation will have a major effect on clinical outcome, and that approaches which inhibit its effect might positively alter that outcome. In considering potential strategies it is important to recognize that the pattern of repopulation after chemotherapy is likely to be more complex than after radiotherapy for several reasons. First, most drugs are cytostatic as well as cytotoxic, and proliferation is likely to be inhibited for a period of time after treatment that will depend on the rate of clearance of the drug. Secondly, as almost all chemotherapeutic drugs are more active against proliferating cells, the potential benefits of inhibiting repopulation between cycles would be lost if tumor cells were rendered effectively resistant to the chemotherapy by being non-proliferative at the time of the next treatment. Any strategy to inhibit repopulation must therefore be discontinued prior to the next cycle. Finally, any effort to inhibit repopulation must be tumor specific, and allow normal tissues such as the bone marrow or intestine to recover between cycles of chemotherapy.

There have been several different approaches to improving response and clinical outcome with chemotherapy that might have an impact on tumor cell repopulation. Increasing dose intensity, either with higher doses or shorter intervals between treatment cycles, shows potential to improve outcome in drug-sensitive malignancies such as leukemia, lymphoma and testicular carcinoma. The limiting factor for this approach is normal tissue tolerance and, despite the use of recombinant hematologic growth factors, there is a limit to the extent that dose intensity can be increased before substantial toxicity occurs. Another approach is prolonged infusional chemotherapy or chronic low dose oral treatment. Although this has the potential to inhibit tumor repopulation, by avoiding the treatment-free period when tumors cells can repopulate, normal tissue tolerance necessitates dose reduction which may reduce tumor cell kill. There are, however, examples where infusional chemotherapy has shown modest improvements in response, such as infusional 5-FU in metastatic colon and breast cancer. More recently, oral formulations have become available that provide equivalent effects with easier administration. Whether the mechanism of improved effect is reduced repopulation or simply better scheduling for this cycle-dependent drug is not known.

There are a number of biological agents that have been shown to inhibit tumor cell proliferation and to induce cytostasis in a variety of malignancies. Examples of such cytostatic "modifiers" that are suitable for testing between cycles of chemotherapy include hormonal agents and inhibitors of growth factors, their receptors or of related signal transduction pathways. The agent chosen should ideally meet the criteria described above, i.e., be tumor specific and have a rapid onset and short duration of action. We are currently undertaking experimental studies of the effect of an epidermal growth factor inhibitor and of a short acting anti-estrogen on tumor cell proliferation following chemotherapy *in vitro* and in animal models and plan to extend this work into clinical trials.

An alternative approach to inducing selective cytostasis in tumors might take advantage of the tumor microenvironment. The mean extracellular pH in many tumors is lower than in normal tissues, and cells survive and proliferate in this environment because of the activity of membrane-based ion exchange mechanisms that maintain cytosolic pH within the normal range[43,44]. New and more selective inhibitors of these pH-regulatory mechanisms are becoming available and might allow equilibration of intracellular and extracellular pH, with a selective fall in intracellular pH within tumors. Cells are able to survive for long periods with a small decrease in their cytoplasmic pH, but generally stop proliferating[45], providing a possible mechanism for putting tumor cells out of cycle.

3. DRUG PENETRATION THROUGH TISSUE

3.1 Methods for Study of Drug Penetration

An absolute requirement for activity of anticancer drugs against solid tumors is penetration to tumor cells in a sufficient concentration to cause lethal activity. Until recently, studies of drug penetration through tumor tissue depended on two methods that are indirect and technically complex:

- Multicellular tumor spheroids can be exposed to fluorescent or radiolabeled drugs, and fluorescence or radiolabel can be related to radial penetration in histologic sections or autoradiographs. This method has been used to demonstrate limited penetration of several anticancer drugs including doxorubicin, methotrexate and vinblastine[46–49]. Recent refinements using confocal laser scanning microscopy have confirmed limited distribution of doxorubicin in larger spheroids[50].
- The vital fluorescent dye, Hoechst 33342, has been used to establish a gradient into tissue from the periphery of spheroids, or from tumor blood vessels. Following treatment with an anticancer drug, the tissue is dissociated, cells are separated on the basis of Hoechst fluorescence by cell sorting, and clonogenic cell survival is estimated as a function of distance into tissue[51,52]. This method has confirmed that drug penetration is a major limitation for doxorubicin, although more uniform cell killing has been observed for 5-FU and for several alkylating agents[52–54]. Although the same factors that lead to slow penetration after acute administration were shown to lead to longer retention after chronic exposure[55], most of the drug administered *in vivo* is likely to be excreted before tissue penetration has occurred.

More recently, a new and conceptually simple technique has been established by Wilson and his colleagues which allows direct assessment of tissue penetration by anticancer drugs[56,57]. Tumor cells are grown on collagen-coated microporous Teflon® membranes as multicellular layers (MCL) that have many of the characteristics of tumor tissue *in vivo*. MCL typically achieve a thickness of ~200 μm, similar to the maximum distance between blood vessels and viable tumor cells in human tumors, and larger MCL may form a layer of central necrosis (Figure 5). We have shown that cells within MCL may establish tight junctions that are characteristic of epithelial tissues *in vivo*, and that they establish an extracellular matrix containing collagen, laminin and other proteins. Variants of this technique have now been established in several laboratories[58–60].

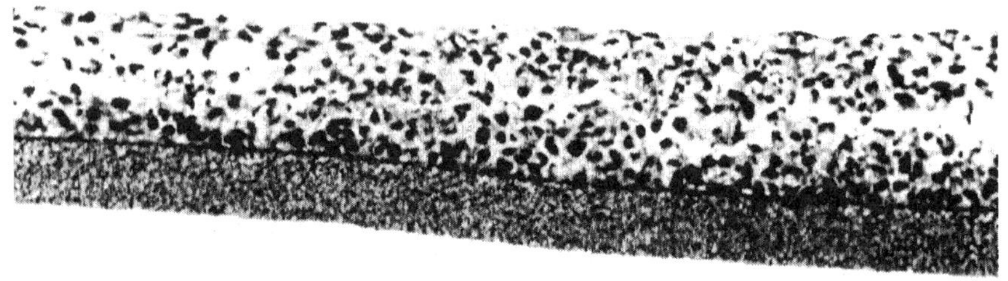

Figure 4. A representative MCL grown from EMT-6 cells.

For studies of tissue penetration, a drug is added to medium on one side of the MCL (compartment 1 in Figure 6) and its time-dependent appearance in medium on the other side of the MCL (compartment 2 in Figure 6) is determined by using appropriate analytical methods. In order to minimize the effects of convection (which *in vivo* will be inhibited by the presence of the blood vessel wall), the drugs are usually added to compartment 1 in dilute agar. We have shown that the rate of penetration of the MCL is minimally influenced by the concentration of agar that is used. The simplest method for analysis of drug penetration is to use drugs that are radiolabeled with tritium or ^{14}C, although it is then possible that one may detect the isotope on drug metabolites rather than on the parent compound. Confirmatory studies using chromatographic or other analytical methods are desirable. It is important to include appropriate controls to ensure consistency between experiments. In our studies, we evaluate concurrently penetration of the anticancer drug through the Teflon-coated membrane in the absence of an MCL and penetration of each MCL by sucrose (labeled with a different radioisotope to the anticancer drug that is being evaluated). We also examine the MCL to ensure that they are of relatively uniform thickness, and dissociate one MCL from a batch to be used in experiments to ensure that the number of cells is within a limited range.

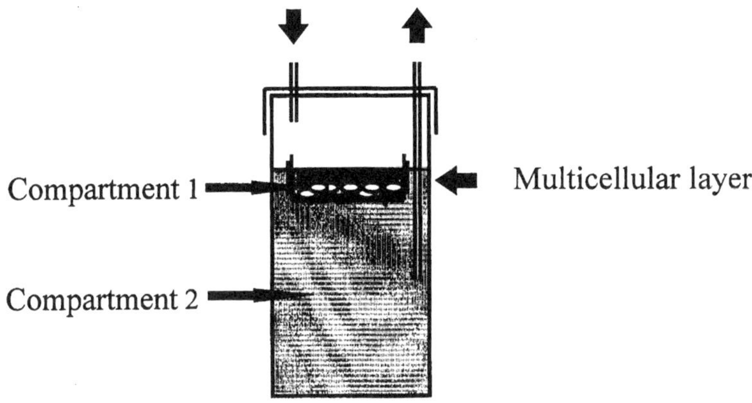

Figure 5. The multi-cellular membrane method. In studies of drug penetration through tissue, drug is added to medium in compartment 1 (above the MCL) and its appearance in compartment 2 (below the MCL) is studied as a function of time.

3.2 Penetration of Tissue by Anticancer Drugs

Using the above methodology we have assessed the penetration through MCL of a representative sample of anticancer drugs that are used commonly to treat patients with solid tumors[59,61]. In these experiments we have generated and studied MCL from murine EMT-6 cells, human breast cancer MCF-7 cells, and human bladder cancer MGH-U1 cells. Although the MCL derived from human cells grow more slowly (about 6 days to establish MCL of thickness 200 μm for the human lines and about 4 days for the murine line), the penetration of drugs through MCL of similar thickness was found to be quite similar. In Figure 7 we illustrate the time-dependent penetration of radiolabeled methotrexate and doxorubicin through MCL derived from EMT-6 cells, in comparison to that through the cell-free Teflon membrane. Here the concentration of drug in compartment 2 (see Figure 6) is expressed as a percentage of the expected concentration when the drug has reached equilibrium between the two compartments (any drug bound in tissue or to the membrane is neglected in this calculation). In Figure 8 is presented a summary of the penetration through MCL (relative to that through the Teflon membrane alone) of all of the drugs that we have studied: cisplatin, doxorubicin, 5-fluorouracil, gemcitabine, methotrexate, mitoxantrone, paclitaxel, etoposide and vinblastine.

Data presented in Figures 7 and 8 illustrate that the MCL acts as a considerable barrier to the penetration of many anticancer drugs: there is a substantial concentration gradient across the cell layers within the MCL that is only slowly dissipated in a period that exceeds 6 hours. The penetration of most of the drugs through the MCL is of the order of 30-50% of that through the Teflon membrane alone, but is particularly poor for doxorubicin and mitoxantrone where it is less than 10% of that through the Teflon membrane. Most of these drugs are given by a short intravenous infusion when they are used *in vivo*, and following an initial peak concentration there is a rapid fall in plasma concentration that is due both to drug distribution and to metabolism and excretion. This decline is likely to be considerably more rapid *in vivo* than that in compartment 1 of the MCL model system, where drug clearance via the blood stream is not a factor. The data from MCL are therefore likely to underestimate the problem of tissue penetration *in vivo*, and suggest strongly that there will be steep gradients of concentration into tissue from blood vessels for almost all of the anticancer drugs in common use. Equilibrium conditions, with a constant concentration in different regions of solid tissue, would only be achieved following prolonged continuous infusion of drugs (as is sometimes done for 5-fluorouracil). Moreover, since tumor vasculature is often poorly formed in comparison with normal tissue, with large inter-capillary distances and variable rates of blood flow, poor penetration of anticancer drugs through solid tissue is likely to lead to selective resistance of tumors to chemotherapy.

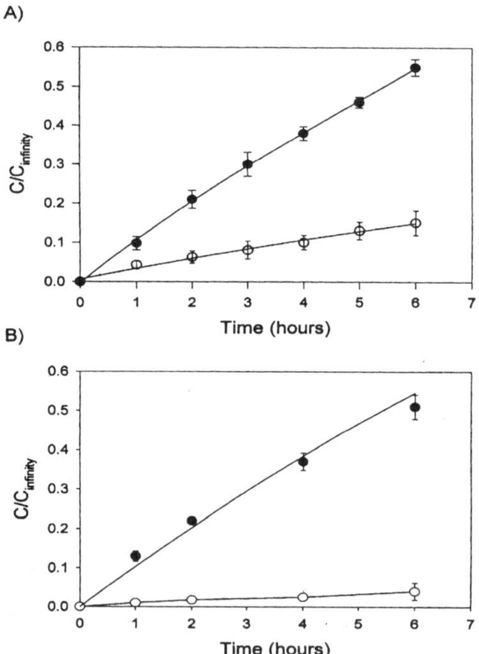

Figure 7. Penetration of (A) methotrexate and (B) doxorubicin through EMT-6 MCL. Solid symbols represent the cell free controls and the open symbols indicate the presence of an MCL. Points represent the mean of at least 3 experiments and error bars are the standard error of that mean. Drug penetration through the MCL as a function of time is presented as the ratio of the measured concentration, C, to that expected at equilibrium, $C_{infinity}$. (From Tunggal *et al.*[59]).

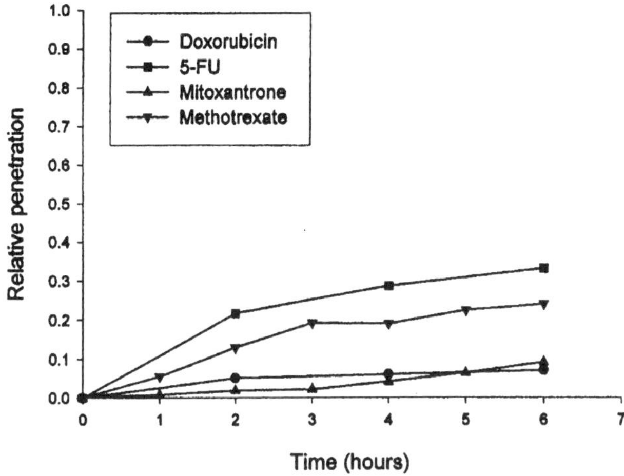

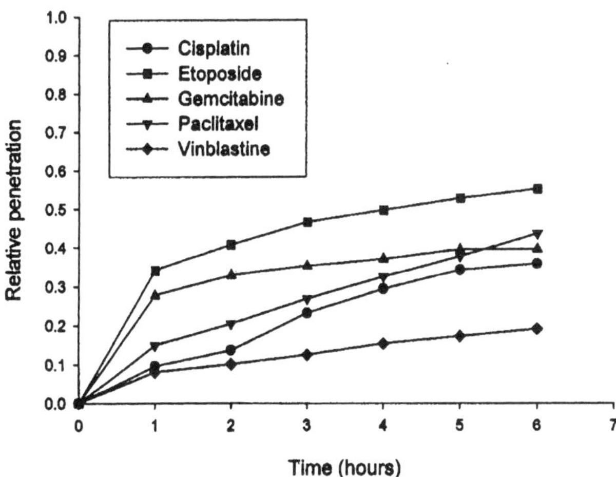

Figure 8. A summary of the relative penetration of the drugs studied in our laboratory.

It is perhaps surprising that drugs such as doxorubicin and mitoxantrone, which have such poor penetration of tissue, have any activity at all against solid tumors. In tumors that are sensitive to these drugs, it is probable that successive layers of peri-vascular cells are killed after sequential administration (rather like peeling an inside-out onion). This effect may lead to tumor response (i.e., shrinkage) if the rate of repopulation from surviving tumor cells is slow and/or a high proportion of more distant cells have lost their clonogenic potential – and hence their ability to repopulate the tumor. Doxorubicin and mitoxantrone are rarely active against rapidly growing tumors in mice, perhaps because such tumors contain a high proportion of clonogenic cells and have a rapid rate of repopulation. Of note is the general finding that the rate of cell proliferation decreases with distance from a blood vessel in both human and experimental tumors[62,63]. The slower rate of cell proliferation makes cells distant from tumor blood vessels more resistant to most anticancer drugs, even in the absence of poor drug penetration, and might reflect a lower clonogenic potential of these cells, especially in human tumors. However, there is substantial evidence that profoundly hypoxic cells can regenerate a tumor after treatment with radiation so that a proportion of cells distant from blood vessels must retain their clonogenic capacity. Penetration of drugs to kill these cells will be required for them to provide long-term control of solid tumors.

3.3 Factors That Influence Penetration of Drugs Through Tissue

Within an MCL (as in tumor tissue) there are several factors that influence drug penetration. These include the concentration gradient across the MCL, which will change with time; the diffusion coefficient through the extra-cellular matrix and through the cells themselves (which will depend on solubility in water and in lipids); and the consumption of drug by the constituent cells. "Consumption" is a complex term, which may include metabolism of the drug (leading to either active or inactive metabolic products), and uptake and binding of the drug to intracellular molecules or compartments. Wilson *et al.*[57–64] have derived a mathematical equation to describe drug penetration in terms of these parameters, and curves such as those in Figures 7 and 8 which describe time-dependent penetration can be fitted to this equation. Unfortunately, the curves that describe penetration of MCL by drugs are not defined with sufficient precision to give reliable information about the different factors that influence the process. They may not differentiate, for example, between slow diffusion and a high rate of uptake and binding in cells as causes of poor drug penetration. These issues are therefore best studied experimentally.

We have undertaken quite detailed studies of some of the factors that influence the penetration of tissue by the drugs doxorubicin and methotrexate. These studies suggest that factors which lead to increased drug uptake into cells have a substantial effect to decrease drug penetration through the MCL, and vice versa. In the study of doxorubicin, we compared tissue penetration across MCL derived from murine EMT-6 or human MCF-7 cells that either did or did not express the drug export pump, P-glycoprotein (P-gp)[65]. As shown in Figure 9A, we found that there was better penetration of doxorubicin across MCL derived from cells that expressed P-gp (with poor uptake of doxorubicin) than across MCL that did not express this drug resistance marker. Moreover, inhibition of the activity of P-gp by either verapamil or the experimental agent GG918 decreased penetration of tissue by doxorubicin, and might therefore be expected to have opposing effects on therapeutic activity through increased drug uptake into proximal cells but decreased penetration to distal cells (Figure 9B). These results, as well as our previous data showing that inhibitors of P-gp lose effectiveness against cells at high cell concentration[66], may in part explain the limited therapeutic benefit for these agents against established solid tumors in animals[67,68], or in randomized controlled trials to treat human cancer[69–71].

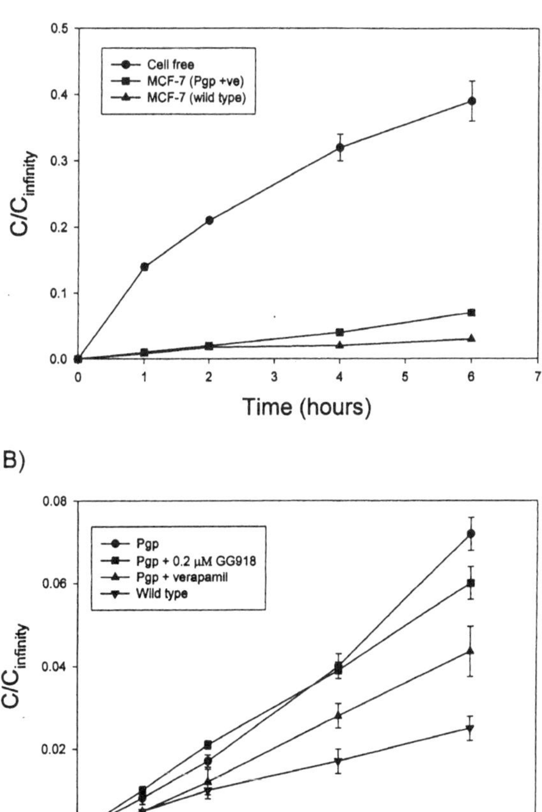

Figure 9. (A) Penetration of doxorubicin through MCL derived from wild-type MCF-7 cells (low or absent P-gp expression), the BC19 sub-line of MCF-7 cells that expresses P-gp, and through the Teflon membrane alone. Note the better penetration in the presence of P-gp expression. (B) Penetration of doxorubicin through MCL derived from wild type MCF-7 cells, the P-gp expressing sub-line, alone, or in the presence of the inhibitors of P-gp function, verapamil and GG918. Note that P-gp reversal leads to poorer tissue penetration. (From Tunggal *et al.*[65]).

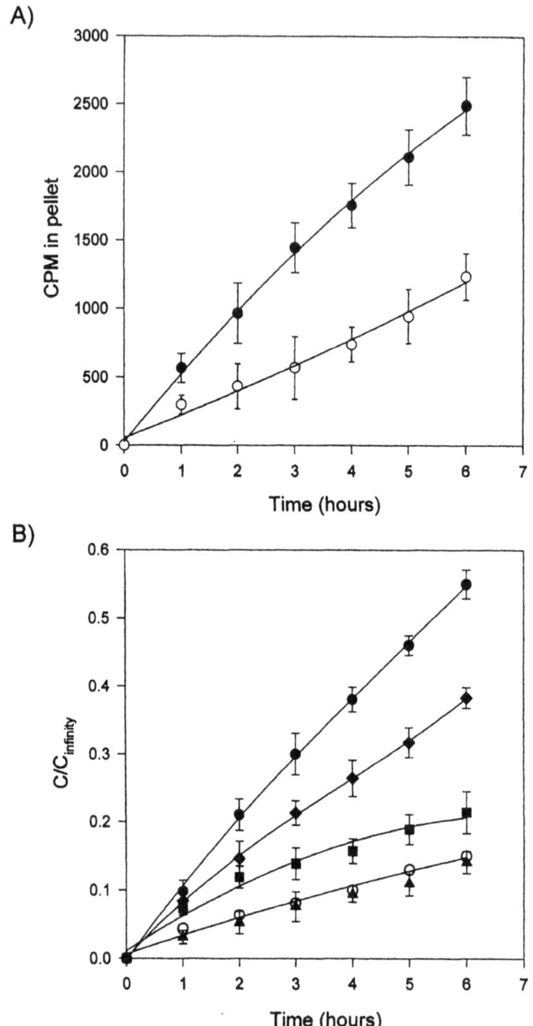

Figure 10. (A) Effect of folic acid on the intracellular uptake of methotrexate. The open and closed circles represent the uptake of methotrexate in the presence and absence of 1 mM folic acid under aerobic exposure conditions. (B) Effect of folic acid on penetration of methotrexate through EMT-6 MCL. Solid circles represent the cell free control and open circles represent methotrexate penetration in the presence of an MCL. Triangles, squares and diamonds represent the co-administration of folic acid at concentrations of 0.1, 0.3 and 1 mM respectively. Points represent the mean of at least 3 experiments and error bars are the standard error of the mean. Drug penetration through the MCL as a function of time is presented as the ratio of the measured concentration (C) to that expected at equilibrium ($C_{infinity}$). (From Cohen *et al.*[61]).

In other studies, we found that exposure of single cells in culture to methotrexate in the presence of increasing concentration of its normal metabolic analog folic acid led to a progressive decrease in cellular uptake of the drug (Figure 10A)[61]. When increasing concentrations of folic acid were added to both compartments of the MCL model system, there was a progressive increase in penetration of methotrexate through the MCL (Figure 10B). Exposure of cells to methotrexate at low pH also decreased cellular uptake of drug, and exposure of MCL to low pH increased its penetration through them. Of note, neither alkaline conditions, nor exposure to folinic acid (citrovorum factor) had any effect on either cellular uptake of methotrexate or its penetration through MCL. These results suggest that drug uptake into cells is the major factor that limits the tissue penetration of this water-soluble drug.

3.4 Factors That Might Influence Drug Penetration

Obtaining information about the factors which lead to limited penetration of anticancer drugs through tissue is important, but even more important is the potential to improve tissue penetration. Inter-capillary distances are usually larger, and stasis and slow blood flow more common, in tumors than in normal tissues[72–74]. Thus, strategies that improve tissue penetration are likely to have a much greater effect on anti-tumor effects than on toxicity to normal tissues, and may be expected to improve the therapeutic index. Inhibition of drug uptake into proximal cells is one strategy that will improve tissue penetration, as described above, but in general is likely to lead also to a decrease in drug activity and not, therefore, to a therapeutic benefit. This would not be the case, however, if inhibition of cellular uptake were achieved by preventing the binding or sequestration of drugs in intra-cellular compartments that are not associated with cellular cytotoxicity.

One strategy that appears appropriate for manipulation is the inhibition of sequestration of basic drugs within acidic endosomes of cells. Cells are known to contain intra-cytoplasmic organelles such as lysosomes and the trans-Golgi network, which have an internal pH that may be as low as 5.0[75,76]. When basic drugs diffuse into such compartments, they will be protonated and hence sequestered, reaching an equilibrium concentration that is very high compared to that in the cytoplasm and dependent on the pH gradient across the organellar membrane. Fluorescence and confocal laser microscopy have been used to demonstrate the sequestration of doxorubicin and other basic drugs in acidic organelles[57,77]. This effect inhibits drugs from reaching their cellular target (usually DNA) and acts as a 'sink' so that drug is absorbed rapidly by cells proximal to blood vessels with consequent inhibition of penetration of tissue. While the first of these effects is likely to apply to all cells, the effect to decrease penetration of tissue is likely to be much more important in tumors with their poorer vascular supply.

Increased drug penetration through tissue should occur if decreasing the pH gradient across the membranes of these organelles inhibits the sequestration of drugs in endosomes. Strong evidence for such an effect was obtained in a proof-of-principle experiment by Hicks *et al.*[57] who used 50 mM ammonium chloride to increase markedly the penetration of a basic experimental drug (DAPA) across MCL, and we have observed similar effects of ammonium chloride on the penetration of doxorubicin and mitoxantrone (unpublished data). While this result is not useful for clinical application, we have reasoned that other strategies could be used to cause partial inhibition of the pH gradient across endosomal membranes. Preliminary data obtained in our laboratory have suggested that two approaches can increase endosomal pH, decrease net cellular uptake of doxorubicin or mitoxantrone, and increase the penetration of these drugs through MCL. These effects have been achieved by the administration of chloroquine, a basic drug that is known to be sequestered in acidic endosomes and to raise the pH within them[78,79], and by omeprazole, an inhibitor of ATPase proton pumps that generate the pH gradient between endosomes and cytoplasm. The effects of these agents on therapeutic benefit due to doxorubicin and mitoxantrone against solid tumors are under investigation. Chloroquine is in clinical use for the treatment of malaria, and omeprazole for the treatment of ulcer disease, so that both drugs are available for study as modulators of chemotherapy in clinical trials.

Another possible approach may be modification of the extra-cellular matrix (ECM), leading to improved penetration of drugs through the extra-cellular space. The ECM of solid tissue contains a complex array of molecules that interact with cells through transmembrane surface receptors, the integrins[80]. Constituents of the ECM are controlled in part by a series of enzymes, the matrix metalloproteinases, that break down extra-cellular molecules such as collagen and fibrinogen, and by a series of inhibitors, the tissue inhibitors of metalloproteinases or TIMPs[81,82]. One type of resistance to alkylating drugs is expressed only when cells are grown in 3-dimensional contact as spheroids, and this type of resistance increases for compact spheroids with a high cell density[83]. This result may be due in part to up-regulation of the cyclin-dependent kinase inhibitor p27 as a result of cellular contact in compact spheroids, leading to a decrease in the rate of cell proliferation and hence of drug sensitivity[84], but may also depend on changes in penetration of drugs through the ECM. Since several pharmacological inhibitors of matrix metalloproteinases have been developed, and are in clinical trials for their putative anti-metastatic and anti-angiogenic properties[85], agents of this type could be administered with chemotherapy in clinical trials if they are found to influence drug penetration.

CONCLUSION

To most scientists and clinical oncologists, the words ‘drug resistance’ are regarded almost synonymously with genetically determined changes in the phenotype of cells that render them individually resistant to anticancer drugs. Exploration of the multiple mechanisms that lead to this type of resistance have contributed substantially to knowledge of tumor biology, and there is some evidence for the presence of such mechanisms in human tumors. However, they are not the only mechanisms that can lead to effective resistance to drugs of human solid tumors, and they may not even be the most common ones. In the present chapter we have presented concepts, along with some supporting data, to suggest that factors relating to tumor physiology can also lead to effective resistance of solid tumors to chemotherapy, even if the cells within them remain individually sensitive.

Repopulation of surviving cells between courses of chemotherapy seems to have been particularly neglected in the scientific and clinical literature, especially as the parallel process during radiation therapy has been characterized extensively. It is likely to be even more important after chemotherapy, where treatments are of necessity given at less frequent intervals to allow normal tissue recovery. If repopulation accelerates during continued treatment, as is seen during radiation therapy and in the few experimental studies that have addressed it following drug treatment, then this process can account for the shrinkage and regrowth of human tumors without development of any intrinsic resistance of the tumor cells. This has been illustrated by the simple modeling shown in Figure 4. Repopulation can also explain why longer courses of adjuvant chemotherapy are not necessarily better than shorter ones, even if there has been no selection of drug-resistant cells. Moreover, the process is readily amenable to manipulation, especially with the current development of biological agents that are tumor-selective and often cytostatic rather than cytotoxic.

Limited penetration of tissue by anticancer drugs as a cause of effective resistance of solid tumors has been investigated only slightly more often. Now, however, the availability of the conceptually simple MCL method makes study of this phenomenon much easier, and work from our and other laboratories has shown consistently that penetration through tissue is a limitation for almost all of the drugs in common clinical use that have been studied. There is a large literature on the pharmacokinetics of available drugs that describes the delivery of drugs to tumor blood vessels (or mean drug concentration in a tumor), often with the implicit assumption that this represents delivery to the tumor cells. Studies of drug penetration described in this chapter show that this is not the case: limited penetration of tissue can lead to very large gradients in drug concentration so that some tumor cells are exposed to adequate concentrations of drug while others are exposed to very little. Moreover, the relatively poor vasculature of tumors (as compared to normal tissue) results in a therapeutic disadvantage because of poor drug penetration. Better understanding of the factors that influence drug penetration through tissue is an important goal of applied cancer research. Strategies to increase tissue penetration by active drugs have the potential to improve substantially the effectiveness of chemotherapy for solid tumors.

REFERENCES

1. Chlebowski RT, Lillington LM. A decade of breast cancer clinical investigation: results as reported in the Program/Proceedings of the American Society of Clinical Oncology. J Clin Oncol, 12:1789-1795, 1994.
2. Withers HR. From Bedside to Bench and Back. Academic Press, New York, NY, 1991.

3. Teicher BA, Herman TS, Holden SA, *et al.* Tumor resistance to alkylating agents conferred by mechanisms operative only in vivo. Science, 247:1457-1461, 1990.
4. Kerbel RS, Rak J, Kobayashi H, *et al.* Multicellular resistance: a new paradigm to explain aspects of acquired drug resistance of solid tumors. Cold Spring Harb Symp Quant Biol, 59:661-672, 1994.
5. Castiglione-Gertsch M, Tattersall M, Hacking A, *et al.* Retreating recurrent breast cancer with the same CMF-containing regimen used as adjuvant therapy. The International Breast Cancer Study Group. Eur J Cancer, 33:2321-2325, 1997.
6. Valagussa P, Tancini G, Bonadonna G. Salvage treatment of patients suffering relapse after adjuvant CMF chemotherapy. Cancer, 58:1411-1417, 1986.
7. Buzdar AU, Legha SS, Hortobagyi GN, *et al.* Management of breast cancer patients failing adjuvant chemotherapy with adriamycin-containing regimens. Cancer, 47:2798-2802, 1981.
8. Steel G. Growth Kinetics of Tumors. Clarendon Press, Oxford, UK, 1977.
9. Tubiana M. Tumor cell proliferation kinetics and tumor growth rate. Acta Oncol, 28:113-121, 1989.
10. Collins V, Loeffler R, Tivey H. Observations on growth rates of human tumors. AJR, 76:988-1000, 1956.
11. Salmon SE. Expansion of the growth fraction in multiple myeloma with alkylating agents. Blood, 45:119-129, 1975.
12. Norton L, Simon R. Tumor size, sensitivity to therapy, and design of treatment schedules. Cancer Treat Rep, 61:1307-1317, 1977.
13. Norton L, Simon R. The Norton-Simon hypothesis revisited. Cancer Treat Rep, 70:163-169, 1986.
14. Begg AC, Hofland I, Kummermehr J. Tumour cell repopulation during fractionated radiotherapy: correlation between flow cytometric and radiobiological data in three murine tumours. Eur J Cancer, 27:537-543, 1991.
15. Abe Y, Urano M, Kenton LA, *et al.* The accelerated repopulation of a murine fibrosarcoma, FSA-II, during the fractionated irradiation and the linear-quadratic model. Int J Radiat Oncol Biol Phys, 21:1529-1534, 1991.
16. Suit H, Urano M. Repair of sublethal radiation injury in hypoxic cells of a C3H mouse mammary carcinoma. Radiat Res, 37:423-434, 1969.
17. Hermens AF, Barendsen GW. Cellular proliferation patterns in an experimental rhabdomyosarcoma in the rat. Eur J Cancer, 3:361-369, 1967.
18. Milas L, Yamada S, Hunter N, *et al.* Changes in TCD50 as a measure of clonogen doubling time in irradiated and unirradiated tumors. Int J Radiat Oncol Biol Phys, 21:1195-1202, 1991.
19. Maciejewski B, Preuss-Bayer G, Trott KR. The influence of the number of fractions and of overall treatment time on local control and late complication rate in squamous cell carcinoma of the larynx. Int J Radiat Oncol Biol Phys, 9:321-328, 1983.
20. Withers HR, Taylor JM, Maciejewski B. The hazard of accelerated tumor clonogen repopulation during radiotherapy. Acta Oncol, 27:131-146, 1988.
21. Bentzen SM, Thames HD. Clinical evidence for tumor clonogen regeneration: interpretations of the data. Radiother Oncol, 22:161-166, 1991.
22. Fyles A, Keane TJ, Barton M, *et al.* The effect of treatment duration in the local control of cervix cancer. Radiother Oncol, 25:273-279, 1992.

23. Lanciano RM, Pajak TF, Martz K, *et al.* The influence of treatment time on outcome for squamous cell cancer of the uterine cervix treated with radiation: a patterns-of-care study. Int J Radiat Oncol Biol Phys, 25:391-397, 1993.
24. Norin T, Onyango J. Radiotherapy in Burkitt's lymphoma: conventional or superfractionated regime--early results. Int J Radiat Oncol Biol Phys, 2:399-406, 1977.
25. Saunders M, Dische S, Barrett A, *et al.* Continuous hyperfractionated accelerated radiotherapy (CHART) versus conventional radiotherapy in non-small-cell lung cancer: a randomised multicentre trial. CHART Steering Committee. Lancet, 350:161-5, 1997.
26. Dische S, Saunders M, Barrett A, *et al.* A randomised multicentre trial of CHART versus conventional radiotherapy in head and neck cancer. Radiother Oncol, 44:123-136, 1997.
27. Saunders MI, Dische S, Barrett A, *et al.* Randomised multicentre trials of CHART vs conventional radiotherapy in head and neck and non-small-cell lung cancer: an interim report. CHART Steering Committee. Br J Cancer, 73:1455-1462, 1996.
28. Hansen O, Overgaard J, Hansen HS, *et al.* Importance of overall treatment time for the outcome of radiotherapy of advanced head and neck carcinoma: dependency on tumor differentiation. Radiother Oncol, 43:47-51, 1997.
29. Skladowski K, Maciejewski B, Golen M, *et al.* Randomized clinical trial on 7-day-continuous accelerated irradiation (CAIR) of head and neck cancer - report on 3-year tumour control and normal tissue toxicity. Radiother Oncol, 55:101-110, 2000.
30. Kinsella TJ, Gould MN, Mulcahy RT, *et al.* Keynote address: integration of cytostatic agents and radiation therapy: a different approach to "proliferating" human tumors. Int J Radiat Oncol Biol Phys, 20:295-302, 1991.
31. Ezekiel MP, Bonner JA, Robert F, *et al.* Phase I trial of chimerized anti-epidermal growth factor receptor (Anti-EGFr) antibody in combination with either once-daily or twice-daily irradiation for locally advanced head and neck malignancies. Proc Amer Soc Clin Oncol, 18:1501, 1999.
32. Stephens TC, Peacock JH. Tumour volume response, initial cell kill and cellular repopulation in B16 melanoma treated with cyclophosphamide and 1-(2-chloroethyl)-3-cyclohexyl-1-nitrosourea. Br J Cancer, 36:313-321, 1977.
33. Rosenblum ML, Knebel KD, Vasquez DA, *et al.* In vivo clonogenic tumor cell kinetics following 1,3-bis(2-chloroethyl)-1-nitrosourea brain tumor therapy. Cancer Res, 36:3718-3725, 1976.
34. Rosenblum ML, Gerosa MA, Dougherty DV, *et al.* Improved treatment of a brain-tumor model. Part 1: Advantages of single-over multiple-dose BCNU schedules. J Neurosurg, 58:177-182, 1983.
35. Milas L, Nakayama T, Hunter N, *et al.* Dynamics of tumor cell clonogen repopulation in a murine sarcoma treated with cyclophosphamide. Radiother Oncol, 30:247-253, 1994.
36. Walter J, Maurer-Schultze B. Tumor cell recruitment in the mouse adenocarcinoma EO 771 directly demonstrated by double labeling with [3H]- and [14C] thymidine and flow cytometry. J Cancer Res Clin Oncol, 115:53-60, 1989.
37. Sutherland RM. Cell and environment interactions in tumor microregions: the multicell spheroid model. Science, 240:177-184, 1988.
38. Durand RE. Multicell spheroids as a model for cell kinetic studies. Cell Tissue Kinet, 23:141-159, 1990.
39. Durand RE, Vanderbyl SL. Tumor resistance to therapy: a genetic or kinetic problem? Cancer Commun, 1:277-283, 1989.
40. Durand RE, Vanderbyl SL. Schedule dependence for cisplatin and etoposide multifraction treatments of spheroids. J Natl Cancer Inst, 82:1841-1845, 1990.

41. Bourhis J, Wilson G, Wibault P, *et al.* Rapid tumor cell proliferation after induction chemotherapy in oropharyngeal cancer. Laryngoscope, 104:468-472, 1994.
42. Tannock IF. Conventional cancer therapy: promise broken or promise delayed? Lancet, 351 Suppl 2:SII9-16, 1998.
43. Tannock IF, Rotin D. Acid pH in tumors and its potential for therapeutic exploitation. Cancer Res, 49:4373-4384, 1989.
44. Lagarde AE, Pouyssegur JM. The Na+:H+ antiport in cancer. Cancer Biochem Biophys, 9:1-14, 1986.
45. Musgrove E, Seaman M, Hedley D. Relationship between cytoplasmic pH and proliferation during exponential growth and cellular quiescence. Exp Cell Res, 172:65-75, 1987.
46. Sutherland RM, Eddy HA, Bareham B, *et al.* Resistance to adriamycin in multicellular spheroids. Int J Radiat Oncol Biol Phys, 5:1225-1230, 1979.
47. West GW, Weichselbaum R, Little JB. Limited penetration of methotrexate into human osteosarcoma spheroids as a proposed model for solid tumor resistance to adjuvant chemotherapy. Cancer Res, 40:3665-3668, 1980.
48. Nederman T, Carlsson J. Penetration and binding of vinblastine and 5-fluorouracil in cellular spheroids. Cancer Chemother Pharmacol, 13:131-135, 1984.
49. Kerr DJ, Kaye SB. Aspects of cytotoxic drug penetration, with particular reference to anthracyclines. Cancer Chemother Pharmacol, 19:1-5, 1987.
50. Wartenberg M, Hescheler J, Acker H, *et al.* Doxorubicin distribution in multicellular prostate cancer spheroids evaluated by confocal laser scanning microscopy and the "optical probe technique". Cytometry, 31:137-145, 1998.
51. Durand RE. Use of Hoechst 33342 for cell selection from multicell systems. J Histochem Cytochem, 30:117-122, 1982.
52. Chaplin DJ, Durand RE, Olive PL. Cell selection from a murine tumour using the fluorescent probe Hoechst 33342. Br J Cancer, 51:569-572, 1985.
53. Durand RE. Chemosensitivity testing in V79 spheroids: drug delivery and cellular microenvironment. J Natl Cancer Inst, 77:247-252, 1986.
54. Durand RE. Distribution and activity of antineoplastic drugs in a tumor model. J Natl Cancer Inst, 81:146-152, 1989.
55. Durand RE. Slow penetration of anthracyclines into spheroids and tumors: a therapeutic advantage? Cancer Chemother Pharmacol, 26:198-204, 1990.
56. Cowan DS, Hicks KO, Wilson WR. Multicellular membranes as an in vitro model for extravascular diffusion in tumours. Br J Cancer Suppl, 27:S28-31, 1996.
57. Hicks KO, Ohms SJ, van Zijl PL, *et al.* An experimental and mathematical model for the extravascular transport of a DNA intercalator in tumours. Br J Cancer, 76:894-903, 1997.
58. Minchinton AI, Wendt KR, Clow KA, *et al.* Multilayers of cells growing on a permeable support. An in vitro tumour model. Acta Oncol, 36:13-16, 1997.
59. Tunggal JK, Cowan DS, Shaikh H, *et al.* Penetration of anticancer drugs through solid tissue: a factor that limits the effectiveness of chemotherapy for solid tumors. Clin Cancer Res, 5:1583-1586, 1999.
60. Phillips RM, Loadman PM, Cronin BP. Evaluation of a novel in vitro assay for assessing drug penetration into avascular regions of tumours. Br J Cancer, 77:2112-2119, 1998.
61. Cowan DSM, Tannock IF. Factors which influence the penetration of methotrexate through solid tissue. Int J Cancer, 91:120-125, 2000.
62. Tannock IF. The relation between cell proliferation and the vascular system in a transplanted mouse mammary tumour. Br J Cancer, 22:258-273, 1968.

63. Hirst DG, Denekamp J. Tumour cell proliferation in relation to the vasculature. Cell Tissue Kinet, 12:31-42, 1979.
64. Wilson WR, Hicks KO. Measurement of extravascular drug diffusion in multicellular layers. Br J Cancer, 79:1623-1626, 1999.
65. Tunggal JK, Melo T, Ballinger JR, *et al.* The influence of expression of P-glycoprotein on the penetration of anticancer drugs through multicellular layers. Int J Cancer, 86:101-107, 2000.
66. Tunggal JK, Ballinger JR, Tannock IF. Influence of cell concentration in limiting the therapeutic benefit of P-glycoprotein reversal agents. Int J Cancer, 81:741-747, 1999.
67. Van de Vrie W, Jonker AM, Marquet RL, *et al.* The chemosensitizer cyclosporin A enhances the toxic side-effects of doxorubicin in the rat. J Cancer Res Clin Oncol, 120:533-538, 1994.
68. Arvelo F, Poupon MF, Bichat F, *et al.* Adding a reverser (verapamil) to combined chemotherapy overrides resistance in small cell lung cancer xenografts. Eur J Cancer, 31A:1862-1868, 1995.
69. Dalton WS, Crowley JJ, Salmon SS, *et al.* A phase III randomized study of oral verapamil as a chemosensitizer to reverse drug resistance in patients with refractory myeloma. A Southwest Oncology Group study. Cancer, 75:815-820, 1995.
70. Wishart GC, Bissett D, Paul J, *et al.* Quinidine as a resistance modulator of epirubicin in advanced breast cancer: mature results of a placebo-controlled randomized trial. J Clin Oncol, 12:1771-1777, 1994.
71. Milroy R. A randomised clinical study of verapamil in addition to combination chemotherapy in small cell lung cancer. West of Scotland Lung Cancer Research Group, and the Aberdeen Oncology Group. Br J Cancer, 68:813-818, 1993.
72. Jain RK. Transport of molecules in the tumor interstitium: a review. Cancer Res, 47:3039-3051, 1987.
73. Helmlinger G, Yuan F, Dellian M, *et al.* Interstitial pH and pO2 gradients in solid tumors in vivo: high-resolution measurements reveal a lack of correlation. Nature Med, 3:177-182, 1997.
74. Minchinton AI, Durand RE, Chaplin DJ. Intermittent blood flow in the KHT sarcoma--flow cytometry studies using Hoechst 33342. Br J Cancer, 62:195-200, 1990.
75. Yamashiro DJ, Maxfield FR. Acidification of endocytic compartments and the intracellular pathways of ligands and receptors. J Cell Biochem, 26:231-246, 1984.
76. Overly CC, Lee KD, Berthiaume E, *et al.* Quantitative measurement of intraorganelle pH in the endosomal-lysosomal pathway in neurons by using ratiometric imaging with pyranine. Proc Natl Acad Sci USA, 92:3156-3160, 1995.
77. Altan N, Chen Y, Schindler M, *et al.* Defective acidification in human breast tumor cells and implications for chemotherapy. J Exp Med, 187:1583-1598, 1998.
78. Thorens B, Vassalli P. Chloroquine and ammonium chloride prevent terminal glycosylation of immunoglobulins in plasma cells without affecting secretion. Nature, 321:618-620, 1986.
79. Pless DD, Wellner RB. In vitro fusion of endocytic vesicles: effects of reagents that alter endosomal pH. J Cell Biochem, 62:27-39, 1996.
80. Dedhar S, Hannigan GE, Rak J, *et al.* The Extracellular Environment and Cancer, 3rd edition, McGraw Hill, New York, NY, 1998.
81. Khokha R, Waterhouse P. The role of tissue inhibitor of metalloproteinase-1 in specific aspects of cancer progression and reproduction. J Neurooncol, 18:123-127, 1994.

82. Gomez DE, Alonso DF, Yoshiji H, *et al.* Tissue inhibitors of metalloproteinases: structure, regulation and biological functions. Eur J Cell Biol, 74:111-122, 1997.
83. Kobayashi H, Man S, Graham CH, *et al.* Acquired multicellular-mediated resistance to alkylating agents in cancer. Proc Natl Acad Sci USA, 90:3294-3298, 1993.
84. St. Croix B, Florenes VA, Rak JW, *et al.* Impact of the cyclin-dependent kinase inhibitor p27Kip1 on resistance of tumor cells to anticancer agents. Nature Med, 2:1204-1210, 1996.
85. Wojtowicz-Praga SM, Dickson RB, Hawkins MJ. Matrix metalloproteinase inhibitors. Invest New Drugs, 15:61-75, 1997.

Chapter 2

THE ROLE OF MEMBRANE TRANSPORTERS IN CELLULAR RESISTANCE TO ANTICANCER NUCLEOSIDE DRUGS

Marilyn L. Clarke[1], John R. Mackey[1,2,6], Stephen A. Baldwin[3], James D. Young[4], and Carol E. Cass[1,5,6]
Departments of [1]Experimental Oncology and [2]Medicine, Cross Cancer Institute, Edmonton, Alberta, Canada
[3]School of Biochemistry and Molecular Biology, University of Leeds, Leeds, United Kingdom
Departments of [4]Physiology, [5]Biochemistry and [6]Oncology, University of Alberta, Edmonton, Alberta, Canada

1. INTRODUCTION

Physiologic nucleosides and most therapeutic nucleoside analogs do not readily cross plasma membranes by passive diffusion due to their low solubility in lipid bilayers, and their cellular uptake is mediated by integral membrane proteins. Nucleoside transporters serve as the cellular entry point for nucleoside salvage pathways. Some cell types use these pathways exclusively because they lack the ability to synthesize purine and pyrimidine nucleotides. Other cell types use salvage pathways in addition to their *de novo* synthesis pathways. Nucleotides are key activated intermediates for many essential cellular biosynthetic pathways, including the synthesis of DNA and RNA.

Inhibition of DNA synthesis in rapidly proliferating cancer cells has been exploited clinically by the use of antimetabolites such as nucleoside analogs. Anticancer nucleoside drugs such as cladribine, cytarabine and fludarabine have proven effective in several hematologic malignancies, and more recently, gemcitabine and capecitabine have shown efficacy against solid tumors. While these agents may induce durable complete remissions, the majority of cancers treated with these drugs eventually exhibit clinical resistance, either by progression during therapy or by relapse after an initial treatment response. Consequently, resistance to nucleoside analogs is a major clinical problem and strategies to avoid or reverse resistance have become important areas for research, with implications for rational drug design and combination therapies. Predictive assays capable of differentiating those patients with nucleoside-sensitive and nucleoside-resistant malignancies would greatly improve patient management by avoiding ineffective therapies and their attendant toxicities.

2. NUCLEOSIDE TRANSPORT PROCESSES

Nucleoside transport processes have recently been given transport classification (TC) numbers based on functional and phylogenetic characteristics[1]. Two distinct, structurally unrelated, nucleoside transport protein families have been identified and both are classified as electrochemical potential-driven porters. The ENT (Equilibrative Nucleoside Transporter; TC 2.A.57) family members in mammals facilitate transport in a bidirectional manner, accept both purine and pyrimidine nucleosides as substrates, and are widely distributed among eucaryotes. The mammalian CNT (Concentrative Nucleoside Transporter; TC 2.A.41) family members are inwardly directed sodium/nucleoside symporters, which are capable of moving nucleosides against the concentration gradient through coupled movement of sodium down its transmembrane electrochemical gradient. CNTs are distributed throughout the bacteria, archea and eucarya[1].

Seven functionally distinct nucleoside transport processes have been described in human cells, of which five have been characterized in molecular terms through isolation and functional expression of cDNAs encoding the transporter proteins in *Xenopus laevis* oocytes, mammalian cells or yeast[2–9]. The classification of nucleoside transport processes is based on functional and pharmacological characteristics, such as permeant selectivities and sensitivity to nanomolar concentrations of nucleoside and non-nucleoside inhibitors[3,10–15].

2.1 Characterized ENT Processes

Equilibrative transporters have been found in most cell types studied and are probably ubiquitous. Two human ENT subtypes (hENT1, hENT2) have been identified by molecular cloning and both are proteins consisting of 456 amino acids (50 kDa) with 11 predicted transmembrane domains (TMDs). The extracellular loop connecting TMDs 1 and 2 is glycosylated and there is a large intracellular loop connecting TMDs 6 and 7. Functional studies with chimeras formed from recombinant ENT proteins suggest that TMDs 3-6 are important for inhibitor interactions[16,17]. These ENT1 and ENT2 subtypes are responsible for processes that have been characterized on the basis of their sensitivity to nitrobenzylmercaptopurine ribonucleoside (NBMPR). The *equilibrative sensitive* (*es*) transport processes are inhibited by low concentrations of NBMPR (K_i 0.1-10 nm), whereas the *equilibrative insensitive* (*ei*) transport processes are unaffected by low concentrations of NBMPR (<1 μM). ENT1 and ENT2 proteins mediate *es* and *ei* processes, respectively, and are often produced in the same cell types. As both equilibrative transporters have broad substrate specificities, the physiological explanation for the co-existence of these two transporters might be found in the ability of the *ei* process to transport the purine nucleobase, hypoxanthine[17,18]. Degradation of purine nucleosides produces hypoxanthine, providing an important source of purines for salvage by cells lacking *de novo* synthesis such as bone marrow, where the concentration of hypoxanthine has been reported to reach 30 μM[17,19].

2.2 The *es* Transporter (hENT1)

hENT1 was first identified by molecular cloning from a human placental cDNA library (GenBank™ accession U81375) by comparison to the N-terminal amino acid sequence of the purified *es* transporter from human erythrocytes[4]. The hENT1 cDNA encodes a protein with a single glycosylation site in the external loop between TMDs 1 and 2[20], and the native human erythrocyte *es* transporter is known to be a heterogeneously glycosylated protein (45-65 kDa)[21]. hENT1 also possesses a number of potential phosphorylation consensus sites, although it has not been determined if hENT1 is phosphorylated *in vivo*. The hENT1 gene has been localized to chromosome 6p21.1-p21.2[22]. Recombinant hENT1 has been produced in *X. laevis* oocytes[4] and shown to mediate transport of uridine (K_m 0.24 mM) and adenosine. Uridine transport in hENT1-producing oocytes is inhibited by physiological purine and pyrimidine nucleosides, and by the nucleoside drugs cladribine, cytarabine, fludarabine, and gemcitabine (Figure 1). Uridine transport by recombinant hENT1 is also inhibited by NBMPR (IC_{50} 3.6 nM; Figure 2) and by the coronary vasodilators dipyridamole, dilazep and draflazine.

The rat homolog (rENT1) has 457 amino acids and 11 predicted TMDs with three potential glycosylation sites in the loop between TMDs 1 and 2[23]. hENT1 and rENT1 are highly conserved, with 78% identity and 88% similarity at the amino acid level. rENT1 is unusual in that it is *insensitive* to inhibition by dipyridamole[11], and studies with recombinant chimeric proteins in which various TMDs of hENT1 and rENT1 were interchanged established that dipyridamole and dilazep bind to a region of hENT1 between TMDs 3 and 6[16]. hENT1 transcripts have been detected by northern analysis in many tissues (see The Institute for Genomic Research, Human Gene Index) and several human cancer cell lines such as K562[24]. Expressed sequence tags (ESTs) with identity to hENT1 from many different normal and neoplastic human tissues have been registered in the data bases.

2.3 The *ei* Transporter (hENT2)

Based on sequence similarity to hENT1 (49% identical and 69% similar), a cDNA encoding hENT2 was isolated from a human placenta cDNA library (GenBank™ accession AF029358)[7]. The hENT2 gene has been localized to chromosome 11 (GenBank™ accession NT_009379; International Human Genome Project). The recombinant hENT2 protein exhibited *ei*-type activity when produced in *X. laevis* oocytes[7]. An identical transporter was identified in cultured HeLa cells by functional expression cloning of HeLa cDNA in an

NT-deficient leukemia cell line[6]. The rat homolog (rENT2), which was isolated from a rat jejunal cDNA library[23], also has 456 amino acids and 11 predicted TMDs. hENT2 and rENT2 are 93% similar and 88% identical at the amino acid level.

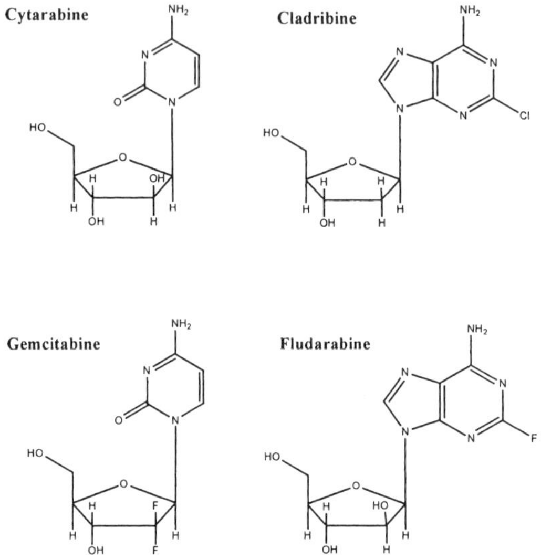

Figure 1. Chemical structures of nucleoside analogs used for treating cancer. Cytarabine and gemcitabine are analogs of the pyrimidine nucleoside, cytidine. Cladribine and fludarabine are analogs of the purine nucleoside, adenosine.

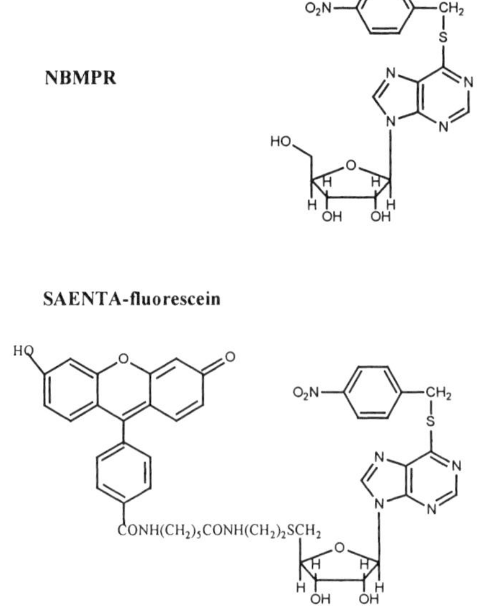

Figure 2. Chemical structures of the hENT1 transport inhibitor NBMPR and its fluorescent derivative, SAENTA-fluorescein.

Recombinant hENT2 exhibits a K_m value for uridine transport of 0.20 mM when produced in *X. laevis* oocytes[7]. In studies undertaken to identify potential permeants and/or inhibitors, in which test compounds (1 mM) were assessed for their ability to block inward transport of 10 μM ^{3}H-uridine[6], complete inhibition of transport was demonstrated with adenosine, inosine, or thymidine, partial inhibition with guanosine, cytidine or hypoxanthine, and no inhibition with adenine or uracil. Partial inhibition of recombinant hENT2 activity was achieved by 1 μM dipyridamole, dilazep or draflazine[6,7]. hENT2 mRNA has been observed in a variety of tissues, including brain, heart, lung, thymus, prostate, pancreas, with the highest levels occurring in skeletal muscle[6]. The physiological role of hENT2 in skeletal muscle has been suggested to be the transport of adenosine metabolites such as inosine and hypoxanthine during and after strenuous exercise[6]. A recent comparison of the biochemical, pharmacologic and kinetic parameters of recombinant hENT1 and hENT2, produced in a transport-deficient swine kidney epithelial cell line, has confirmed that hENT2 is a low affinity transporter compared to hENT1[25]. However, the study also revealed that hENT2 has a 4-fold higher affinity than hENT1 for inosine, and is consistent with a putative role for hENT2 during physical exercise[6,25].

2.4 The hENT3 Transporter

A recent search of the GenBank™ database resulted in the discovery of novel mammalian ENTs that have only been partially characterized[26]. cDNA of the human homolog (hENT3) was amplified from a placental cDNA library and encoded a 475-residue protein that was 73% identical to the putative mouse protein (mENT3) but had low sequence identity with either hENT1 or hENT2 (30-33%). The hENT3 gene (GenBank™ accession AF326987) is located on chromosome 10. Analysis of the human EST database has shown that the ENT3 mRNA is expressed in a range of normal and neoplastic human tissues, including kidney, placenta, breast, colon, testes, fetal liver and spleen. The relevance of this putative transporter to cancer chemotherapy and resistance cannot be determined until the hENT3 substrate specificity has been characterized.

2.5 Characterized CNT Processes

Sodium-dependent concentrative nucleoside transport processes of human cells comprise five functional subtypes (*cit*, concentrative, insensitive to NBMPR and thymidine selective; *cif*, concentrative, insensitive to NBMPR and formycin B-selective; *cib*, concentrative, insensitive to NBMPR and broadly selective; *csg*, concentrative, sensitive to NBMPR and guanosine selective; *cs*, concentrative and sensitive to NBMPR) that differ in their substrate selectivities, inhibitor profiles and tissue distributions. The three characterized CNTs have been divided phylogenetically into two groups: CNT1/CNT2 and CNT3 subfamilies. The hCNT1 and hCNT2 genes both map to chromosome 15, have a Na^+-uridine coupling ratio of 1:1, and are usually found in more specialized cell types such as in the kidney, intestine, heart and liver. The hCNT3 transporter maps to chromosome 9, has a Na^+-uridine coupling ratio of at least 2:1, and has a broader tissue distribution.

Although classified into two different subfamilies, the known vertebrate CNTs appear to share a similar topology. Initial hydropathy analysis predicted a structure with 14 TMDs, but recent studies with rCNT1 have shown that the C-terminal tail of rCNT1 is glycosylated and therefore extracellular, suggesting that CNTs have 13 TMDs with an intracellular N-terminus[2,17,27]. Recent studies with recombinant chimeras comprised of regions of the hCNT1 and hCNT2 proteins indicate that TMDs 7-9 contain the region of permeant selectivity. There is an 85% amino acid identity between the transporters in TMDs 7-9, and mutagenesis of just two or four amino acids of hCNT1 to the corresponding hCNT2 residues produced chimeric proteins with *cib*-like or *cif*-like activities, respectively[28].

There is increasing evidence that CNT processes are highly regulated. Sodium-dependent transport activity can be induced in cultured human leukemia cells upon activation by stimuli such as phorbol esters[2,29,30], lipopolysaccharides[29] and anti-CD3[30] antibodies. Although the proteins involved in regulation have yet to be characterized, it is expected that they soon will be, due to the recent advances in molecular cloning techniques and availability of genetic data bases for sequence comparisons. Understanding the regulatory pathways involved may well have implications for the rational design of anticancer drugs and combination treatment regimens.

2.6 The *cit* Transporter (hCNT1)

The *cit* process was first described in freshly isolated mouse intestinal epithelial cells as *concentrative*, *insensitive* to inhibition by NBMPR and capable of transporting *thymidine*[31]. Nucleoside transport processes with *cit*-type activity exhibit a preference for pyrimidine nucleosides and, although they are inhibited by low concentrations of adenosine, do not transport adenosine well[10,11]. The protein responsible for the *cit* process was identified when cDNA isolated from rat jejunum was expressed and its functionality tested in *X. laevis* oocytes[32,33]. Recombinant rCNT1 mediates the transport of the antiviral nucleosides, zidovudine and zalcitabine (K_m 0.5 mM)[32,34]. Cladribine and cytarabine, both anticancer drugs, inhibited rCNT1-mediated thymidine transport with IC_{50} values of 61 μM and 88 μM respectively[13]. Recombinant rCNT1 was also assessed in transiently transfected COS cells[35] in studies where the relative abilities of several nucleoside analogs to inhibit uridine transport were: 5-fluoro-2'-deoxyuridine > 5-iodo-2'-deoxyuridine > zidovudine > zalcitabine > cytarabine > gemcitabine. Additional studies in transfected mammalian cells showed that gemcitabine, 5-fluoro-2'-deoxyuridine and 5-fluorouridine are relatively good permeants whereas cytarabine is a poor permeant of rCNT1[36,37].

hCNT1 was subsequently identified by hybridization/RT-PCR cloning and functional expression in *X. laevis* oocytes of two almost identical cDNAs from human kidney[5]. The two human cDNAs encoded similar proteins designated hCNT1a and hCNT1b that were >99% identical (650 versus 648 amino acids, 71 kDa). These minor differences in protein sequence were attributed to genetic polymorphisms and/or errors induced during PCR amplification and are both considered to represent functional hCNT1 (GenBank™ accession U62966)[5]. Since hCNT1 has 83% amino acid sequence identity with rCNT1, it is expected to have a similar topology with 13, rather than 14, TMDs. The hCNT1 gene maps to chromosome 15q25-26[5].

Recombinant hCNT1 produced in *X. laevis* oocytes exhibits *cit*-type activity, has a K_m for uridine uptake of 42 μM, mediates uptake of zidovudine, zalcitabine and gemcitabine, and is inhibited by adenosine, thymidine, cytidine, and uridine but not by guanosine or inosine[5,38]. Adenosine binds with high affinity to hCNT1, yet is transported at low rates compared to uridine. Since physiologic adenosine concentrations rarely exceed 5-10 μM, it is possible that adenosine regulates hCNT1 activity *in vivo*, acting to inhibit transport of pyrimidine nucleosides such as uridine. Recombinant hCNT1 produced in transiently transfected HeLa cells mediated the transport of uridine (K_m 59 μM), cytidine (K_m 140 μM), deoxycytidine (K_m 150 μM)[39], and gemcitabine (K_m 18 μM)[37].

Structural determinants of nucleosides important for recognition by rCNT1 in *X. laevis* oocytes have recently been reported[40]. Electrophysiology has been used to directly examine the effects of modifying nucleosides at various positions on transport. The 6-position of the pyrimidine ring was found to be important for successful transport of uridine and cytidine analogs, whereas modifications could be made to the 3-, 4- and 5-position, or to the 5'-hydroxyl group of the sugar without affecting transportability.

2.7 The *cif* Transporter (hCNT2)

The *cif* process was first described in freshly isolated mouse intestinal epithelial cells[31] as *concentrative*, *insensitive* to inhibition by NBMPR and capable of transporting *formycin B* (the C-nucleoside analog of inosine). Nucleoside transport processes with *cif*-type activity were subsequently shown to be capable of transporting purine nucleosides in addition to uridine[10,11]. cDNAs encoding *cif*-type transporters were first isolated from rat liver (SPNT)[41] by functional expression cloning in *X. laevis* oocytes and subsequently by RT-PCR from rat jejunum (rCNT2)[42]. Although SPNT and rCNT2 differ by two conservative amino acid substitutions, they have similar transport properties and are therefore considered to be functionally the same. rCNT2 is predicted to have 659 amino acids (72 kDa) and is 64% identical to rCNT1 with five glycosylation sites and several possible phosphorylation sites, suggesting the potential for regulation by protein kinase-dependent mechanisms.

cDNAs encoding the human homologs of SPNT and rCNT2 were isolated from kidney (hSPNT1)[8] and intestine (hCNT2)[9] by hybridization/RT-PCR cloning. The human homologs were identical (658 amino acids), with the exception of a single, conservative amino acid substitution, and are hereafter referred to as hCNT2 (GenBank™ accession AF036109). The hCNT2 gene is located on chromosome 15[8,9]. Northern analyses suggest expression of hCNT2 mRNA in a variety of human tissues, including heart, liver, skeletal muscle, kidney, intestine, pancreas, placenta, brain, and lung. Recombinant hCNT2 produced in *X. laevis* oocytes exhibited K_m values of 4, 8, and 40 μM, respectively, for inward transport of inosine, adenosine and uridine[8,9]. Other hCNT2 permeants include adenosine, 2'-deoxyadenosine, guanosine and didanosine, but not thymidine, cytidine, uracil, zidovudine or zalcitabine[9]. A *cif* process has been described in the NB4 acute promyelocytic leukemia cell line[43] with K_m values, respectively, of 10 μM and 30 μM for adenosine and uridine. However, it is not known if hCNT2 is the protein responsible for this activity.

2.8 The *cib* Transporter (hCNT3)

The *cib* process is *concentrative*, *insensitive* to NBMPR, and possesses *broad* permeant selectivity for both purine and pyrimidine nucleosides. It was first described in freshly isolated human leukemic blasts[44] and human colon cancer CaCo-2 cells[45]. Despite the technical difficulties in functionally distinguishing between the various concentrative transporter types when multiple activities are present in single tissues or cells, the *cib* transporter protein has recently been identified in both mouse and human cells based on its relationship to a *cib* transporter of a primitive vertebrate[2].

The protein responsible for *cib* activity in the hagfish (hfCNT) was identified by molecular cloning and functional expression of its cDNA[2]. When the hagfish cDNA sequence was compared to the EST database, partial matches were found with sequences from human and mouse mammary gland and human colon adenocarcinoma. The human and mouse *cib* transporters were subsequently identified by molecular cloning of cDNAs from differentiated HL-60 cells and mammary gland (hCNT3), and from mouse liver (mCNT3). hCNT3/mCNT3 are 79% identical and comprised of 691 and 703 amino acid residues, respectively. The hCNT3 gene (GenBank™ accession AF305210) has an upstream phorbol ester response element and is located on chromosome 9q22.2[2].

Functional studies of recombinant hCNT3 in *X. laevis* oocytes confirmed that transport activity was *cib*-like with broad permeant selectivity for purines and pyrimidines with apparent K_m values of 15-53 μM (cytosine, adenosine < uridine, thymidine < guanosine, inosine). Anticancer and antiviral nucleoside analogs were also transported: 5-fluoruridine > 5-fluoro 2'-deoxyuridine > cladribine > zebularine > gemcitabine > fludarabine > zidovudine > 2',3'-dideoxyinosine > 2',3'-dideoxycytosine[2].

2.9 Concentrative Nucleoside Transport Processes Mediated by Unknown Proteins

There are additional CNT-like activities that have been described in human cells, but the proteins responsible have not been identified. Until the permeant selectivities and tissue distribution have been fully characterized, it will be difficult to define the relevance of these activities to cancer chemotherapy.

An atypical *cit*–type activity that accepts guanosine, adenosine and pyrimidine nucleosides as substrates has been described in human brush-border membrane vesicles[13]. Another atypical *cit*-type activity has recently been described in CD3-activated human peripheral blood mononuclear cells[30]. The *csg* process, which is *concentrative*, *sensitive* to NBMPR and selective for *guanosine*, has been reported in NB4 acute promyelocytic leukemia cells[46] and in human B-cell lines (Raji and BLS-1) after activation with phorbol esters or lipopolysaccharide[29]. Tumor necrosis factor-α may be involved in mediating these effects, which include down-regulation of the *es* transport activity[29]. The *cs* process is *concentrative* and *sensitive* to NBMPR and has been reported in freshly isolated chronic lymphocytic leukemia (CLL) cells and acute myelogenous leukemia (AML) cells, in which it mediates cellular uptake of cladribine and fludarabine[47].

3. THE ROLE OF NUCLEOSIDE TRANSPORT IN ANTICANCER NUCLEOSIDE ACTIVITY AND CELLULAR RESISTANCE

3.1 Transport Processes and Cytotoxicity

Anticancer nucleoside drugs in general clinical use are cladribine, cytarabine, fludarabine, gemcitabine and capecitabine. Because the pharmacologic targets of these drugs are usually intracellular, mediated transport across plasma membranes is a prerequisite step for inducing cytotoxicity[10]. The structural differences among these compounds (Figure 1) result in marked differences in their interactions with nucleoside transporter proteins, which contribute to the differing cellular and tissue specificities of these drugs.

Nucleoside transport may contribute to the relative selectivity of nucleoside chemotherapy for malignant cells. High cellular proliferation rates have been associated with high levels of *es* transport activity, NBMPR-binding sites (a measure of transporter abundance) and hENT1 protein. The number of *es* transporters increased when human leukemia cells were stimulated to proliferate with growth factors[48] and mitotic rates were correlated to the number of NBMPR-binding sites in human thymocytes[49] and myeloblasts[50]. Recently, hENT1 abundance determined by immunohistochemistry was observed to be higher in breast carcinoma cells than in normal breast epithelia[51]. The *es*-mediated process is the primary mode of inwardly directed transport of nucleoside drugs in many cell types, and it is not surprising that cellular hENT1 abundance has been correlated with sensitivity to nucleoside drugs[37,51,52].

3.2 Transporter-Mediated Mechanisms of Drug Resistance

Since anticancer nucleoside drugs must enter cells to cause cytotoxicity, reduced inwardly directed transport will slow the intracellular accumulation of nucleosides, potentially conferring resistance. Cell types with intrinsically low nucleoside transport activity will be inherently resistant to short exposures to nucleoside drugs, as has been demonstrated with *es*-deficient myeloblasts[50]. Whether acquired clinical nucleoside resistance is due to the down-regulation of nucleoside transport activity, or to the selection of neoplastic cells with transport-deficient phenotypes, remains to be determined.

Because equilibrative transporters (*es* and *ei*) are bi-directional and depend on chemical concentration gradients, drug efflux is also potentially involved in resistance. A recent study has demonstrated that cladribine exits cultured acute lymphocytic leukemia (ALL) cells after short-term drug exposure, and cytotoxicity was enhanced by post-cladribine exposure to inhibitors of the bi-directional equilibrative transporters to prevent efflux[53]. The contribution of drug efflux to cellular nucleoside exposure *in vivo* is unknown, but is unlikely to substantially reduce cellular accumulation of cytarabine or cladribine, which are delivered using prolonged continuous intravenous infusions.

Transport of nucleosides may potentially affect the pharmacokinetics of anticancer nucleoside drugs. Organic ion transporters in the kidney have been recently implicated in the renal secretion of nucleosides[54]. Differential activity of such transporters could contribute to inter-patient variability in the serum half-life of these drugs, and might result in some patients receiving sub-optimal drug exposure.

3.2.1 Resistance to nucleoside analogs in cultured cancer cell lines

Transport-related resistance to nucleosides and synthetic analogs in cultured cells was first studied in AE_1 cells, a variant of the S49 murine T-cell lymphoma cell line[55]. The AE_1 clone was produced by chemical mutagenesis and a single-step selection with a cytotoxic concentration of adenosine in the presence of the adenosine deaminase inhibitor, erythro-9-(2-hydroxy-3-nonyl) adenine. The resulting cell line exhibited reduced uptake of both purine and pyrimidine nucleosides that was not related to loss of metabolic enzyme activity, but rather due to the loss of functional nucleoside transport activity mediated by a single carrier protein[55]. Further characterization of the AE_1 cell line showed that the loss of nucleoside transport activity was accompanied by a loss of high affinity NBMPR-binding sites[56]. AE_1 cells are cross resistant to the anticancer nucleoside analogs cytarabine, 5-fluorouridine, 5-fluoro-2'-deoxyuridine[55] and gemcitabine[37].

The first human cell line exhibiting transport-related resistance was produced in a similar manner to that used to generate the mouse AE_1 clone. Parental CCRF-CEM cells, exhibiting primarily *es*-mediated transport activity, were chemically mutagenized to produce a hypoxanthine guanine phosphoribosyltransferase deficient clone and then selected for growth in the presence of 8 μM cytarabine. The resulting clone (CEM/ARAC8C) was deficient in *es* activity, lacked high affinity NBMPR-binding sites and was cross resistant to several cytotoxic nucleosides[57,58].

Transport-related resistance has also been observed in the absence of chemical mutagenesis[59]. Exposure of murine erythroleukemia cells to increasing concentrations of periodate-oxidized adenosine yielded cells with genetically stable high-level resistance and a 20-fold decrease in NBMPR binding sites, suggesting a loss of hENT1 protein. In human HCT-8 colon cancer cells[60], resistance (700-fold) was obtained by exposure to increasing concentrations of 5-fluoro 2'-deoxyuridine. Resistant cells exhibited no measurable uptake of 5-fluoro 2'-deoxyuridine or NBMPR binding. These studies clearly demonstrate that the absence of *es*-transport activity, presumably due to altered hENT1 protein expression and/or function, confers high level-resistance to nucleoside analogs.

3.3 Clinical Evidence for Transport-Related Resistance to Nucleoside Analogs

Although *in vitro* studies have shown the importance of facilitated transport for nucleoside antimetabolites to achieve a therapeutic effect, the relevance of transport deficiency in clinical drug resistance is still under investigation. This is mainly due to the difficulty of performing transport studies on malignant cells derived from clinical specimens, and the problems associated with quantifying nucleoside transporter proteins in malignant clones admixed with normal cells. However, there is strong evidence that clinical resistance to cytarabine can be mediated by a transport deficiency.

3.3.1 Cytarabine

Cytarabine (ara-C, 1-β-D-arabinofuranosyl cytosine, Cytosar-U®) is a pyrimidine nucleoside analog that has played a major role in the curative therapy of AML for many years. When cytarabine is administered as a single agent, remissions are produced in about 30% of patients[61]. Improved responses are usually observed, however, when cytarabine is used in combination with other chemotherapy agents such as anthracyclines (e.g., daunorubicin or idarubicin) for standard induction, consolidation, maintenance, and intensification regimens for patients with AML. Combinations including cytarabine are also used for the treatment of chronic myelogenous leukemia (CML), multiple myeloma, Hodgkin's lymphoma[62] and non-Hodgkin's lymphomas[63]. Cytarabine has low activity against solid tumors. Adverse reactions include fever, nausea, alopecia and myelosuppression[64].

Cytarabine permeates cells primarily by *es*-mediated transport processes in human leukemia cells[65] and is activated by enzymes of the nucleoside salvage pathways. Intracellular activation of cytarabine is initiated by deoxycytidine kinase to produce the monophosphate derivative. Subsequent phosphorylation steps produce the cytotoxic triphosphate metabolite (ara-CTP). Ara-CTP is incorporated into DNA and, because it is a potent inhibitor of DNA polymerases α and β, causes premature chain termination, DNA fragmentation and apoptosis[66–68]. The relationship between ara-CTP accumulation, incorporation of ara-CTP into DNA and treatment efficacy has been clearly demonstrated in leukemic cells[69,70].

Mediated inward transport of cytarabine is the major determinant of ara-CTP accumulation at low cytarabine concentrations (<1 μM) achieved by standard dose regimens (e.g., 100-200 mg/m^2/day)[71]. The efficiency of cytarabine uptake by leukemic blast cells has been related to clinical outcome in AML patients receiving standard doses, where three patients that failed therapy exhibited the lowest rates of cytarabine uptake and NBMPR-binding sites (as a measure of functional *es* transporters)[72]. The development of transport-related resistance during treatment with cytarabine has been described in a patient with T-cell ALL, whose blasts prior to therapy had rapid cytarabine uptake, ara-CTP accumulation and high numbers of NBMPR-binding sites[73]. This patient initially responded to standard-dose treatment, but presented at the time of disease relapse with cells exhibiting an ~75% decrease of NBMPR-binding site number and ara-CTP accumulation rate.

Uptake of cytarabine is primarily by *es*-activity (a process presumably mediated by the hENT1 protein) and can be measured indirectly by binding of SAENTA-fluorescein (5'-S-(2-aminoethyl)-N6-(4-nitrobenzyl)-5'-thioadenosine-fluorescein, an impermeant fluorescent analog of NBMPR). Because there is a positive correlation between the number of NBMPR-binding sites, cytarabine influx and cytotoxity[52,65,74,75], SAENTA-fluorescein may be a useful tool for detecting the presence of inherent resistance (low number of NBMPR-binding sites at initial diagnosis).

To avoid transport-related resistance, anticancer nucleoside drugs administered at high doses will enter cells by passive diffusion, where the phosphorylation capacity of deoxycytidine kinase becomes the rate-limiting step[65,76,77]. High-dose cytarabine regimens (e.g., 3 g/m^2/day) produce remissions in some patients refractory to standard doses and generate plasma levels above 50 μM[78]. Two randomized studies have also shown the benefit of using high-dose induction treatment regimens by demonstrating that, although remission rates were similar to those obtained with standard doses, superior disease-free survival rates were seen in the high-dose groups[79,80].

3.3.2 Fludarabine

Fludarabine (9-β-D-arabinosyl-2-fluoroadenine, F-ara-A, Fludara®) is a purine nucleoside analog that is the most active single agent in the treatment of CLL[81]. Fludarabine also has activity in: (i) low-grade non-Hodgkin's lymphoma inducing partial responses in ~50% of patients with relapsed or refractory disease and complete responses in ~40% of patients receiving fludarabine as the initial treatment[82,83]; (ii) Waldenström's macroglobulinemia; and (iii) other hematologic malignancies[82,84]. Fludarabine has little solid tumor activity[85]. Adverse reactions include cell-mediated immunodeficiency characterized by reduced CD4/CD8 counts and opportunistic infections, and dose-limiting myelosuppression[64,86].

Following intravenous administration as fludarabine 5'-monophosphate, it is rapidly dephosphorylated extracellularly to fludarabine by plasma phosphatases and ecto-5' nucleotidase. Intracellularly, fludarabine is rephosphorylated by deoxycytidine kinase and further phosphorylated to F-ara-ATP, which induces toxicity through incorporation into DNA and RNA, and inhibition of ribonucleotide reductase, DNA polymerase-α, DNA primase, and DNA ligase[85,87–89].

Fludarabine enters cells by *es*[52], *cib*[2] and *cs*[47]-mediated processes. In lymphoblasts harvested from ALL patients, fludarabine sensitivity *in vitro* correlated with *es* transporter (i.e., hENT1) abundance in the plasma membrane, as determined by SAENTA-fluorescein binding[52].

3.3.3 Cladribine

Cladribine (CdA, 2-chloro-2'-deoxyadenosine, Leustatin®) is a purine nucleoside analog that achieves durable complete remissions in the majority of patients with hairy cell leukemia, and short-lived remissions in CLL and non-Hodgkin's lymphoma[82]. Cladribine has minimal solid tumor activity. Adverse effects include fever, myelosuppression and profound cell-mediated immunosuppression[64].

Cladribine enters cells by *es*[90], *ei*[90], *cib*[2] and *cs*[47]-mediated processes. Transport by the *es* and *ei* processes was demonstrated by NBMPR and dipyridamole protection studies in human hematopoietic cancer cell lines[91]. Transport kinetics of radiolabeled cladribine have been determined for the *es*, *ei* and *cif*-mediated processes in several leukemic cell lines where the degree of cytotoxicity was directly correlated with the efficiency of transport[90]. In freshly harvested ALL lymphoblasts, *in vitro* sensitivity to cladribine correlated with *es* transporter (i.e., hENT1) protein abundance in plasma membranes as determined by SAENTA-fluorescein binding[52].

3.3.4 Gemcitabine

Gemcitabine (2', 2'-difluorodeoxycytidine, dFdC, Gemzar®) is a pyrimidine nucleoside drug that has activity against solid tumors, including non-small cell lung, breast, bladder, ovarian, and head and neck cancers[63]. Adverse reactions include fever, alopecia and myelosuppression[62].

Gemcitabine is first converted intracellularly to gemcitabine 5'-monophosphate by deoxycytidine kinase, and subsequently phosphorylated to the 5-diphosphate and 5'-triphosphate derivatives by pyrimidine monophosphate and diphosphate kinases[92]. dFdCDP inhibits ribonucleotide reductase, while dFdCTP is incorporated into DNA and RNA[93]. Although the relative contributions of these effects to cytotoxicity are not known, gemcitabine exhibits the property of self-potentiation in that dFdCTP inhibits deoxycytidine monophosphate deaminase, thereby decreasing its own catabolic degradation[92]. Studies in Chinese hamster ovary cells showed that the rates of inward transport of gemcitabine and cytarabine were similar, and the observed differences in cytotoxicity of the two drugs were attributed to gemcitabine's higher affinity for deoxycytidine kinase and the longer intracellular retention of dFdCTP compared to ara-CTP[94].

The transportability of gemcitabine, and its importance in gemcitabine cytotoxicity, has been examined in detail in studies with both native and recombinant transport proteins[2,37,38]. A complete deficiency in transport activity, produced either pharmacologically or genetically, confers two to three-log resistance of cultured cells to gemcitabine cytotoxicity. Kinetic studies with a panel of murine and human cell lines with defined nucleoside transport processes demonstrated that gemcitabine uptake is mediated by *es, ei, cit* and *cib*, but not by *cif*. The most efficient processes were those mediated by *es* and *cit*, although the rates of gemcitabine transport were ~10% of uridine. Cellular gemcitabine transport capacity appears to be an important determinant of clinical activity, as it is typically administered as a short bolus and is rapidly degraded in plasma, producing short-term drug exposures.

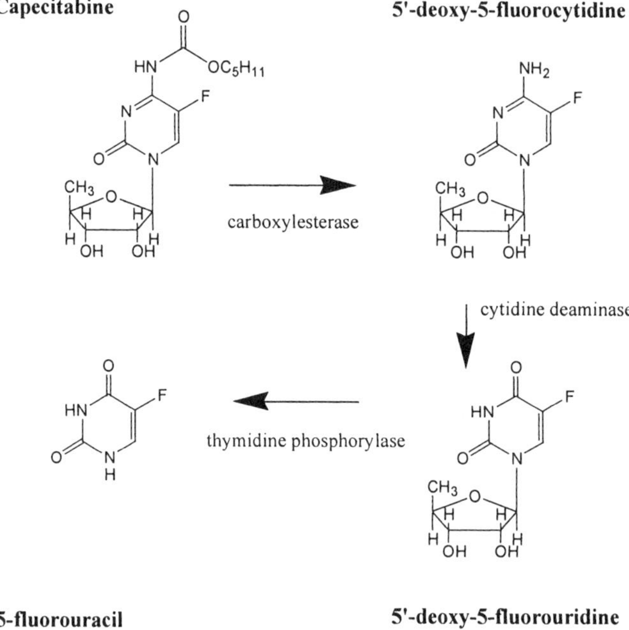

Figure 3. Chemical structures of capecitabine and its metabolites. The enzymes involved in the metabolic pathway of capecitabine are indicated.

3.3.5 Capecitabine

Capecitabine (5'-Deoxy-5-N-[(pentoxy)carbonyl]-cytidine, Xeloda®) is an oral prodrug of 5-fluorouracil (Figure 3). Capecitabine has substantial activity in patients with colon cancer and in patients with advanced breast cancer with prior exposure to taxane or anthracycline chemotherapy[95]. Toxic effects include palmar-plantar erythrodysesthesia, mucositis, and diarrhea.

Capecitabine is rapidly and extensively absorbed, metabolised in the liver by carboxylesterase to 5'-deoxy-5-fluorocytidine, then converted to 5'-deoxy-5-fluorouridine by cytidine deaminase in both liver and tumor tissues. Finally, 5'-deoxy-5-fluorouridine is converted to 5-fluorouracil by thymidine phosphorylase, an enzyme found at high levels in many tumor tissues[96]. The uptake of 5'-deoxy-5-fluorouridine is mediated predominantly by hENT1, since the presence of the transport inhibitor, NBMPR, conferred a 5.5-fold protection against the cytotoxic effects of drug exposure[51]. 5-Fluorouracil is metabolized to produce three cytotoxic compounds: (i) 5-fluorodeoxyuridine monophosphate that inhibits thymidylate synthase; (ii) 5-fluoruridine triphosphate that is incorporated into RNA; and (iii) 5-fluorodeoxyuridine triphosphate that is incorporated into DNA[97].

3.4 Measuring Nucleoside Drug Uptake as a Resistance Marker

The nucleoside transport capability of tumor cells may be a determinant of the clinical outcome of treatment regimens using nucleoside drugs. Presently, leukemia cells can be tested by flow cytometry with SAENTA-fluorescein[52] to assess the abundance of NBMPR-binding sites (i.e., hENT1) protein on the cell surface. In the case of standard-dose cytarabine treatment of adult AML, this result appears to be predictive of clinical outcome. However, until recently, there was no way to assess the nucleoside transport capability of malignant cells within solid tumors. We have developed an immunohistochemical method to assess hENT1 abundance of malignant cells in breast tumors[51] in which frozen sections of 33 primary breast cancers were stained with monoclonal antibodies raised against a synthetic peptide derived from the large intracellular loop of hENT1[98]. Staining intensity varied markedly among the breast samples and at least nine were hENT1 deficient, suggesting that this method will be helpful for screening biopsy tissue samples to predict nucleoside drug uptake. Future studies will determine whether immunohistochemistry with hENT1 antibodies has broader applications to other solid tumors.

CONCLUSION

Nucleoside analogs are an important class of antimetabolites used to treat cancer either as single agents or in combination regimens. Ultimately, their effectiveness is limited by drug resistance. Nucleoside prodrugs enter cells primarily by hENT1-mediated processes, and the loss of functional transporters represents a mechanism of acquired resistance that has been documented for cytarabine chemotherapy. However, the importance of transport-related resistance to treatment failure of other clinically-relevant nucleoside drugs, gemcitabine, capecitabine, fludarabine and cladribine has yet to be determined.

The differential uptake and cytotoxicities of nucleoside drugs in various tissues will most likely be a function of the relative distribution of equilibrative and concentrative transporters present and the ability of drugs to gain access to their intracellular targets. It is therefore important to fully document the relative tissue distribution of nucleoside transporters. Elucidation of the structural determinants required for transport will allow nucleoside analogs to be rationally designed to target specific tissues with defined nucleoside-transport profiles. Although little is known about the regulatory mechanisms of nucleoside transporters, the downregulation of equilibrative, and the upregulation of concentrative, transporters observed when cells are induced to differentiate (e.g., with Bryostatin 1), is already being exploited clinically to enhance the cytotoxicity of nucleoside drugs[99,100].

ACKNOWLEDGEMENTS

We thank Linda Harris (Librarian) for assistance with the preparation of this manuscript. This work was supported by the Alberta Cancer Board, the Canadian Institutes of Health Research, the National Cancer Institute of Canada, Medical Research Council, UK and the Wellcome Trust, UK. JDY is a Heritage Medical Scientist of the Alberta Heritage Foundation for Medical Research.

REFERENCES

1. Saier MH. A functional-phylogenetic classification system for transmembrane solute transporters. Microbiol Mol Biol Rev, 64:354-411, 2000.
2. Ritzel MWL, Ng AML, Yao SYM, *et al.* Molecular identification and characterization of novel human and mouse concentrative Na^+-nucleoside cotransporter proteins (hCNT3 and mCNT3) broadly selective for purine and pyrimidine nucleosides (System cib). J Biol Chem, 276:2914-2927, 2001.
3. Vickers MF, Young JD, Baldwin SA, *et al.* Nucleoside transporter proteins: emerging targets for drug discovery. Emerging Therapeutic Targets, 4:515-539, 2000.
4. Griffiths M, Beaumont N, Yao SY, *et al.* Cloning of a human nucleoside transporter implicated in the cellular uptake of adenosine and chemotherapeutic drugs. Nature Med, 3:89-93, 1997.
5. Ritzel MWL, Yao SYM, Huang MY, *et al.* Molecular cloning and functional expression of cDNAs encoding a human Na+-nucleoside cotransporter (hCNT1). Amer J Physiol, 272:C707-C714, 1997.
6. Crawford CR, Patel DH, Naeve C, Belt JA. Cloning of the human equilibrative, nitrobenzylmercaptopurine riboside (NBMPR)-insensitive nucleoside transporter ei by functional expression in a transport-deficient cell line. J Biol Chem, 273:5288-5293, 1998.
7. Griffiths M, Yao SYM, Abidi F, *et al.* Molecular cloning and characterization of a nitrobenzylthioinosine-insensitive (ei) equilibrative nucleoside transporter from human placenta. Biochem J, 328:739-743, 1997.
8. Wang J, Su S-F, Dresser MJ, *et al.* Na+-dependent purine nucleoside transporter from human kidney: cloning and functional characterization. Amer J Physiol, 273:F1058-F1065, 1997.
9. Ritzel MW, Yao SY, Ng AM, *et al.* Molecular cloning, functional expression and chromosomal localization of a cDNA encoding a human Na+/nucleoside cotransporter (hCNT2) selective for purine nucleosides and uridine. Mol Membr Biol, 15:203-211, 1998.
10. Cass CE. Nucleoside transport. *In*: Drug Transport in Antimicrobial Therapy and Anticancer Therapy. NH Georgopapadakou (ed.), Marcel Dekker, New York, NY, 1995.

11. Griffith DA, Jarvis SM. Nucleoside and nucleobase transport systems of mammalian cells. Biochim Biophys Acta, 1286:153-181, 1996.
12. Buolamwini JK. Nucleoside transport inhibitors: Structure-activity relationships and potential therapeutic applications. Curr Med Chem, 4:35-66, 1997.
13. Wang J, Schaner ME, Thomassen S, *et al.* Functional and molecular characteristics of Na(+)-dependent nucleoside transporters. Pharm Res, 14:1524-1532, 1997.
14. Che M, Gatmaitan Z, Arias IM. Ectonucleotidases, purine nucleoside transporter, and function of the bile canalicular plasma membrane of the hepatocyte. FASEB J, 11:101-108, 1997.
15. Thorn JA, Jarvis SM. Adenosine transporters. Gen Pharmacol, 27:613-620, 1996.
16. Sundaram M, Yao SY, Ng AM, *et al.* Chimeric constructs between human and rat equilibrative nucleoside transporters (hENT1 and rENT1) reveal hENT1 structural domains interacting with coronary vasoactive drugs. J Biol Chem, 273:21519-21525, 1998.
17. Baldwin SA, Mackey JR, Cass CE, Young JD. Nucleoside transporters: molecular biology and implications for therapeutic development. Mol Med Today, 5:216-224, 1999.
18. Osses N, Pearson JD, Yudilevich DL, Jarvis SM. Hypoxanthine enters human vascular endothelial cells (ECV 304) via the nitrobenzylthioinosine-insensitive equilibrative nucleoside transporter. Biochem J, 317:843-848, 1996.
19. Tattersall MH, Slowiaczek P, De Fazio A. Regional variation in human extracellular purine levels. J Lab Clin Med, 102:411-420, 1983.
20. Vickers MF, Mani RS, Sundaram M, *et al.* Functional production and reconstitution of the human equilibrative nucleoside transporter (hENT1) in Saccharomyces cerevisiae. Interaction of inhibitors of nucleoside transport with recombinant hENT1 and a glycosylation-defective derivative (hENT1/N48Q). Biochem J, 339:21-32, 1999.
21. Kwong FY, Wu JS, Shi MM, *et al.* Enzymic cleavage as a probe of the molecular structures of mammalian equilibrative nucleoside transporters. J Biol Chem, 268:22127-22134, 1993.
22. Coe IR, Griffiths M, Young JD, *et al.* Assignment of the human equilibrative nucleoside transporter (hENT1) to 6p21.1-p21.2. Genomics, 45:459-460, 1997.
23. Yao SY, Ng AM, Muzyka WR, *et al.* Molecular cloning and functional characterization of nitrobenzylthioinosine (NBMPR)-sensitive (es) and NBMPR-insensitive (ei) equilibrative nucleoside transporter proteins (rENT1 and rENT2) from rat tissues. J Biol Chem, 272:28423-28430, 1997.
24. Boleti H, Coe IR, Baldwin SA, *et al.* Molecular identification of the equilibrative NBMPR-sensitive (es) nucleoside transporter and demonstration of an equilibrative NBMPR-insensitive (ei) transport activity in human erythroleukemia (K562) cells. Neuropharmacol, 36:1167-1179, 1997.
25. Ward JL, Sherali A, Mo ZP, Tse CM. Kinetic and pharmacological properties of cloned human equilibrative nucleoside transporters, ENT1 and ENT2, stably expressed in nucleoside transporter-deficient PK15 cells. ENT2 exhibits a low affinity for guanosine and cytidine but a high affinity for inosine. J Biol Chem, 275:8375-8381, 2000.
26. Hyde RJ, Cass CE, Young JD, Baldwin SA. The ENT family of eukaryote nucleoside transporters: recent advances in the investigation of structure/function relationships and the identification of novel isoforms. Mol Membr Biol, 18:53-63, 2001.
27. Hamilton SR, Yao SYM, Ingram JC, *et al.* Sub-cellular distribution and membrane topology of the rat concentrative Na^+-nucleoside co-transporter rCNT1. J Biol Chem, 276:27981-27988, 2001.

28. Loewen SK, Ng AM, Yao SY, *et al.* Identification of amino acid residues responsible for the pyrimidine and purine nucleoside specificities of human concentrative Na(+) nucleoside cotransporters hCNT1 and hCNT2. J Biol Chem, 274:24475-24484, 1999.
29. Soler C, Felipe A, Mata JF, *et al.* Regulation of nucleoside transport by lipopolysaccharide, phorbol esters, and tumour necrosis factor-α in human B-lymphocytes. J Biol Chem, 273:26939-26945, 1998.
30. Kichenin K, Pignede G, Fudelej F, Seman M. CD3 activation induces concentrative nucleoside transport in human T lymphocytes. Eur J Immunol, 30:366-370, 2000.
31. Vijayalakshmi D, Belt JA. Sodium-dependent nucleoside transport in mouse intestinal epithelial cells. Two transport systems with differing substrate specificities. J Biol Chem, 263:19419-19423, 1988.
32. Huang QQ, Yao SY, Ritzel MW, *et al.* Cloning and functional expression of a complementary DNA encoding a mammalian nucleoside transport protein. J Biol Chem, 269:17757-17760, 1994.
33. Huang QQ, Harvey CM, Paterson AR, *et al.* Functional expression of Na(+)-dependent nucleoside transport systems of rat intestine in isolated oocytes of Xenopus laevis. Demonstration that rat jejunum expresses the purine-selective system N1 (cif) and a second, novel system N3 having broad specificity for purine and pyrimidine nucleosides. J Biol Chem, 268:20613-20619, 1993.
34. Yao SY, Cass CE, Young JD. Transport of the antiviral nucleoside analogs 3'-azido-3'-deoxythymidine and 2',3'-dideoxycytidine by a recombinant nucleoside transporter (rCNT) expressed in Xenopus laevis oocytes. Mol Pharmacol, 50:388-393, 1996.
35. Fang X, Parkinson FE, Mowles DA, *et al.* Functional characterization of a recombinant sodium-dependent nucleoside transporter with selectivity for pyrimidine nucleosides (cNT1rat) by transient expression in cultured mammalian cells. Biochem J, 317:457-465, 1996.
36. Crawford CR, Cass CE, Young JD, Belt JA. Stable expression of a recombinant sodium-dependent, pyrimidine-selective nucleoside transporter (CNT1) in a transport-deficient mouse leukemia cell line. Biochem Cell Biol, 76:843-851, 1998.
37. Mackey JR, Mani RS, Selner M, *et al.* Functional nucleoside transporters are required for gemcitabine influx and manifestation of toxicity in cancer cell lines. Cancer Res, 58:4349-4357, 1998.
38. Mackey JR, Yao SY, Smith KM, *et al.* Gemcitabine transport in xenopus oocytes expressing recombinant plasma membrane mammalian nucleoside transporters. J Natl Cancer Inst, 91:1876-1881, 1999.
39. Graham KA, Leithoff J, Coe IR, *et al.* Differential transport of cytosine-containing nucleosides by recombinant human concentrative nucleoside transporter protein hCNT1. Nucleosides Nucleotides Nucleic Acids, 19:415-434, 2000.
40. Dresser MJ, Gerstin KM, Gray AT, *et al.* Electrophysiological analysis of the substrate selectivity of a sodium-coupled nucleoside transporter (rCNT1) expressed in Xenopus laevis oocytes. Drug Metabolism and Disposition, 28:1135-1140, 2000.
41. Che M, Ortiz DF, Arias IM. Primary structure and functional expression of a cDNA encoding the bile canalicular, purine-specific Na+-nucleoside cotransporter. J Biol Chem, 270:13596-13599, 1995.
42. Yao SY, Ng AM, Ritzel MW, *et al.* Transport of adenosine by recombinant purine- and pyrimidine-selective sodium/nucleoside cotransporters from rat jejunum expressed in Xenopus laevis oocytes. Mol Pharmacol, 50:1529-1535, 1996.
43. Roovers KI, Meckling-Gill KA. Characterization of equilibrative and concentrative Na+-dependent (cif) nucleoside transport in acute promyelocytic leukemia NB4 cells. J Cell Physiol, 166:593-600, 1996.

44. Belt JA, Harper EH, Byl JA, Noel LD. Sodium-dependent nucleoside transport in human myeloid leukemic cell lines and freshly isolated myeloblasts. Proc Amer Assoc Cancer Res, 33:20, 1992.
45. Belt JA, Marina NM, Phelps DA, Crawford CR. Nucleoside transport in normal and neoplastic cells. Adv Enzyme Regul, 33:235-252, 1993.
46. Flanagan SA, Mecklinggill KA. Characterization of a novel Na+ dependent, guanosine specific, nitrobenzylthioinosine sensitive transporter in acute promyelocytic leukemia cells. J Biol Chem, 272:18026-18032, 1997.
47. Paterson AR, Gati WP, Vijayalakshmi D, *et al.* Inhibitor-sensitive, Na(+)-linked transport of nucleoside analogs in leukemia cells from patients. Proc Amer Assoc Cancer Res, 34:A84, 1993.
48. Wiley JS, Cebon JS, Jamieson GP, *et al.* Assessment of proliferative responses to granulocyte-macrophage colony-stimulating factor (GM-CSF) in acute myeloid leukaemia using a fluorescent ligand for the nucleoside transporter. Leukemia, 8:181-185, 1994.
49. Smith CL, Pilarski LM, Egerton ML, Wiley JS. Nucleoside transport and proliferative rate in human thymocytes and lymphocytes. Blood, 74:2038-2042, 1989.
50. Wiley JS, Snook MB, Jamieson GP. Nucleoside transport in acute leukaemia and lymphoma: close relation to proliferative rate. Br J Haematol, 71:203-207, 1989.
51. Mackey JR, Jennings LL, Clarke ML, *et al.* Immunohistochemical variation of human equilibrative nucleoside transporter 1 (hENT1) protein in primary breast cancers. Clin Cancer Res, 1:110-116, 2002.
52. Gati WP, Paterson AR, Belch AR, *et al.* Es nucleoside transporter content of acute leukemia cells: role in cell sensitivity to cytarabine (araC). Leuk Lymphoma, 32:45-54, 1998.
53. Wright AM, Gati WP, Paterson AR. Enhancement of retention and cytotoxicity of 2-chlorodeoxyadenosine in cultured human leukemic lymphoblasts by nitrobenzylthioinosine, an inhibitor of equilibrative nucleoside transport. Leukemia, 14:52-60, 2000.
54. Chen R, Nelson JA. Role of organic cation transporters in the renal secretion of nucleosides. Biochem Pharmacol, 60:215-219, 2000.
55. Cohen A, Ullman B, Martin DW, Jr. Characterization of a mutant mouse lymphoma cell with deficient transport of purine and pyrimidine nucleosides. J Biol Chem, 254:112-116, 1979.
56. Cass CE, Kolassa N, Uehara Y, *et al.* Absence of binding sites for the transport inhibitor nitrobenzylthioinosine on nucleoside transport-deficient mouse lymphoma cells. Biochim Biophys Acta, 649:769-777, 1981.
57. Ullman B, Coons T, Rockwell S, McCartan K. Genetic analysis of 2',3'-dideoxycytidine incorporation into cultured human T lymphoblasts. J Biol Chem, 263:12391-12396, 1988.
58. Ullman B. Dideoxycytidine metabolism in wild type and mutant CEM cells deficient in nucleoside transport or deoxycytidine kinase. Adv Exp Med Biol, 253B:415-420, 1989.
59. Hoffman J. Murine erythroleukemia cells resistant to periodate-oxidized adenosine have lowered levels of nucleoside transporter. Adv Exp Med Biol, 309A:443-446, 1991.
60. Sobrero AF, Handschumacher RE, Bertino JR. Highly selective drug combinations for human colon cancer cells resistant in vitro to 5-fluoro-2'-deoxyuridine. Cancer Res, 45:3161-3163, 1985.
61. Ellison RR, Holland JF, Weil M, *et al.* Arabinosyl cytosine: a useful agent in the treatment of acute leukemia in adults. Blood, 32:507-523, 1968.
62. Solimando DA, Bressler LR, Kintzel PE, Geraci M. Drug Information Handbook for Oncology. Lexi-Comp Inc., Hudson (Cleveland), Ohio, 1999.

63. Allegra CJ, Grem JL. Antimetabolites. *In*: Cancer: Principles and Practice of Oncology. 5th edition, VT DeVita Jr (ed.), Lippincott-Raven, Philadelphia, PA, 1997.
64. Skeel RT. Handbook of Cancer Chemotherapy, 5th edition, Lippincott Williams and Wilkins, New York, NY, 1999.
65. Wiley JS, Jones SP, Sawyer WH. Cytosine arabinoside transport by human leukaemic cells. Eur J Cancer Clin Oncol, 19:1067-1074, 1983.
66. Yoshida S, Yamada M, Masaki S. Inhibition of DNA polymerase α and β of calf thymus by 1-β-D-arabinofuranosylcytosine 5' triphosphate. Biochim Biophys Acta, 477:144-150, 1977.
67. Dijkwel PA, Wanka F. Enhanced release of nascent single strands from DNA synthesized in the presence of arabinosylcytosine. Biochim Biophys Acta, 520:461-471, 1978.
68. Gunji H, Kharbanda S, Kufe D. Induction of internucleosomal DNA fragmentation in human myeloid leukemia cells by 1-β-D-arabinofuranosylcytosine. Cancer Res, 51:741-743, 1991.
69. Kufe D, Spriggs D, Egan EM, Munroe D. Relationships among ara-CTP pools, formation of (ara-C)DNA, and cytotoxicity of human leukemic cells. Blood, 64:54-58, 1984.
70. Rustum YM, Preisler HD. Correlation between leukemic cell retention of 1-β-D-arabinofuranosylcytosine 5'-triphosphate and response to therapy. Cancer Res, 39:42-49, 1979.
71. Ho DHW, Frei E. Clinical pharmacology of 1-β-D-arabinofuranosyl cytosine. Clin Pharmacol Ther, 12:944-954, 1971.
72. Wiley JS, Jones SP, Sawyer WH, Paterson AR. Cytosine arabinoside influx and nucleoside transport sites in acute leukemia. J Clin Invest, 69:479-489, 1982.
73. Wiley JS, Woodruff RK, Jamieson GP, *et al.* Cytosine arabinoside in the treatment of T-cell acute lymphoblastic leukemia. Aust N Z J Med, 7;17:379-386, 1987.
74. Wiley JS, Taupin J, Jamieson GP, *et al.* Cytosine arabinoside transport and metabolism in acute leukemias and T cell lymphoblastic lymphoma. J Clin Invest, 75:632-642, 1985.
75. Gati WP, Paterson AR, Larratt LM, *et al.* Sensitivity of acute leukemia cells to cytarabine is a correlate of cellular es nucleoside transporter site content measured by flow cytometry with SAENTA-fluorescein. Blood, 90:346-353, 1997.
76. White JC, Rathmell JP, Capizzi RL. Membrane transport influences the rate of accumulation of cytosine arabinoside in human leukemia cells. J Clin Invest, 79:380-387, 1987.
77. Jamieson GP, Snook MB, Wiley JS. Saturation of intracellular cytosine arabinoside triphosphate accumulation in human leukemic blast cells. Leuk Res, 14:475-479, 1990.
78. Capizzi RL, Yang JL, Cheng E, *et al.* Alteration of the pharmacokinetics of high-dose ara-C by its metabolite, high ara-U in patients with acute leukemia. J Clin Oncol, 1:763-771, 1983.
79. Bishop JF, Matthews JP, Young GA, *et al.* A randomized study of high-dose cytarabine in induction in acute myeloid leukemia. Blood, 87:1710-1717, 1996.
80. Weick JK, Kopecky KJ, Appelbaum FR, *et al.* A randomized investigation of high-dose versus standard-dose cytosine arabinoside with daunorubicin in patients with previously untreated acute myeloid leukemia: a Southwest Oncology Group study. Blood, 88:2841-2851, 1996.
81. Grever MR, Kopecky KJ, Coltman CA, *et al.* Fludarabine monophosphate: a potentially useful agent in chronic lymphocytic leukemia. Nouv Rev Fr Hematol, 30:457-459, 1988.
82. Cheson BD. New prospects in the treatment of indolent lymphomas with purine analogues. Cancer J, 4:S27-S36, 1998.
83. Leiby JM, Snider KM, Kraut EH, *et al.* Phase II trial of 9-β-D-arabinofuranosyl-2-fluoroadenine 5'-monophosphate in non-Hodgkin's lymphoma: prospective comparison of response with deoxycytidine kinase activity. Cancer Res, 47:2719-2722, 1987.

84. Plunkett W, Saunders PP. Metabolism and action of purine nucleoside analogs. Pharmacol Ther, 49:239-268, 1991.
85. Cheson BD. Miscellaneous chemotherapeutic agents. *In*: Cancer: Principles and Practice of Oncology, 5th edition, VT DeVita Jr (ed.), Lippincott-Raven, Philadelphia, PA, 1997.
86. Ross SR, McTavish D, Faulds D. Fludarabine. A review of its pharmacological properties and therapeutic potential in malignancy. Drugs, 45:737-759, 1993.
87. Plunkett W, Chubb S, Alexander L, Montgomery JA. Comparison of the toxicity and metabolism of 9-β-D-arabinofuranosyl-2-fluoroadenine and 9-β-D-arabinofuranosyladenine in human lymphoblastoid cells. Cancer Res, 40:2349-2355, 1980.
88. Huang P, Plunkett W. Fludarabine- and gemcitabine-induced apoptosis: incorporation of analogs into DNA is a critical event. Cancer Chemother Pharmacol, 36:181-188, 1995.
89. Huang P, Plunkett W. Action of 9-β-D-arabinofuranosyl-2-fluoroadenine on RNA metabolism. Mol Pharmacol, 39:449-455, 1991.
90. King KM, Cass CE. Membrane transport of 2-chloro-2'-deoxyadenosine and 2-chloro-2'-arabinofluoro-2'-deoxyadenosine is required for cytotoxicity. Proc Amer Assoc Cancer Res, 35:A3436, 1994.
91. Avery TL, Rehg JE, Lumm WC, *et al.* Biochemical pharmacology of 2-chlorodeoxyadenosine in malignant human hematopoietic cell lines and therapeutic effects of 2-bromodeoxyadenosine in drug combinations in mice. Cancer Res, 49:4972-4978, 1989.
92. Heinemann V, Xu YZ, Chubb S, *et al.* Cellular elimination of 2',2'-difluorodeoxycytidine 5'-triphosphate: a mechanism of self-potentiation. Cancer Res, 52:533-539, 1992.
93. Baker CH, Banzon J, Bollinger JM, *et al.* 2'-Deoxy-2'-methylenecytidine and 2'-deoxy-2',2'-difluorocytidine 5'- diphosphates: potent mechanism-based inhibitors of ribonucleotide reductase. J Med Chem, 34:1879-1884, 1991.
94. Heinemann V, Hertel LW, Grindey GB, Plunkett W. Comparison of the cellular pharmacokinetics and toxicity of 2',2'-difluorodeoxycytidine and 1-beta-D-arabinofuranosylcytosine. Cancer Res, 48:4024-4031, 1988.
95. Blum JL, Jones SE, Buzdar AU, *et al.* Multicenter phase II study of capecitabine in paclitaxel-refractory metastatic breast cancer. J Clin Oncol, 17:485-493, 1999.
96. Ishikawa T, Utoh M, Sawada N, *et al.* Tumor selective delivery of 5-fluorouracil by capecitabine, a new oral fluoropyrimidine carbamate, in human cancer xenografts. Biochem Pharmacol, 55:1091-1097, 1998.
97. Schmoll H-J, Buchele T, Grothey A, Dempke W. Where do we stand with 5-fluorouracil? Semin Oncol, 26:589-605, 1999.
98. Jennings LL, Hao C, Cabrita MA, *et al.* Distinct regional distribution of human equilibrative nucleoside transporter proteins 1 and 2 (hENT1 and hENT2) in the central nervous system. Neuropharmacol, 40:722-731, 2001.
99. Ahmad I, Al-Katib AM, Beck FW, Mohammad RM. Sequential treatment of a resistant chronic lymphocytic leukemia patient with bryostatin 1 followed by 2-chlorodeoxyadenosine: case report. Clin Cancer Res, 6:1328-1332, 2000.
100. Beck FW, Al-Katib AM, Ahmad I, *et al.* Bryostatin 1-induced modulation of nucleoside transporters and 2-chlorodeoxyadenosine influx in WSU-CLL cells. Int J Mol Med, 5:341-347, 2000.

Chapter 3

MDR AND MRP GENE FAMILIES AS CELLULAR DETERMINANT FACTORS FOR RESISTANCE TO CLINICAL ANTICANCER AGENTS

Lei Deng[1], Shigaru Tatebe[1], Yen-Chiu Lin-Lee[1], Toshihisa Ishikawa[2] and M. Tien Kuo[1]
[1]Department of Molecular Pathology, The University of Texas MD Anderson Cancer Center Houston, Texas, USA
[2]Department of Biomolecular Engineering, Graduate School of Bioscience and Biotechnology, Tokyo Institute of Technology, Yokohama, Japan

1. INTRODUCTION

The constant threat by a countless array of environmental poisons, natural products and synthetic agents, over evolutionary time has led living organisms to develop many elaborate mechanisms that combat the toxic effects of these insults. Among such mechanisms is one that decreases the intracellular accumulation of a toxic substance by directly pumping toxic molecules out of the cells, and another that modifies the metabolism of the toxic substances and effluxes the metabolized compounds. The former mechanism is typified by the mammalian multidrug resistance system mediated by P-glycoproteins (P-gp) that are encoded by the MDR gene family. The second mechanism is exemplified by the multidrug resistance protein (MRP). Both P-gp and MRP contain ATP-binding cassettes and therefore belong to the ABC superfamily of membrane transporters.

Both MDR and MRP systems have been studied extensively over the past several years, and many review articles have been published[1–4]. In this chapter, rather than covering every aspect of both transport systems, we will focus on their clinical relevance. The basic biology of the system that is relevant to their clinical aspects will be briefly discussed. A summary of many important aspects of the MDR and MRP gene families is presented in Table 1.

Table 1. Summary of MDR and MRP gene family.

Family	Member	Chromosome Location	Main Location of Expression	Endogenous Substrates	Frequently Over-expressed In MDR Cells	Conferred MDR Phenotype	Drug Resistance Profile	Phenotype in Knockout Mice
MDR	MDR1	7q21.1	Many tissues	?	+	+	Vincristine, vinblastine, doxorubicin, etc.	Mdrla(-/-) mdr1b (-/-) apparently normal
	MDR2	7q21.1	Liver	Phosphatidyl Choline	-	-	-	Impaired phospholipid transport
MRP	MRP1	16p13	Ubiquitous	GSH-conjugates, leukotrienes, steroids, glucuronides, GSSG	+	+	Etoposide, doxorubicin, etc.	Accumulation of LTC4 in mast cells, impaired in inflammatory response
	MRP2	10q24	Liver, kidney	GSH-conjugates multispecific organic anions, GSSG	+	+	Etoposide, MTX, cisplatin	Hyperbilirubinema
	MRP3	17q21	Liver, kidney, colon, adrenal gland	GSH-conjugates	+	+	MTX, etoposide, teniposide	?
	MRP4	13q31-32	Widely expressed, high in pancreas, kidney, prostate	?	?	?	?	?
	MRP5	3q27	Many tissues, high in prostate, lung, muscle, pancreas, testes	?	+	?	?	?
	MRP6	16p13	Liver, kidney	?	+	?	?	?

2. MDR

2.1 Biology of the MDR System

Juliano and Ling[5] discovered that a 170-kDa protein was overproduced in MDR cells. They called it P-glycoprotein (P-gp) for permeability glycoprotein, though later it was shown that the permeability of these MDR cells was not altered. P-gp is a membrane protein that acts as an energy-dependent efflux pump. In humans, two classes of MDR genes encode P-gp. MDR1 is involved in multidrug resistance and MDR2 transports phosphatidylcholine into bile. In rodents, mdr1a and mdr1b (also known as mdr3 and mdr1, respectively) confer drug resistance, whereas mdr2 is homologous to the human MDR2.

Knockout analysis demonstrated that animals carrying either mdr1a(-/-) or mdr1a(-/-) mdr1b(-/-) backgrounds are apparently normal[6]. When antitumor agents of known P-gp substrates were injected into these animals, accumulation of these agents in certain organs was evident, especially in the blood-brain barrier where P-gp is normally over-expressed[7]. These findings suggested that the primary function of P-gp is to protect against toxic xenobiotics by limiting the uptake of the toxic compounds. These findings also suggest that P-gp may have important implication in clinical drug resistance. Thus, the regulation of P-gp expression levels in tumor cells seems to be an important parameter associated with multidrug resistance.

2.2 Regulation of MDR Gene Expression and P-glycoprotein Activity

MDR1 gene expression and function can be regulated by at least four layers of mechanisms: [i] In chronic selection of drug-resistant cell lines, P-gp may be overproduced through the amplification of *MDR1* genes, thereby increasing its copy number in cells[8]. However, amplification of *MDR1* is uncommon in clinical tumor samples. [ii] Stabilization of *MDR* mRNA represents the second mechanism by which P-gp could be up-regulated[9]. The stability of *MDR1* mRNA seems to be controlled by the presence of AU-rich sequences located at the 3' untranslated region, which occur in many mRNAs with short half-lives[10]. [iii] Post-translational modifications such as N-glycosylation and phosphorylation of P-gp may affect its affinity for certain drugs and change the velocity of drug transport[11,12]. Alternatively, glycosylation and phosphorylation may also affect the stability of P-gp. (iv) Perhaps the most important regulatory mechanism of *MDR1* gene expression occurs at the transcriptional level. The *MDR1* gene appears to be regulated by an upstream and downstream promoter[13]. Studies with the human *MDR1* promoter have mainly focused on the downstream promoter. Several cis-acting elements controlling basal and inducible expression of *MDR1* by various extracellular influences have been identified[14]. Of particular interest is the Y-box that controls basal expression. In 27 out of 27 untreated primary breast cancer samples, YB-1 protein, the transcription factor recognizing the Y-box, was found in the cytoplasm. However, in a subset of tumors in which P-gp expression was elevated, YB-1 was predominantly localized in the nucleus. These results suggest that translocation of the transcription activator YB-1 from the cytoplasmic compartment into the nuclear compartment is correlated to the increased P-gp[15]. The underlying mechanisms associated with transcription factor translocation are not yet determined.

2.3 Clinical Relevance of MDR1 in Cancer Chemotherapy

The role of MDR1 expression in conferring drug resistance has been conclusively demonstrated in cultured cell systems. However, its clinical relevance in cancer chemotherapy has not yet been as conclusive. Correlation between levels of *MDR1* gene expression in tumors and treatment outcome for patients has often been used as a first criterion to assess the clinical relevance. Yet, multiple layers of complexity are associated with this general approach. First, a reliably qualitative and quantitative method has to be employed. The probes used should detect MDR1 without cross-reaction with MDR2, which confers no resistance to antitumor agents. As most detection methods have strengths and weaknesses in their own right, it is advisable to use combined detection methods so that the results can be cross referenced. Second, sequential samples prior to and after chemotherapy have to be used. This approach would establish correlation between P-gp expression with response rates of chemotherapy. Unfortunately, many published studies in the literature relied on static, single point in time analyses. To substantiate the role of MDR1 in clinical drug resistance, it is also necessary to determine whether modulation of MDR1 expression would alter drug sensitivity in clinical trials using MDR1 reversal agents.

2.3.1 Significance of MDR1 expression in hematological neoplasms

There is a significant association of MDR1 expression with poor outcome of chemotherapy in the treatment of acute myeloblastic leukemia (AML), multiple myeloma (MM), and non-Hodgkin's lymphoma. Many studies have documented a positive correlation between MDR1 expression and either decreased remission rates or refractory disease in AML[16,17]. P-gp-mediated drug resistance may be particularly important in the mediation of chemotherapy responses in older patients with AML, a subpopulation that traditionally responds poorly to chemotherapy. An analysis of 211 patients with AML aged older than 55 years showed that both MDR1 protein expression and altered drug efflux frequently occurred in leukemia cells[18]. In several publications, the MDR phenotype is also linked with an increase in early deaths during treatment[19]. The MDR phenotype is more frequently seen in $CD34^+$ leukemias, and co-expression of P-gp and CD34 identifies a subgroup with very poor prognosis[20,21].

In acute lymphoblastic leukemia (ALL) patients, the incidence of MDR1 over-expression is relatively low compared with that of AML, with a conservative estimate of 10-15% at diagnosis and 34% at relapse[22]. Although the MDR phenotype is not common among ALL patients, it occurs in certain poor prognostic subgroups of ALL, including adult ALL[23]. The majority of studies have concluded that MDR1 expression is not predictive of treatment failure. However, a recent study with 102 newly diagnosed childhood ALL cases found that P-gp expression is an independent prognostic parameter of dismal outcome[24].

Although several MDR mechanisms exist in MM, a correlation of MDR1 over-expression and failure of chemotherapy has been observed in most studies with MM[25,26]. The incidence of P-gp over-expression usually is low at diagnosis in MM, but increases with preceding anthracycline-vinca alkaloid treatment. After eight cycles of VAD (vincristine/adriamycin/dexamethasone) treatment, 85% of MM patients became P-gp positive and 96% of VAD-refractory patients expressed the MDR phenotype[19,27]. For this reason, MM is regarded as a model of the drug-induced MDR phenotype and is widely used to test the effects of P-gp reversal agents.

2.3.2 Significance of MDR1 expression in solid tumors

It is a challenge to determine the correlation of P-gp expression with outcome of treatment in solid tumors, as solid tumors usually contain heterogeneous cell populations. Moreover, accurate assessment of drug accumulation in solid tumor cells is more difficult than in hematological cells. In organs that normally express high levels of MDR1 proteins such as liver, colon, kidney and adrenal glands, tumors developed in these organs are usually resistant and have a poor response to chemotherapy[28]. In other tumors, such as breast cancer, ovarian cancer and sarcomas, which derive from tissues that normally do not express a significant amount of MDR1, the initial levels of P-gp are usually low and the primary tumors are responsive to chemotherapy. However, an unacceptable portion of patients eventually experience disease recurrence as the tumor cells become highly resistant. In this group of cancers, multidrug resistance is often an adverse prognostic indicator[28,29]. A disease-oriented review of the correlation of MDR1 expression and clinical drug resistance in several major solid tumors is presented below.

In lung cancer, the most common malignancy in North America, most patients initially respond to chemotherapy but ultimately relapse and have a poor response to salvage regimens. Yokoyama *et al.*[30] immunohistochemically examined P-gp expression in 159 non-small cell lung cancers and found a significant association of poor prognosis and P-gp expression. An earlier study[31] of sequential samples of 31 small-cell lung cancer patients also reached a similar conclusion. In contrast, the result of a Japanese study of 87 lung cancer patients suggested that MDR1 gene is not associated with tumor progression and drug resistance[32]. Most patients with metastatic non-small cell lung cancer do not respond to a regimen containing etoposide and cisplatin, which are not P-gp substrates. This suggests the existence of alternative drug resistance mechanisms. Consistent with this is the finding that MRP is generally involved in drug resistance in lung cancers[33].

As in lung cancer, the clinical significance of MDR1 expression in breast cancer is also a topic of great controversy. Studies with samples from 127 primary and 8 locally relapsed breast cancer patients[34] and a meta-analysis[29] agreed that MDR1 expression in breast cancer is associated with a poor response to chemotherapy. Based on immunochemical analysis with three monoclonal antibodies and RNAse protection analysis of 92 primary and 12 metastatic breast cancers, Linn *et al.*[35] also concluded that P-gp expression in tumor cells has prognostic value in primary breast cancer and is likely to be a marker of a more malignant phenotype. Similarly, Gregorcyk *et al.*[36] also found that P-gp is frequently expressed in patients with untreated breast cancer, with P-gp positive patients being at significantly greater risk of disease recurrence. However, a well controlled study by Lizard-Nacol *et al.*[37] with sequential tumor samples from 75 patients could not establish an association between MDR1 expression and clinical outcomes. The report of Hegewisch-Becker *et al.*[38] suggests that the contamination of lymphocytes, which express P-gp, can be a potential problem with those studies using RT-PCR as their principle approach to measure MDR1 expression.

Studies of hepatocellular carcinoma generally agree that the chemotherapy response is inversely related to P-gp expression[39]. Childhood solid tumors, including sarcoma and neuroblastoma, have provided the best evidence for a strong correlation of the expression of P-gp with chemotherapeutic outcome[40].

2.3.3 Clinical trials using P-glycoprotein reversal agents

Since over-expression of P-gp was identified as a drug resistance mechanism, a variety of compounds have been investigated for their ability to reverse the P-gp-mediated MDR phenotype. These compounds are mostly substrates of P-gp, thereby competing with the available P-gp in transporting antitumor agents.

The first generation of MDR reversal agents, such as verapamil, quinine and cyclosporines, have been shown to greatly increase the sensitivity of resistant leukemia cells to cytotoxic agents both *in vitro* and *in vivo*. However, serious cardiac effects or immunosuppressive actions limit the utility of these MDR modulators[41].

The second generation of MDR-reversing agents, exemplified by R-verapamil and PSC-833 (also known as valspodar, a cyclosporin analogue), are much more potent MDR inhibitors, but have less side-effects than their parental compounds. Early studies using R-verapamil in Hodgkin's or non-Hodgkin's lymphoma patients showed remarkable improvement in response to chemotherapy[42,43]. *In vitro* experiments indicated that PSC-833 interacts directly with P-gp with high affinity and probably interferes with the ATPase activity of P-gp[44]. Phase I/II trials with PSC-833 showed that it could be safely administered in combination with different chemotherapy regimens after dose adjustments of cytotoxic drugs that are P-gp substrates[44]. PSC-833 has been intensively tested in patients with AML, MM, and non-Hodgkin's lymphoma, and the results are quite promising. In 1999 alone, there were about 30 reports dealing with the clinical testing results of PSC-833, with most of them focused on the effect of this compound on hematological neoplasms. In a multicenter study[45], 37 patients with poor-risk types of AML were treated with PSC-833 plus mitoxantrone, etoposide, and cytarabine (PSC-MEC). Overall, post-chemotherapy marrow hypoplasia was achieved in 33 patients. Of these, 12 patients (32%) achieved complete remission and 4 achieved partial remission. The results from a Southwest Oncology Group Trial in patients with poor-prognostic acute leukemia are also encouraging. In this trial, 226 patients were randomized to receive chemotherapy with or without the P-gp antagonist cyclosporin A[46]. In patients treated with cyclosporin A, the relapse-free survival at 3 years demonstrated a significant improvement (43% versus 10%, P=0.033). However, definitive clinical benefits of using MDR modulators in hematological malignancies still awaits the results of ongoing randomized Phase III trials.

In solid tumors, the clinical trial results have been largely disappointing[47]. MDR modulators could reverse the MDR phenotype in cultured multicellular tumor spheroids[48]; but the results of clinical tests in renal cancer, colorectal cancer and breast cancer patients have been mostly negative[47,49,50]. Among solid tumors, perhaps the most promising data are for ovarian cancer. Two studies involving patients with refractory ovarian cancer have shown some benefits of PSC-833[51,52].

There is an appealing opinion that a strategy aimed at preventing the emergence of drug resistance is more likely to be successful than MDR reversal interventions. Consistent with this concept are reports by several research groups[53,54] that the addition of P-gp antagonists in the initial treatment of cancer showed an advantage in preventing the MDR phenotype.

In addition to its role in cancer chemotherapy, the expression of MDR1 may have prognostic value: [i] Baldini *et al.*[55] reported that increased levels of P-gp in osteosarcoma were significantly associated with the decreased probability of patients' remaining event-free after diagnosis. These investigators also reported that patients whose tumors had high levels of P-gp had a 2-fold higher relapse rate than those with P-gp-negative tumors. In other studies, it has been reported that the incidence of P-gp over-expression was higher among patients with localized disease at clinical onset than in patients with evidence of metastases[56,57]. [ii] Elevated P-gp expression has been correlated with a subpopulation of colorectal cancer patients who developed vessel invasion and lymph node metastases[58]. [iii] In primary breast cancer, elevated expression of P-gp has been associated with shorter survival of patients with locally advanced breast cancer[59]. [iv] From a study to determine whether P-gp over-expression has a cause-effect relationship with the reduced metastatic potential of tumor cells, Scotlandi *et al.*[60] reported that *MDR1*-transfected osteosarcoma cells were completely unable to grow as lung metastases in athymic mice, in contrast to the untransfected controls. These results suggested that P-gp over-expression is causally related to the low malignant potential of osteosarcoma cells. [v] According to Takanishi *et al.*[61], P-gp expression was inversely correlated with the proliferative activity of human hepatocellular carcinoma (HCC). These investigators reported that human HCC presenting higher levels of Ki-67 expression had low levels of P-gp expression; whereas in those showing low levels of Ki-67, levels of P-gp expression were high. These observations, if proven, bear important clinical implications. P-gp levels may be a prognostic marker for selecting a subgroup of cancer patients who require more aggressive chemotherapy; also the idea of using P-gp modulators to enhance chemotherapeutic efficacy may have to take into account that down-regulation of P-gp may alter a tumor's aggressive potential. Further investigations in these areas are warranted.

Finally, it is important to note that the clinical MDR phenotype may involve multiple mechanisms that could co-exist in solid tumors. Only by careful determination of the expression of P-gp at various stages of the treatment, and by combined pharmacokinetic analyses of MDR modulators and antitumor drugs, can treatment outcomes be evaluated for the effects of P-gp expression. Nonetheless, the results thus far collected suggest that P-gp expression may play a role in the treatment of certain types of cancers, depending upon tumor types, treatment regimens, and patient population.

3. MULTIDRUG RESISTANCE-ASSOCIATED PROTEIN (MRP)

3.1 The Biology of MRP

Over-expression of MRP1 has been identified by molecular cloning from a non-P-gp MDR phenotype in cultured cells[3,4]. In addition to *MRP1*, other *MRP* homologues designated *MRP2-6* have been identified by expressed sequence tags or by using low-stringency hybridization screening conditions.

MRP1 transports drug conjugates including glutathione (GSH), glucuronate, and sulfate moieties[62]. These findings suggest that *MRP1* is functionally related to the GS-X (ATP-dependent GSH S-conjugate export) pump[63]. Endogenous GS-X compounds such as LTC4 are transported by MRP1. Following homozygous deletion of *mrp1*, mice exhibit accumulation of intracellular LTC4 in bone marrow-derived leukocytes[64]. These animals suffer from impairment of inflammatory response.

MRP2, which is mainly expressed in the canalicular membrane of hepatocytes, encodes canalicular multispecific organic anion transporter (cMOAT) for hepatobiliary excretion of bilirubin glucuronides and other multivalent organic anions, including GSH S-conjugates[65,66]. Like *MRP1*-transfected cells, transfection of *MRP2* into cultured cells was found to confer elevated resistance to various antitumor agents[67,68]. MRP3, which is the closest homologue of MRP1 in the MRP family, shares 58% amino acid identity with MRP1[69,70]. Although *MRP3*-transfected cells displayed resistance to antitumor agents (etoposide and methotrexate), these cells did not show increased GSH export[70]. Over-expression of MRP4 was associated with resistance to antiviral acyclic nucleoside analogues[71]. MRP5 and MRP6 share 36% and 45%, respectively, of their amino acid identities with MRP1[72]. MRP5 is expressed in many human tissues, with relatively high levels of expression in skeletal muscles and brain, whereas expression of MRP6 is relatively restricted, with elevated levels of expression found in liver and kidney[73].

The identification of these members of the MRP gene family has been performed only in the recent years. Investigations into the function of each encoded isoform has been progressing rapidly. However, several important aspects of those genes, particularly *MRP3* to *MRP6*, remain to be investigated (Table 1).

3.2 Regulation of MRP Function

It has been demonstrated that GSH levels play an important role in the regulation of MRP1 expression, since MRP1 is functionally related to the GS-X pump[74]. The γ-glutamylcysteine synthetase (γ-GCS) catalyzes the synthesis of glutamylcysteine, which is the rate-limiting step in overall GSH biosynthesis. Thus, the cellular GSH level is substantially regulated by γ-GCS[75]. In a number of cell lines, expression of MRP1 and γ-GCS heavy chain (γ-GCSh, the catalytic subunit of γ-GCS) can be co-induced by treatment with pro-oxidants, e.g., *t*-butylhydroquinone, 2,3-dimethyoxy-1,4-naphthoquinone and menadione. These observations suggest that regulation of MRP1 and γ-GCSh may be oxidative stress-sensitive. Consistent with this idea, over-expression of the physiological antioxidant GSH in γ-GCSh-transfected cells down-regulates MRP1 and γ-GCSh expression[76]. These findings suggest that a dynamic GSH homeostasis may be associated with response to cancer chemotherapy. Since other MRP members, e.g., MRP2, MRP3 and MRP5, also exhibit GS-X pump activity, the altered GSH content may have a broad effect on the overall function of the MRP family. However, the effects of GSH homeostasis on the function of these MRP members require further demonstrations. These findings, if proven, may have clinical relevance to trials in which modulators of MRP and GSH function are considered. The cytotoxic effects of antitumor agents may induce transient expression of MRP1 and γ-GCSh. Elevated MRP1 expression may facilitate the elimination of antitumor agents at the expense of GSH consumption, resulting in depletion of the GSH pool and subsequent downregulation of MRP1-mediated drug resistance.

As in MDR1, multiple mechanisms are likely to be involved in the regulation of MRP1 expression. Zhu and Center[77] reported that the SP1 binding sites located between -29 and -12 are involved in basal MRP1 gene expression. Gomi *et al.*[78] reported that a post-transcriptional mechanism may also be involved in the regulation of MRP1 induced by antitumor alkylating agents. Wang and Beck[79] demonstrated that wild-type p53 could suppress the transcriptional expression of MRP1 gene expression by diminishing SP1 activity. Using immunohistochemical or flow cytometric analysis, MRP1 expression was correlated with mutated p53 protein expression in human non-small cell lung cancer, colorectal cancer and acute myeloid leukemia[80,81]. The suppressive effect of wild-type p53 on MRP1 was also demonstrated in a prostate cancer cell line[82].

3.3.1 Clinical relevance of MRP in cancer chemotherapy

The clinical relevance of MRP in resistance to cancer chemotherapy has not been thoroughly investigated. The investigations are likely to be more complex than that of MDR1 because: [i] Co-expression of multiple MRP isoforms is often observed in MDR cell lines selected with a single antitumor agent; therefore, reliable methodologies to differentiate the contribution from each member are desirable. To this end, isoform-specific probes for individual members have to be used. Given the fact that many MRP transporters have similar substrate spectra, although affinities toward the same substrate differ among the isoforms, modulators of individual MRP isoforms may not be readily available. Monoclonal antibodies that recognize specific MRP isoforms have been produced[83,84]. Alternatively, it may be possible to explore neutralizing antisense oligonucleotides to specific *MRP* mRNAs without cross-reacting with other isoforms[85]. [ii] In tumor cells, cellular locations of expressed MRP may not be membrane-located or properly spanned into the membrane lipid bilayer. Thus, measurement of MRP expression by biochemical means needs to be coupled to immunohistochemical determination. [iii] MRP-mediated transport of antitumor agents requires

GSH or other organo-anionic constituents. Thus, measurable levels of MRP expression may not actually reflect the transport activities.

Despite these difficulties, some progress has been noted. Expression of *MRP1* mRNA and MRP1 was detected in a wide spectrum of human cancers[86]. Sullivan *et al.*[87] showed that MRP1 expression was more frequent in prostate cancer than in benign glandular elements, and Fukushima *et al.*[81] showed that the frequency of MRP1 expression in colorectal carcinoma was significantly higher than in adenoma. Previously we demonstrated that the expression level of *MRP1* mRNA was higher in human colorectal carcinoma than in the matched non-tumor specimens[88]. These findings suggest that MRP1 expression is up-regulated during carcinogenesis.

Several studies have found expression levels of MRP1 to be of prognostic significance. In non-small cell lung cancer patients who underwent postoperative chemotherapy, Oshika *et al.*[80] showed that the prognosis of patients with MRP1-positive tumors was significantly worse than that of patients with MRP1-negative lesions. Studying breast cancer patients with small tumors (<2 cm) and negative lymph node metastasis, Nooter *et al.*[89] showed that the prognosis of patients with MRP1-positive tumors was significantly poorer than that of patients with MRP1-negative tumors.

Endo *et al.*[90] investigated the relationship between MRP1 expression and chemosensitivity to cisplatin, doxorubicin, etoposide, and mitomycin C in 75 patients with gastric cancer. The MTT assays showed that MRP1 positive gastric cancer tissue was less sensitive to cisplatin, doxorubicin, and mitomycin C compared with MRP1 negative tissue. A similar tendency was noted with etoposide. Campling *et al.*[33] demonstrated a significant correlation between doxorubicin resistance and MRP1 expression levels, but found no correlation between MRP1 expression levels and sensitivity to cisplatin, etoposide or vincristine.

Young *et al.*[91] studied the relationship between *MRP2-5* mRNA expressions and chemosensitivity in 23 human lung cancer cell lines. They noted a significant correlation between *MRP3* expression levels and drug resistance to doxorubicin, etoposide, vincristine and cisplatin. In addition, there was a significant correlation between *MRP3* and *MRP1* mRNA expression levels. Like MRP1, MRP3 may contribute to the drug-resistance phenotype of human lung cancer cells.

Several compounds have been reported to modulate drug resistance in MRP1 over-expressing cell lines. These include the calcium channel blockers verapamil and nicardipine, the tiapanmil analogue, the cyclosporin analogue PSC-833, tyrosine kinase inhibitors, and others[74]. The specificity of these modulators have not been conclusively demonstrated. Moreover, their clinical utilities have not been explored.

CONCLUSION

P-gp was the first human ABC transporter protein cloned. The discovery of MRP1 expands our understanding of the molecular basis of multidrug resistance. MDR and MRP are among the most intensively studied ABC transporter proteins because multidrug resistance is a major cause of cancer chemotherapy failure. We have learned a great deal about the biology of these two drug transporters, particularly in cultured cell systems. Major efforts have also been devoted to the investigation of whether expression of MDR and MRP plays a role in clinical drug resistance in cancer chemotherapy, and from these studies we hope to develop strategies that may circumvent multidrug resistance by modulating MDR and MRP expression.

In light of the MDR and MRP gene families' function as transporters of many antitumor agents, their frequent up-regulation in human neoplasms, and the association between their expression and treatment efficacies in certain human malignancies, make it likely that MDR and MRP play an important role in clinical drug resistance, at least in certain forms of cancer. Likewise, the expression of these transporters may be a prognostic predicator of the treatment outcomes. However, the challenge remains the development of effective strategies to circumvent MDR- and MRP-mediated drug resistance in clinical settings.

Finally, more than 40 ABC transporter sequences have been identified in the human genome, and perhaps as many remain to be explored. These yet-to-be identified ABC transporters may also contribute to resistance to cancer chemotherapy. By exploiting the entire spectrum of drug resistance mechanisms, we will learn the overall complexity of the MDR phenotype. These studies may eventually enable us to design better strategies to combat drug resistance in cancer treatment.

ACKNOWLEDGEMENTS

Work in the authors' laboratories is supported by grants CA72404 and CA79085 from the National Institute of Health.

REFERENCES

1. Gottesman MM, Pastan I, Ambudkar SV. P-glycoprotein and multidrug resistance. Curr Opinion Genet Dev, 6:610-617, 1996.
2. Ling V. Multidrug resistance: molecular mechanisms and clinical relevance. Cancer Chemother Pharmacol, 40 Suppl:S3-8, 1997.
3. Cole SP, Deeley RG. Multidrug resistance mediated by the ATP-binding cassette transporter protein MRP. BioEssays, 20: 931-940, 1998.

4. Borst P, Evers R, Kool M, Wijnholds J. The multidrug resistance protein family. Biochim Biophys Acta, 1461:347-357, 1999.
5. Juliano RL, Ling V. A surface glycoprotein modulating drug permeability in Chinese hamster ovary cell mutants. Biochim Biophys Acta, 455:152-162, 1976.
6. Borst P, Schinkel AH. What have we learnt thus far from mice with disrupted P-glycoprotein genes? Eur J Cancer, 32A:985-990, 1996.
7. Zhang ZJ, Saito T, Kimura Y, *et al.* Disruption of mdr1a P-glycoprotein gene results in dysfunction of blood-inner ear barrier in mice. Brain Res, 852:116-216, 2000.
8. Capranico G, De Isabella P, Castelli C, *et al.* P-glycoprotein gene amplification and expression in multidrug-resistant murine P388 and B16 cell lines. Br J Cancer, 59:682-685, 1989.
9. Kuo MT, Julian J, Husain F, *et al.* Regulation of multidrug resistance gene mdr1b/mdr1 expression in isolated mouse uterine epithelial cells. J Cell Physiol, 164:132-141, 1995.
10. Jackson RJ. Cytoplasmic regulation of mRNA function: the importance of the 3' untranslated region. Cell, 74:9-14, 1993.
11. Center MS. Evidence that adriamycin resistance in Chinese hamster lung cells is regulated by phosphorylation of a plasma membrane glycoprotein. Biochem Biophys Res Commun, 115:159-166, 1983.
12. Kramer R, Weber TK, Arceci R, *et al.* Inhibition of N-linked glycosylation of P-glycoprotein by tunicamycin results in a reduced multidrug resistance phenotype. Br J Cancer, 71:670-675, 1995.
13. Gottesman MM, Pastan I. Biochemistry of multidrug resistance mediated by the multidrug transporter. Annu Rev Biochem, 62:385-427, 1993.
14. Chin KV, Ueda K, Pastan I, Gottesman MM. Modulation of activity of the promoter of the human MDR1 gene by Ras and p53. Science, 255:459-462, 1992.
15. Bargou RC, Jurchott K, Wagener C, *et al.* Nuclear localization and increased levels of transcription factor YB-1 in primary human breast cancers are associated with intrinsic MDR1 gene expression. Nature Med, 3:447-450, 1997.
16. Del Poeta G, Venditti A, Aronica G, *et al.* P-glycoprotein expression in de novo acute myeloid leukemia. Leukemia Lymphoma, 27:257-274, 1997.
17. Senent L, Jarque I, Martin G, *et al.* P-glycoprotein expression and prognostic value in acute myeloid leukemia. Haematologica, 83:783-787, 1998.
18. Leith CP, Kopecky KJ, Godwin J, *et al.* Acute myeloid leukemia in the elderly: assessment of multidrug resistance (MDR1) and cytogenetics distinguishes biologic subgroups with remarkably distinct responses to standard chemotherapy. A Southwest Oncology Group study. Blood, 89:3323-3329, 1997.
19. Marie JP, Zhou DC, Gurbuxani S, *et al.* MDR1/P-glycoprotein in haematological neoplasms. Eur J Cancer, 32A:1034-1038, 1996.
20. te Boekhorst PA, de Leeuw K, Schoester M, *et al.* Predominance of functional multidrug resistance (MDR-1) phenotype in CD34+ acute myeloid leukemia cells. Blood, 82:3157-3162, 1993.

21. Guerci A, Merlin JL, Missoum N, *et al.* Predictive value for treatment outcome in acute myeloid leukemia of cellular daunorubicin accumulation and P-glycoprotein expression simultaneously determined by flow cytometry. Blood, 85:2147-2153, 1995.
22. Moscow JA, Schneider E, Ivy SP, Cowan KH. Multidrug resistance. Cancer Chemother Biol Response Modif, 17:139-177, 1997.
23. Goasguen J, Dossot J, Fardel O. Expression of the multidrug resistance-associated P-glycoprotein (P-170) in 59 cases of de novo acute lymphoblastic leukemia: prognostic implications. Blood, 81:2394-2398, 1993.
24. Dhooge C, De Moerloose B. Clinical significance of P-glycoprotein (P-gp) expression in childhood acute lymphoblastic leukemia. Results of a 6-year prospective study. Adv Exp Med Biol, 457:11-19, 1999.
25. Rossi JF. Chemoresistance and multiple myeloma: from biological to clinical aspects. Stem Cells, 13 Suppl 2:64-71, 1995.
26. Sonneveld P. Modulation of multidrug resistance in multiple myeloma. Baillieres Clin Haematol, 84:831-844, 1995.
27. Hegewisch-Becker S, Hossfeld DK. The MDR phenotype in hematologic malignancies: prognostic relevance and future perspectives. Ann Hematol, 72:105-117, 1996.
28. Baldini N. Multidrug resistance--a multiplex phenomenon. Nature Med, 3:378-380, 1997.
29. Trock BJ, Leonessa F, Clarke RJ. Multidrug resistance in breast cancer: a meta-analysis of MDR1/gp170 expression and its possible functional significance. J Natl Cancer Inst, 89:917-931, 1997.
30. Yokoyama H, Ishida T, Sugio K, *et al.* Immunohistochemical evidence that P-glycoprotein in non-small cell lung cancers is associated with shorter survival. Surg Today, 29:1141-1147, 1999.
31. Savaraj N, Wu CJ, Xu R, *et al.* Multidrug-resistant gene expression in small-cell lung cancer. Amer J Clin Oncol, 20:398-403, 1997.
32. Oka M, Fukuda M, Sakamoto A, *et al.* The clinical role of MDR1 gene expression in human lung cancer. Anticancer Res, 17:721-724, 1997.
33. Campling BG, Young LC, Baer KA, *et al.* Expression of the MRP and MDR1 multidrug resistance genes in small cell lung cancer. Clin Cancer Res, 3:115-122, 1997.
34. Punyammalee B, Manoromana S, Purisa W, *et al.* Association of mdr1 gene expression with other prognostic factors and clinical outcome in human breast cancer. J Med Assoc Thai, 80:S162-173, 1997.
35. Linn SC, Giaccone G, van Diest PJ, *et al.* Prognostic relevance of P-glycoprotein expression in breast cancer. Ann Oncol, 6:679-685, 1995.
36. Gregorcyk S, Kang Y, Brandt D, *et al.* P-glycoprotein expression as a predictor of breast cancer recurrence. Ann Surg Oncol, 3:8-14, 1996.
37. Lizard-Nacol S, Genne P, Coudert B, *et al.* MDR1 and thymidylate synthase (TS) gene expressions in advanced breast cancer: relationships to drug exposure, p53 mutations, and clinical outcome of the patients. Anticancer Res, 19:3575-3581, 1999.
38. Hegewisch-Becker S, Staib F, Loning T, *et al.* No evidence of significant activity of the multidrug resistance gene product in primary human breast cancer. Ann Oncol, 9:85-93, 1998.
39. Ng IO, Liu CL, Fan ST, Ng M. Expression of P-glycoprotein in hepatocellular carcinoma. A determinant of chemotherapy response. Amer J Clin Pathol, 113:355-363, 2000.

40. Goldstein LJ. MDR1 gene expression in solid tumours. Eur J Cancer, 32A:1039-1050, 1996.
41. Raderer M, Scheithauer W. Clinical trials of agents that reverse multidrug resistance. A literature review. Cancer, 72:3553-3563, 1993.
42. Wilson WH, Jamis-Dow C, Bryant G, *et al.* Phase I and pharmacokinetic study of the multidrug resistance modulator dexverapamil with EPOCH chemotherapy. J Clin Oncol, 13:1985-1994, 1995.
43. Wilson WH, Bates SE, Fojo A, Chabner BA. Modulation of multidrug resistance by dexverapamil in EPOCH-refractory lymphomas. J Cancer Res Clin Oncol, 121 Suppl 3:R25-29, 1995.
44. Atadja P, Watanabe T, Xu H, Cohen D. PSC-833, a frontier in modulation of P-glycoprotein mediated multidrug resistance. Cancer Metastasis Rev, 17:163-168, 1998.
45. Advani R, Saba HI, Tallman MS, *et al.* Treatment of refractory and relapsed acute myelogenous leukemia with combination chemotherapy plus the multidrug resistance modulator PSC 833 (Valspodar). Blood, 93:787-795, 1999.
46. List AF, Kopecky KJ, Willman CL, *et al.* Benefit of cyclosporine modulation of drug resistance in patients with poor-risk acute myeloid leukemia: a Southwest Oncology Group study. Blood, 98:3212-3220, 2001.
47. Ferry DR, Traunecker H, Kerr DJ. Clinical trials of P-glycoprotein reversal in solid tumours. Eur J Cancer, 32A:1070-1081, 1996.
48. Ehrlich PH, Moustafa ZA, Archinal-Mattheis AE, *et al.* The reversal of multidrug resistance in multicellular tumor spheroids by SDZ PSC 833. Anticancer Res, 17:129-133, 1997.
49. Rodenburg CJ, Nooter KL, Herweijer H, *et al.* Phase II study of combining vinblastine and cyclosporin-A to circumvent multidrug resistance in renal cell cancer. Ann Oncol, 2:305-306, 1991.
50. Verweij J, Herweijer H, Oosterom R, *et al.* A phase II study of epidoxorubicin in colorectal cancer and the use of cyclosporin-A in an attempt to reverse multidrug resistance. Br J Cancer, 64:361-364, 1991.
51. Baekelandt MM, Holm R, Nesland JM, *et al.* P-glycoprotein expression is a marker for chemotherapy resistance and prognosis in advanced ovarian cancer. Anticancer Res, 20:1061-1067, 2000.
52. Fields A, Hochster H, Runowicz C, *et al.* PSC833: initial clinical results in refractory ovarian cancer patients. Curr Opinion Oncol, 10 Suppl 1:S21, 1998.
53. Beketic-Oreskovic L, Duran GE, Chen G, *et al.* Decreased mutation rate for cellular resistance to doxorubicin and suppression of mdr1 gene activation by the cyclosporin PSC 833. J Natl Cancer Inst, 87:1593-1602, 1995.
54. Sikic BI, Fisher GA, Lum BL, *et al.* Modulation and prevention of multidrug resistance by inhibitors of P-glycoprotein. Cancer Chemother Pharmacol, 40 Suppl:S13-19, 1997.
55. Baldini N, Scotlandi K, Barbanti-Brodano B, *et al.* Expression of P-glycoprotein in high-grade osteosarcomas in relation to clinical outcome. New Engl J Med, 333:1380-1385, 1995.

56. Pinedo HM, Giaccone G. P-glycoprotein–a marker of cancer-cell behavior. New Engl J Med, 333:1417-1419, 1995.
57. Scotlandi K, Serra M, Nicoletti G, *et al.* Multidrug resistance and malignancy in human osteosarcoma. Cancer Res, 56:2434-2439, 1996.
58. Weinstein RS, Jakate SM, Dominguez JM, *et al.* Relationship of the expression of the multidrug resistance gene product (P-glycoprotein) in human colon carcinoma to local tumor aggressiveness and lymph node metastasis. Cancer Res, 51:2720-2726, 1991.
59. Chevillard S, Lebeau J, Pouillart P, *et al.* Biological and clinical significance of concurrent p53 gene alterations, MDR1 gene expression, and S-phase fraction analyses in breast cancer patients treated with primary chemotherapy or radiotherapy. Clin Cancer Res, 3:2471-2478, 1997.
60. Scotlandi K, Manara MC, Serra M, *et al.* The expression of P-glycoprotein is causally related to a less aggressive phenotype in human osteosarcoma cells. Oncogene, 18:739-746, 1999.
61. Takanishi K, Miyazaki M, Ohtsuka M, Nakajima N. Inverse relationship between P-glycoprotein expression and its proliferative activity in hepatocellular carcinoma. Oncol, 54:231-237, 1997.
62. Jedlitschky G, Leier I, Buchholz U, *et al.* ATP-dependent glutathione disulphide transport mediated by the MRP gene-encoded conjugate export pump. Cancer Res, 56:988-994, 1996.
63. Ishikawa T. The ATP-dependent glutathione S-conjugate export pump. Trends Biochem Sci, 17:463-468, 1992.
64. Wijnholds J, Evers R, van Leusden MR, *et al.* Increased sensitivity to anticancer drugs and decreased inflammatory response in mice lacking the multidrug resistance-associated protein. Nature Med, 3:1275-1279, 1997.
65. Büchler M, König J, Brom M, *et al.* cDNA cloning of the hepatocyte canalicular isoform of the multidrug resistance protein, cMrp, reveals a novel conjugate export pump deficient in hyperbilirubinemic mutant rats. J Biol Chem, 271:15091-15118, 1996.
66. Taniguchi K, Wada M, Kohno K, *et al.* A human canalicular multispecific organic anion transporter (cMOAT) gene is overexpressed in cisplatin-resistant human cancer cell lines with decreased drug accumulation. Cancer Res, 56:4124-4129, 1996.
67. Cui Y, Konig J, Buchholz JK, *et al.* Drug resistance and ATP-dependent conjugate transport mediated by the apical multidrug resistance protein, MRP2, permanently expressed in human and canine cells. Mol Pharmacol, 55:929-937, 1999.
68. Evers R, Kool M, van Deemter L, *et al.* Drug export activity of the human canalicular multispecific organic anion transporter in polarized kidney MDCK cells expressing cMOAT (MRP2) cDNA. J Clin Invest, 101:1310-1319, 1998.
69. Hirohashi TH, Suzuki H, Sugiyama Y. Characterization of the transport properties of cloned rat multidrug resistance-associated protein 3(MRP3). J Biol Chem, 274:15181-15185, 1999.
70. Kool M, van-der-Linden M, de Haas M, *et al.* MRP3, an organic anion transporter able to transport anti-cancer drugs. Proc Natl Acad Sci USA, 96:6914-6919, 1999.
71. Schuetz JD, Connelly MC, Sun D, *et al.* MRP4: A previously unidentified factor in resistance to nucleoside-based antiviral drugs. Nature Med, 5:1048-1051, 1999.

72. Kool M, de Haas M, Scheffer GL, *et al.* Analysis of expression of cMOAT (MRP2), MRP3, MRP4, and MRP5, homologues of the multidrug resistance-associated protein gene (MRP1), in human cancer cell lines. Cancer Res, 57:3537-3547, 1997.
73. Kool M, van der Linden M, de Haas M, *et al.* Expression of human MRP6, a homologue of the multidrug resistance protein gene MRP1, in tissues and cancer cells. Cancer Res, 59:175-182, 1999.
74. Loe DW, Deeley RG, Cole SP. Biology of the multidrug resistance-associated protein, MRP. Eur J Cancer, 32A:945-957, 1996.
75. Meister A. Glutathione metabolism and its selective modification. J Biol Chem, 263:17205-17208, 1988.
76. Yamane Y, Furuichi M, Song R, *et al.* Expression of multidrug resistance protein/GS-X pump and gamma-glutamylcysteine synthetase genes is regulated by oxidative stress. J Biol Chem, 273:31075-31085, 1998.
77. Zhu Q, Center MS. Evidence that SP1 modulates transcriptional activity of the multidrug resistance-associated protein gene. DNA Cell Biol, 15:105-111, 1996.
78. Gomi A, Masuzawa T, Ishikawa T, Kuo MT. Posttranscriptional regulation of MRP/GS-X pump and gamma-glutamylcysteine synthetase expression by 1-(4-amino-2-methyl-5-pyrimidinyl) methyl-3-(2-chloroethyl)-3-nitrosourea and by cycloheximide in human glioma cells. Biochem Biophys Res Commun, 239:51-56, 1997.
79. Wang Q, Beck WT. Transcriptional suppression of multidrug resistance-associated protein (MRP) gene expression by wild-type p53. Cancer Res, 58:5762-5769, 1998.
80. Oshika Y, Nakamura M, Tokunaga T, *et al.* Multidrug resistance-associated protein and mutant p53 protein expression in non-small cell lung cancer. Mod Pathol, 11:1059-1063, 1998.
81. Fukushima Y, Oshika Y, Tokunaga T, *et al.* Multidrug resistance-associated protein (MRP) expression is correlated with expression of aberrant p53 protein in colorectal cancer. Eur J Cancer, 35:935-938, 1999.
82. Sullivan GF, Yang JM, Vassil A, *et al.* Regulation of expression of the multidrug resistance protein MRP1 by p53 in human prostate cancer cells. J Clin Invest, 105:1261-1267, 2000.
83. Hipfner DR, Gauldie SD, Deeley RG, Cole SP. Detection of the M(r) 190,000 multidrug resistance protein, MRP, with monoclonal antibodies. Cancer Res, 54:5788-5792, 1994.
84. Flens MJ, Izquierdo MA, Scheffer GL, *et al.* Immunochemical detection of the multidrug resistance-associated protein MRP in human multidrug-resistant tumor cells by monoclonal antibodies. Cancer Res, 54:4557-4563, 1994.
85. Stewart AJ, Canitrot Y, Baracchini E, *et al.* Reduction of expression of the multidrug resistance protein (MRP) in human tumor cells by antisense phosphorothioate oligonucleotides. Biochem Pharmacol, 51:461-469, 1996.
86. Nooter K, Westerman AM, Flens MJ, *et al.* Expression of the multidrug resistance-associated protein (MRP) gene in human cancers. Clin Cancer Res, 1:1301-1310, 1995.
87. Sullivan GF, Amenta PS, Villanueva JD, *et al.* The expression of drug resistance gene products during the progression of human prostate cancer. Clin Cancer Res, 4:1393-1403, 1998.

88. Kuo MT, Bao JJ, Curley SA, *et al.* Frequent coordinated overexpression of the MRP/GS-X pump and gamma-glutamylcysteine synthetase genes in human colorectal cancers. Cancer Res, 56:3642-3644, 1996.
89. Nooter K, Brutel de la Riviere G, Look MP, *et al.* The prognostic significance of expression of the multidrug resistance-associated protein (MRP) in primary breast cancer. Br J Cancer, 76:486-493, 1997.
90. Endo K, Maehara Y, Ichiyoshi Y, *et al.* Multidrug resistance-associated protein expression in clinical gastric carcinoma. Cancer, Suppl 77:1681-1687, 1996.
91. Young LC, Campling BG, Voskoglou-Nomikos T, *et al.* Expression of multidrug resistance protein-related genes in lung cancer: correlation with drug response. Clin Cancer Res, 5:673-680, 1999.

Chapter 4

THE GLUTATHIONE SYSTEM IN ALKYLATOR RESISTANCE

David Hamilton[1], Nasser Fotouhi-Ardakani[2] and Gerald Batist[3]
[1]Department of Pharmacology and Therapeutics, [2]Department of Experimental Medicine, [3]The Center for Translational Research in Cancer, McGill University and Lady Davis Institute for Medical Research, Sir Mortimer B Davis-Jewish General Hospital, Montréal, Québec, Canada

1. INTRODUCTION

One of the greatest obstacles in the effective chemotherapy of neoplastic disease is the presence of tumor chemoresistance. In some instances, a tumor can be intrinsically resistant to chemotherapy or, in other cases, develop resistance during the course of antineoplastic treatment. This acquired resistance is thought to occur through the selection of a subpopulation of resistant tumor cells as the tumor is exposed to chemotherapy. To complicate chemotherapeutic drug selection, it has been found that once a tumor demonstrates resistance to one class of drugs, it will often be resistant to other classes that share structural or functional homology.

Alkylating drugs are antitumor agents that exert their cytotoxic effect through the covalent bonding of alkyl groups to cellular molecules[1]. Evidence shows that the formation of interstrand DNA cross-links is the major cytotoxic event and antitumor effect[2]. These drugs have a long history of clinical usage in cancer treatment and have been utilised in the therapy of malignancies such as acute leukemia, lymphomas and breast and ovarian cancer. Despite their clinical importance and efficacy, tumor resistance to alkylating agents is an increasing concern. Melphalan (L-phenylalanine mustard, L-PAM) is a commonly used alkylator that exemplifies much of the pharmacology of the whole class of nitrogen mustards in current clinical use (e.g., cyclophosphamide)[3]. As a result, it has been extensively studied to try and elucidate the cellular and biochemical mechanisms underlying cancer alkylator chemoresistance.

Through such research, the following cellular changes have been reported to exist in chemoresistant tumors: (a) enhanced repair of DNA damage including DNA mono adducts and cross-links[4], (b) alterations in drug transport[5], (c) elevated levels of glutathione (GSH)[6–8] and (d) elevated glutathione-S-transferase (GST) activity[9–11]. In this chapter, we will focus on the role of GSH and its associated enzymes in tumor resistance to alkylating drugs. We will outline the cellular function and biochemistry of GSH and review some of the more prevalent changes associated with this detoxification system in cancer, particularly in resistant tumor lines. Finally, we will discuss therapeutic approaches to alter the balance of the GSH system in host and cancer cells to achieve a better clinical response to chemotherapy.

2. THE GLUTATHIONE SYSTEM

Glutathione (L-γ-glutamyl-L-cysteinyl-glycine; GSH) is an important intracellular antioxidant and represents the major cellular non-protein thiol (>90%). It is involved in a wide range of cellular reactions such as amino acid transport and protection of cells from damage by oxygen intermediates, free radicals, peroxides and toxins of both endogenous and exogenous origin. As well, it can act as a source of cysteine for protein formation, it reduces disulfides to sulfides, and is involved in the formation of deoxyribonucleotides from ribonucleotides[12–14].

2.1 Glutathione Biosynthesis

The intracellular bioformation of GSH is illustrated in Figure 1. As shown, GSH is synthesized through the action of two enzymes, γ-glutamylcysteine synthetase (γ-GCS) and glutathione synthetase. γ-GCS catalyses the amide linkage between cysteine and the γ-carboxyl group of glutamate in an ATP dependent manner to form the dipeptide γ-glutamylcysteine. This reaction is the rate-limiting step in the formation of GSH. Next, glycine is added to the cysteine carboxyl group of γ-glutamylcysteine to form the tripeptide γ-glutamylcysteinyl-glycine (glutathione, GSH). This reaction is catalysed by the enzyme glutathione synthetase and again utilises ATP.

Once formed, GSH can act in a number of biochemical reactions. Some of the more important cellular pathways include: [1] the reduction of peroxides through the enzymatic action of glutathione peroxidase, [2] the conjugation to a wide variety of electrophilic drugs and compounds, catalysed by the glutathione-S-transferases (GSTs), to effectively eliminate them from the cell, and [3] involvement in DNA repair through interaction with enzymes such as DNA ligases and polymerases[15,16].

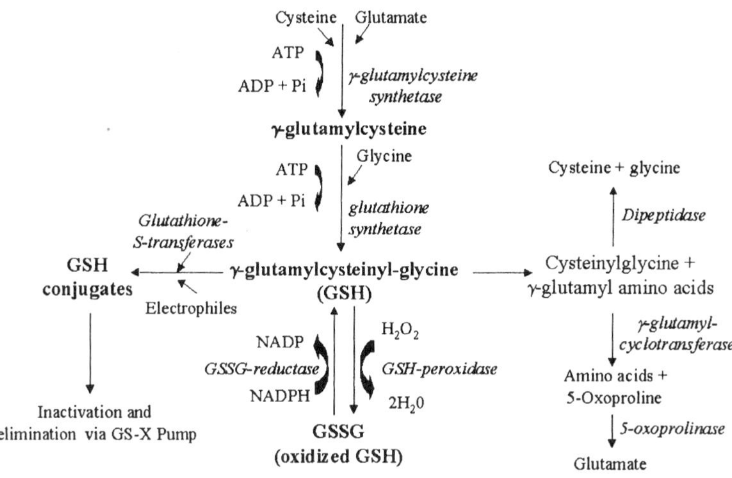

Figure 1. Glutathione biosynthesis and metabolism.

Intracellular GSH levels are typically high (up to 10 mM in hepatocytes) while extracellular concentrations are low (2-10 μM in plasma). It is usually present in a reduced form (GSH) but can become oxidized to glutathione disulfide (GSSG) either through glutathione peroxidase or nonenzymatically through reaction with compounds such as hydroxyl radical, N_2O_3, and peroxynitrite[17]. The high intracellular ratio (100:1) of GSH to GSSG is maintained by NADPH-dependent GSSG reductase.

2.2 γ-Glutamylcysteine Synthetase and Glutathione Synthetase

As mentioned, γ-GCS and glutathione synthetase are the two enzymes involved in the formation of GSH. Each one acts in an ATP dependent manner and is sensitive to its cellular environment, especially oxidative stresses. γ-GCS has been the most studied of the two enzymes, as the reaction it catalyses is the rate limiting step in GSH formation. γ-GCS is a heterodimer composed of a heavy subunit (γ-GCS_h) and a light subunit (γ-GCS_l). The heavy subunit (73-kDa) contains all the catalytic activity for the enzyme and is encoded by a gene located on chromosome 6p12. The light subunit (28-kDa) serves a regulatory function, increasing the affinity of γ-GCS for glutamate and cysteine. It is encoded by a gene on chromosome 1p21.

The subunits associate to form γ-GCS through the formation of a disulfide bond between two molecules of cysteine, one located in each subunit. Of the fourteen cysteine residues present in the γ-GCS_h protein, cysteine-553 has been identified as having an important involvement in heterodimer formation between the two γ-GCS subunits[18]. The ability to respond, through disulfide bond formation, to changes in the redox status of the cellular milieu makes γ-GCS an important enzyme involved in maintaining the reducing thiol-disulfide status of the cytosol. In fact, other enzymes that share a similar function often respond to oxidative stress in the same way. For example, two bacterial proteins, transcription factor OxyR and heat shock protein 33 (Hsp33), are both activated through the oxidation of cysteine residues to disulfide bonds[19]. In *E. coli*, OxyR responds to elevated peroxide concentrations in the cell and then induces the expression of a number of genes, notably glutathione peroxidase[20]. Thus it would appear that disulfide bond formation in enzymes involved in monitoring cellular redox potential is an important and conserved biochemical pathway throughout evolution.

Several regulatory elements have been identified in the 5' and promoter regions of γ-GCS. Both subunit genes contain multiple AP1 and AP1-like binding sites as well as metal and electrophile response elements (MREs and EpREs respectively). An oxidative stress-response element (ORE) has also been identified distal to the heavy subunit promoter[21]. Some studies have implicated members of the AP-1 family of transcriptional activators (JunB, JunD, c-Fos, Fra1, Fra2) and members of the NF-E2 family (Nrf1, Nrf2) as regulators of expression in genes containing EpRE promoter sequences[22]. The γ-GCS_h subunit gene also contains a consensus site for the transcription factor NF-κB, but this is lacking in the γ-GCS_l gene[23]. NF-κB has been shown to be induced by ionizing radiation and therefore acts as a *trans*-regulatory element activating γ-GCS, leading to increased GSH production[24]. The presence of these response elements allows γ-GCS the ability to respond to a wide array of drugs (e.g., cisplatin, cyclohexamide), toxins (cigarette smoke), endogenous metabolites (lipid peroxides, free radicals, oxygen intermediates) and environmental stresses (hypoxia, hypoglycemia, heat shock)[23].

A number of polymorphisms and mutations have been reported in the γ-GCS_h subunit gene. A series of GAG repeats has been identified in the 5' untranslated region (UTR) located 10-30 base pairs upstream from the ATG translational start codon[25]. Three alleles have been reported, each with a different frequency of occurrence: A1; 7 GAGs (f=0.54), A2; 8 GAGs (f=0.11), and A3; 9 GAGs (f=0.35). As well, a polymorphic tetranucleotide insertion (CAGC) has been reported in the 3' UTR, located at cDNA nucleotide 1972, 61 base pairs 3' to the TAG stop codon[26]. This insertion appears to be very common as it was found in 22 of 26 normal people screened and, in fact, it is likely that the tetranucleotide repeat represents the normal sequence and that the polymorphism is actually a tetranucleotide *deletion*.

To date, two mutations in the γ-GCS_h gene have been reported. Both of these mutations were discovered in patients suffering from γ-GCS deficiency. The first is an adenine-to-thymine transversion at cDNA nucleotide 1109[26]. This predicts a histidine-to-leucine amino acid 370 change. The second mutation is a cytosine-to-thymine substitution at cDNA nucleotide 473, predicting a change at amino acid 158 from proline to leucine[27]. The impact of these polymorphisms and mutations on the cellular propensity to carcinogenesis and, as well, cellular ability to respond to stress, detoxify drugs or chemotherapeutics is not known as, to date, little research has been done studying the functional consequences of these abnormalities in the γ-GCS$_h$ gene.

2.3 Glutathione-S-Transferases

The glutathione-S-transferases (GSTs) are a multigene family of enzymes that catalyze the conjugation of GSH with toxic endogenous and xenobiotic compounds. They are part of a phase II detoxification system in which they react with compounds either directly, or after they have undergone phase I activation via cytochrome P450. GSTs catalyse the addition of the thiol group of reduced GSH to a wide variety of electrophilic chemicals containing various functional groups such as chloronitrobenzenes[28], hydroxyalkenals[29], o-quinones[30] and α, β-unsaturated aldehydes[31]. GSTs also bind to hydrophobic compounds such as bilirubin, dexamethasone, heme, and polycyclic aromatic hydrocarbons[32] resulting in decreased toxicity and more easily excretable metabolites.

The GSTs have gone through several classifications since their first discovery in 1975. Currently, three groups of GST enzymes have been identified: [1] the mammalian soluble or cytosolic GSTs, [2] membrane bound GST and [3] the metalloglutathione transferases. The cytosolic GSTs are the best characterised and studied. The have been divided into at least 7 classes, namely, alpha (α), kappa (κ), mu (μ), pi (π), sigma (σ), theta (θ) and zeta (ζ) based on substrate specificity and sequence similarity[32]. The GST members in each class appear to contain distinct gene structures and chromosomal localizations. Each GST class consists of several subunits. The active GST enzymes form homo- or hetero-dimeric combinations of the subunits within each class evolving distinct substrate specificities.

The membrane-bound GSTs include microsomal GST and leukotriene C4 synthase[33,34]. Neither of these GSTs share sequence homology with the cytosolic GST enzymes[35,36]. Microsomal GST is involved in the detoxification of xenobiotic compounds while leukotriene C4 synthase conjugates leukotriene A4 with GSH.

The metalloglutathione transferases are represented by a bacterial GST (FosA), which is involved in resistance to the antibiotic fosfomycin[37]. This superfamily of GSTs has diverse catalytic members including FosA, FosB, glycolase I and estradiol dioxygenases.

As mentioned, the cytosolic GSTs are dimeric enzymes. Each subunit has a complete active site, which does not appear to contribute to the catalytic active site of its neighboring subunit[38]. Each active site has a binding site for GSH (G site) and an adjacent partly hydrophobic site for electrophilic binding (H site)[32]. The basic GST chemistry involves the generation of the thiolate anion (GS^-) of GSH increasing its nucleophilicity towards the electrophilic center of hydrophobic substrates, binding with them through the formation of a thioether bond. Many anticancer alkylating drugs and their metabolites, such as melphalan[39], cyclophosphamide[40] and chlorambucil[41] are potent electrophilic agents, which have been shown to be substrates for GST.

GST expression is very tissue dependent. Normal tissues exhibit qualitative and quantitative differences in GST content[42] and, as well, the different GST isoenzymes appear to have distinct functions as they exhibit different catalytic activities. Given that GSTs represent approximately 1% of the total cellular protein and about 5% of the cytosolic protein in hepatocytes, this suggests that GSTs may be a contributing factor in tissue-specific susceptibility to the carcinogenic process and drug effects[43].

2.4 GS-X Pump/MRP

The multidrug resistance-associated protein (MRP) is a 190-kDa membrane glycoprotein that was discovered in a doxorubicin-selected human lung cancer cell line that demonstrated multidrug resistance but lacked P-glycoprotein[44]. It is a member of the superfamily ABC-type cassette transporters, of which there is one other member, the MDR1-encoded 170-kDa P-glycoprotein (P-gp: see also chapter 3 in this volume by Dr. L. Deng and colleagues).

Subsequent research on the MRP gene showed that it encodes the previously described glutathione S-conjugate export (GS-X) pump[45], and is responsible for the efflux of glutathione conjugates from the cell. It also exports oxidised GSH (GSSG), thus playing an important role in maintaining the reduced status of intracellular thiols under oxidative stress[46], and has been shown to export endogenous compounds such as steroid conjugates, bile salts and some cysteinyl and cysteinylglycine metabolites[47]. Several physiological functions of MRP have been suggested, including: a) protection against heavy metal oxyanions, b) ion channel activity modulation, c) transport of leukotriene C_4 and conjugates of GSH, glucuronate and sulfate, and d) GSH transport through a co-transport mechanism[48].

3. THE GLUTATHIONE SYSTEM IN CANCER AND CHEMORESISTANCE

Much research has focused on the role of the glutathione system in tumor response to chemotherapy and chemoresistance. The elements of this system that have received the greatest amount of attention and research are the GSTs, γ-GCS, MRP/GS-X and GSH itself. This section will outline much of what is known about the role of each of these in carcinogenesis and, in particular, alkylator resistance.

3.1 GSTs

A widely regarded initial step in the chemical carcinogenesis process is the covalent binding of carcinogen-derived electrophilic compounds to DNA and other macromolecules. As most chemotherapeutics themselves are electrophile-producing agents, the GSTs have an important function in the cellular response to chemotherapy. Many antimetabolite anticancer drugs bind target protein or DNA and their GST-mediated conjugation with GSH may interfere with this binding. Given, as mentioned, the high intracellular concentration of GSH (1-10 mM), this interference of action of anticancer drugs can be significant.

Several alkylating agents have been shown to interact with GSH to form stable conjugates. These include melphalan[39,49], chlorambucil[41,50], mechlorethamine[51], cyclophosphamide[40] and ifosfamide[52]. A common characteristic of these drugs is the electrophilic nature of their cytotoxic moieties, allowing them to interact with thiols of reduced GSH to form a thioether, which can then be more easily excreted[53].

Numerous studies have looked at GST levels in cancer cell lines made chemoresistant through chronic exposure to the cytotoxic drug in study. This affords a reliable way to measure cellular biochemical differences in the same cell line prior to and after the development of chemoresistance. From this research, it appears that GSTπ is the subtype most often expressed in tumor tissue. For example, Kotoh *et al.*[54] showed that human bladder cancer cells (KK47) had increased GST activity and gene expression for GSTπ once the cells were made resistant to cisplatin. As well, these cells showed multidrug resistance (mitomycin C, doxorubicin, vinblastin, and etoposide), increased GSH content and γ-GCS gene over-expression[54]. Saburi *et al.*[55] studied a cisplatin-resistant Chinese hamster ovary cell line and found cross resistance to carboplatin, melphalan and $CdSO_4$. Despite having no gene amplification, mRNA levels for GSTπ was 5 times higher in the resistant cell line compared to parent cells, and there was no change in expression for GST μ or α. On the other hand, they found no GST activity differences in a cisplatin-resistant prostate cell line (P/CDP-5), suggesting that mechanisms other than increased GSTπ activity could lead to cisplatin resistance in tumor cell lines.

Goto *et al.*[56] also studied cisplatin resistance in colonic cancer HCT8 cells. They showed that GSTπ was responsible for the formation of cisplatin-glutathione adducts and that cisplatin-resistant HCT8 cells had increased expression of GSTπ mRNA. Adduct formation was abolished upon prior treatment of the cells with ethacrynic acid or ketoprofen, both inhibitors of GSTπ. Ban *et al.*[57] used antisense technology to study the role of GSTπ in drug sensitivity in a colon cancer cell line (M7609). They found that transfection of GSTπ antisense oligonucleotides into M7609 cells caused a ~50% decrease in cellular GSTπ concentrations and this was associated with increased sensitivity to doxorubicin (3.3 fold), cisplatin (2.3 fold), melphalan (2.2 fold) and etoposide (2.1 fold) compared to parent cells[57]. As well, transfection of GSTπ antisense cDNA into an doxorubicin-resistant M7609 cell line (M7609/ADR) caused a similar reduction in GSTπ concentration and decreased the chemoresistance of this cell line towards doxorubicin (4.4 fold)[57].

Another research method to elucidate the role of the GSTs in drug sensitivity has been the use of transfection studies. Many researchers have transfected the cDNAs for the various GSTs into cancer and fibroblast cell lines to determine the change in drug sensitivity or resistance. Human GSTπ cDNA transfection into NIH3T3 cells conferred a low level of resistance against ethacrynic acid[58] and this effect was also demonstrated in MCF-7 cells[59]. Transfection of GST Yc (rat GSTα) cDNA into rat mammary carcinoma cells (MatB) conferred increased resistance to melphalan (6-12 fold), mechlorethamine (10-16 fold) and chlorambucil (7-30 fold)[60], while retrovirus-mediated transfer of GST Yc cDNA into NIH3T3 cells conferred a 5.8-fold resistance to chlorambucil and ~10-fold resistance to mechlorethamine but unaltered sensitivity to methotrexate[61]. Doroshow *et al.*[62] utilised a similar technique in which they transduced NIH3T3 cells with a retrovirus carrying the cDNA for GSTπ and MDR1 (multidrug resistance gene). This combination conferred resistance to doxorubicin (100 fold), colchicine (10 fold), ethacrynic acid (4-5 fold) and 1-chloro-2,4-dinitrobenzene (4-5 fold)[62].

3.2 γ-GCS and GSH

Given that γ-GCS is the rate-limiting enzyme in the formation of GSH, cells having an increased γ-GCS expression could have a selective advantage for drug metabolism and detoxification. As a result, tumors and cancer cell lines have been studied to determine levels of γ-GCS expression and GSH concentration and if this is correlated with drug resistance. Godwin *et al.*[63] measured γ-GCS, GSH, γ-glutamyl transpeptidase and GST levels in human ovarian tumor cell lines made resistant to cisplatin. They found that the development of resistance was correlated with increased expression of mRNAs for γ-GCS and γ-glutamyl transpeptidase and these cells had a significant increase in the level of GSH (13-50 fold). GST levels were unchanged between resistant and parent cells. Further experiments demonstrated that resistance to cisplatin was associated with an increase in the transcriptional rate of γ-GCS and not with RNA stability[64]. Mulcahy *et al.*[65] studied melphalan resistance in human prostate carcinoma cells (DU 145/M4.5). They found resistance to melphalan was associated with increased GSH levels, γ-GCS enzyme activity and γ-GCS mRNA levels[65]. Finally, Iida *et al.*[66] studied the expression of γ-GCS_h and γ-GCS_l in cisplatin-resistant human colon cancer cells (HCT8DDP) and human ovarian cancer cells (A2780DDP), and doxorubicin-resistant human lung cancer cells

(A529DOX). They found that each resistant cell line had increased mRNA and protein expression of both γ-GCS subunits and increased intracellular levels of GSH. Further work proved that the stimulation of expression of γ-GCS_h by doxorubicin and cisplatin was mediated by AP-1[66].

Again, transfection experiments have provided further insight into the role of γ-GCS and GSH in cancer and drug resistance. Mulcahy *et al.*[67] transfected the cDNAs for γ-GCS_h and γ-GCS_l into COS-7 cells and found increased γ-GCS activity and GSH levels, which correlated with a melphalan-resistant phenotype. Kurokawa *et al.*[68] transfected the γ-GCS_h gene into a human small-cell lung cancer cell line (SBC-3) and subsequently found that this transfected cell line had twice the amount of GSH than the parent cells, had increased GS-X pump activity and had a 7.4 fold decreased intracellular cisplatin accumulation. They concluded that γ-GCS gene over-expression leads to an increased intracellular GSH level, which in turn increases GS-X pump activity.

3.3 GS-X Pump

Increased efflux of drug from the cytosol is another mechanism through which a tumor can demonstrate resistance to a chemotherapeutic agent. Numerous studies have looked at the role of the GS-X pump in tumor chemoresistance and how the export pump's activity correlates with other components of the glutathione system.

Some chemoresistant cell lines have been studied to determine their levels of MRP gene expression and GS-X pump activity. Ishikawa *et al.*[69,70] found that the MRP gene is expressed at higher levels in cisplatin-resistant human leukemia (HL-60/R-CP) cells than in sensitive cells and this induction is not due to gene amplification. As well, γ-GCS gene expression in the cisplatin-resistant cells was induced within 24 h of exposure to cisplatin, leading to a significant increase in intracellular GSH levels[69]. These cisplatin-resistant cells were also found to be cross resistant to melphalan and chlorambucil, suggesting that the coordinated action of γ-GCS and the GS-X pump may be important factors in alkylator resistance. The authors further studied the relationship between γ-GCS and the GS-X pump in human colorectal tumor tissue biopsies. They found increased mRNA levels of MRP and γ-GCS genes in 50% and 62%, respectively, of tumor samples. Most importantly, 100% of MRP over-expressing tumor samples had increased γ-GCS mRNA levels, a significant difference compared to normal, matched specimens[71]. This research demonstrates the intimate relationship between GS-X pump activity and cellular GSH levels.

Ogretmen *et al.*[72] also identified an additive interaction between MRP and γ-GCS with regards to doxorubicin resistance. They found increased mRNA levels of MRP and γ-GCS_h in a mesothelioma cell line (Met-5A), compared to normal mesothelial cells, and, as well, expression of MRP correlated with doxorubicin resistance.

Again, transfection studies have added a great deal of information regarding the role of the GS-X pump in cancer chemoresistance. Morrow *et al.*[73] studied the relationship between the GS-X pump and the GSTs in MCF7 cells. They found that MRP1 expression alone confers resistance to many drugs that represent the multidrug resistance phenotype (doxorubicin, vincristine, etoposide, mitoxantrone) but co-expression of MRP1 and GSTA1-1, M1-1 or P1-1 failed to augment MRP1-associated resistance[73]. However, co-expression of MRP1 and GST A1-1 conferred a 4-fold resistance to chlorambucil, whereas no resistance was observed with MRP1 expression alone[73]. This was the first demonstration showing that GST A1-1 and MRP1 can act in synergy to affect cellular resistance to chlorambucil.

Zaman *et al.*[74] transfected non-small lung cancer cells (SW-1573/S1) with a MRP cDNA expression vector and then treated the cells with buthionine sulfoximine (BSO), a γ-GCS inhibitor, to lower intracellular GSH levels. They found that BSO treatment completely reversed resistance to doxorubicin, danorubicin, vincristine and VP-16 in these transfected cells, but had less of an effect when these cells were co-transfected with a MDR1 cDNA vector encoding P-gp[74], demonstrating that the GS-X pump specifically requires GSH for drug transport.

4. MANIPULATION OF THE GLUTATHIONE SYSTEM IN CANCER TREATMENT

Given the role and importance of the glutathione system in drug detoxification and cancer chemotherapy resistance, it would seem a good therapeutic strategy to manipulate the enzymes and substrates of glutathione detoxification in order to achieve a better antineoplastic effect. Several strategies have already been attempted and some are even being used in phase II clinical trials on patients. This section will outline some of the more common and promising GSH modulating compounds and report the effect of these on cancer chemoresistance.

4.1 Buthionine Sulfoximine (BSO)

As defined above, buthionine-(SR)-sulfoximine (L-BSO, BSO) is an irreversible inhibitor of γ-GCS[75] and is the most potent modulator of glutathione. With the use of BSO, no further *de novo* synthesis of GSH is permitted while allowing the ongoing reactions of GSH utilisation and efflux to deplete cellular stores[76]. BSO acts as an inhibitor of GSH formation via binding to the glutamate and cysteine binding sites of γ-GCS, thus preventing the association of the two amino acids necessary for the initial step in the production of GSH[77]. It has been shown that following administration of BSO to mice, marked decreases (10-20% of controls) in cellular GSH can be achieved in most tissues. Kidney, liver, and pancreas cells deplete very quickly ($t_{½}$ = 30-60 min) while most other tissues take several hours to deplete significantly. Red blood cells, which have a slow GSH turnover, deplete gradually ($t_{½}$ ~4 days)[76].

BSO has been extensively studied to determine the effects of GSH depletion on tumor responsiveness to chemotherapy and, as well, to determine the effectiveness of BSO in reversing the chemoresistant phenotype of some forms of cancer. The first pre-clinical experiments were performed in chemoresistant tumor-bearing mice. Following BSO administration, it was found that GSH levels decreased in most normal and tumor tissues, but a greater effect was seen in the neoplastic tissue. BSO itself was non-toxic and was associated with minimal side effects. As well, it appeared that the tumor cells were more sensitive than normal cells to the effects of BSO as tumor GSH levels did not recover as fast following the cessation of treatment[77].

Next, studies that combined BSO treatment and chemotherapy were carried out. In one experiment, mice were inoculated with murine L1210 leukemia cells resistant to the alkylating drug melphalan. After a repeated series of injections of BSO, it was found that GSH concentrations decreased in most tissues by 60-70% and the LD_{50} for melphalan decreased from 22 to 14 mg/kg[78]. As well, it was found that GSH levels depleted more rapidly in the resistant tumor cells compared to sensitive normal cells.

Following a positive response to BSO in animal models, phase I clinical trials were proposed. The results from these trials showed that effective doses of BSO could be administered without significant side effects and with minimal toxicity[79]. Most side effects were limited to nausea and vomiting and it was found that GSH levels in peripheral blood leukocytes showed a variable depletion ranging from 60-90% of starting values[80].

Further phase I trials studied the effect of continuous BSO infusion on GSH levels in normal and tumor tissue[81]. It was found that continuous BSO infusion itself produced minimal toxic effects, although combination with melphalan produced severe myelosuppression in some cases, and frequent low-grade nausea/vomiting. This treatment also produced a consistent and profound depletion in GSH levels (<10% of pretreatment values), and this effect was greater in tumor sections than in peripheral blood lymphocytes[81].

In early phase II clinical trials, patients were initially treated with BSO (every 12 h x 6 doses), followed by the administration of melphalan after the fifth BSO dose[82]. Patients included in the study had been diagnosed with cancer and all had undergone standard treatment regimens for their type of cancer but had exhausted any further treatment options. Results showed that the administration of non-toxic doses of BSO resulted in GSH depletion to levels below 20% of starting values in approximately 50% of treated patients[80]. In the mouse model, utilising murine L1210 leukemia cells, this level of GSH depletion was associated with a two to threefold sensitization to melphalan[78]. There was however an enhanced toxic bone marrow effect with the combination of BSO and melphalan than either drug given alone[82,83].

We have just completed a phase II clinical trial of BSO, administered by continuous infusion for 72 h with melphalan administered at the 48 h time point, in patients with metastatic melanoma with skin lesions that could be serially biopsied. The study again showed myelotoxicity as the principal side effect and cutaneous melanoma metastases demonstrated significant GSH depletion and inhibition of γ-GCS activity. Interestingly, for a given level of γ-GCS inhibition, the degree of GSH depletion was greater in tumor tissue than in peripheral blood mononuclear cells, suggesting greater GSH turnover in tumor cells compared to at least this normal cell type. This has been previously suggested in animal studies. Although there was no comparison between the level of MRP protein (GS-X pump) in the peripheral mononuclear cells versus tumor, MRP protein appeared to be increased after 48 h of BSO exposure[84].

4.2 OTZ

GSH cannot be administered with the aim of increasing intracellular levels, since it's uptake is very inefficient[85]. GSH is broken down by γ-glutamyltranspepidase and dipeptidase into dipeptides and amino acids for the transport and resynthesis of GSH[85], basically making direct GSH administration a cysteine delivery system[86]. Cysteine is the rate-limiting precursor in the formation of GSH as intracellular levels are consistently lower than the levels of glutamate or glycine. As a result, only a small pool of L-cysteine is available to sustain a much larger and metabolically active pool of GSH[76]. Therefore, a mechanism to increase intracellular L-cysteine levels would drive GSH synthesis; however, the direct administration of L-cysteine is associated with toxicity and poor absorption. OTZ (L-2-oxothiazolidine-4-carboxylate, procysteine, OTC) is a prodrug that is converted to S-carboxyl-L-cysteine by 5-oxoprolinase, one of the enzymes in the glutathione system (see Figure 1). Intracellular cysteine is subsequently released following spontaneous decarboxylation. Thus, the use of OTZ affords a mechanism to deliver intracellular cysteine while avoiding the toxic effects of direct delivery of L-cysteine.

Russo *et al.*[87,88] have demonstrated a paradoxical effect of OTZ, in that it increases cellular GSH in normal tissues while at the same time either not affecting levels in tumor tissue or even causing a decrease. This effect has also been demonstrated through *in vivo* work in our laboratory using a rat mammary tumor model[89,90] as well as in cell culture[91]. It was found that the levels of 5-oxoprolinase were 4 times lower in tumor tissue than normal. Experimentally, OTZ was found to effectively increase tumor responsiveness to melphalan when administered surrounding melphalan injection[89], while not being associated with any further bone marrow suppressive effects, as is often the case with BSO usage. To achieve an optimal anti-tumor effect when combining OTZ with chemotherapeutic agents, one must consider both the extent *and* duration of tumor GSH depletion, as cellular repair processes may depend on the availability of GSH[92].

4.3 Oltipraz

Oltipraz [5-(2-pyrazinyl)-4-methyl-1,2-dithole-3-thione] (OPZ) is a synthetic derivative of the plant product 1,2-dithiole-3-thione (D3T) which was developed as a human antischistosomal agent[93]. Oltipraz is a potent inducer of phase II detoxification enzymes, most importantly the GSTs. As well, it has been reported as an enhancer of glucose-6-phosphate dehydrogenase, glutathione reductase and glucuronyl transferase[94]. A lot of research surrounding the use and effects of oltipraz centers on its role in protection from aflatoxin B_1-induced hepatocellular carcinoma (HCC). It has been shown in rats that oltipraz inhibits enzymes of activation, particularly CYP1A and CYP2B[95], while at the same time inducing enzymes of detoxification, particularly GSTα[96]. Our laboratory has shown that HepG2 cells transfected with hepatitis B virus (HBV) have decreased levels of both rat and human GSTα (A5) subunit and, as a result, are hypersensitive to the effects of some alkylating chemotherapeutic agents including melphalan, cisplatin and BCNU[96]. Treatment with oltipraz overcame the effect of HBV on GST α subunit levels, but it was not determined if this decreased alkylator drug sensitivity[96]. The precise mechanism of these effects is the subject of ongoing studies of the GSTα gene promoter.

4.4 Ethacrynic Acid

Ethacrynic acid (EA) is a plant phenolic acid. It has an α, β-unsaturated carboxyl moiety, which results in binding to cellular nucleophiles[97]. EA is conjugated to GSH via GST catalysis and both EA and the EA-GSH conjugate are reversible inhibitors (non-competitive and competitive, respectively) of all the GST classes[98,99]. It has been shown that the GST α mediated conjugation of chlorambucil and GSH is inhibited by EA[41], supporting the notion that GST inhibitors could modify the efficacy of alkylating agents through interruption of their GST-catalyzed conjugation with GSH. EA has been shown to restore the sensitivity of resistant tumor cells to drugs such as doxorubicin[100], melphalan[101], and mitomycin C[102] and to potentiate the toxicity of chlorambucil in rat and human cell lines[103]. Paradoxically, it has been demonstrated that some tumor cells are able to acquire resistance to EA through increased GST expression and activity[104]. As well, chronic exposure to EA results in enhancement in MRP and γ-GCS expression, which leads to increased efflux of the EA-GSH conjugate in EA resistant cells[97]. This is thought to be due to EA interaction with antioxidant response element sequences in promoter regions leading to induction.

Phase I clinical trials using EA have been performed, studying the effects in 27 patients with various forms of cancer. Patients were given EA (25-75

mg/m^2 p.o. every 6 h for 3 doses) and thiotepa (30-55 mg/m^2 i.v., 1 h after the second dose of EA)[105]. The major EA toxic effect observed at every dose level was diuresis, and severe metabolic abnormalities (hyperglycemia, hypocalcemia, hypomagnesemia) occurred at the 75 mg/m^2 dose. It was found that the 50 mg/m^2 EA dose was associated with a 37% decrease in GST activity and the clearance of thiotepa was approximately one half of the value obtained in studies using single agent thiotepa[105].

4.5 Other GSH System Modulators

Some other modulators of the glutathione system exist and have been employed to try and achieve an increased chemotherapeutic response in drug resistant tumors. The MRP/GS-X pump in particular has been targeted. Through research using MRP knockout mice, it has been shown that MRP gene deletion is still compatible with life and fertility[106]. Therefore to try and block this protein or to down-regulate its level in cancer tissue should not be associated with serious host side effects. Verapamil and the cyclosporins have been shown to reverse resistance in MDR cells over-expressing P-gp[107], but in experiments utilizing human large cell lung cancer cells expressing MRP, the resistant cells showed only a slight sensitization to vincristine and daunorubicin following treatment with cyclosporin A or PSC 833 (a cyclosporin analogue) and verapamil was only slightly more efficacious[108]. Further research is investigating the efficacy of other cyclosporins and calcium channel blockers in GS-X pump modulation.

LTC_4, a GSH conjugate of leukotriene A_4, has been shown to be transported extracellularly via the GS-X pump/MRP[109]. MK571, a LTD_4 receptor antagonist, is able to block MRP transport of LTC_4[107] and has been shown to modulate drug resistance in MRP over-expressing cell lines[110]. This effect however did not occur in cell lines co-expressing P-gp.

Antisense technology has also been utilised in targeting MRP over-expressing drug-resistant tumors. Endo *et al.*[111] showed that sensitivity to doxorubicin could be increased following treatment of MRP-positive gastric cancer tissue with antisense oligonucleotides targeted to the coding region of the MRP mRNA, however, no increased sensitivity to mitomycin C or cisplatin was observed.

GSH has been shown to be transported between cells through gap junctions, which are intercellular channels that are formed from members of a family of proteins, the connexins (Cxs). Cancer, and in particular breast cancer, often has a lack of Cx43 gap junctions compared to normal surrounding tissue[112]. As a result, the cancer cells are able to maintain higher levels of GSH than normal cells. In fact, cells sensitive to a chemotherapeutic agent can have an increased resistance to the same agent simply from GSH transfer from neighboring drug-resistant cells[113]. Therefore a good therapeutic strategy to try and decrease intracellular tumor GSH levels is to upregulate the number of gap junctions present in tumor cell membranes. Recent work in our laboratory has demonstrated that dibutyryl-cyclic AMP (db-cAMP) treatment of neuroblastoma cells can lead to an upregulation of gap junctional intercellular communication and Cx43 expression and phosphorylation. This was associated with significant increases in cytotoxic response to a number of chemotherapy agents (doxorubicin, melphalan, BCNU) and it was determined that this effect was accomplished through a significant reduction in intracellular tumor GSH levels[114].

CONCLUSION

As is evident throughout this chapter, the glutathione system is an important determinant in drug detoxification and neoplastic chemotherapy resistance. However, each component of this system does not act in an "all or nothing" fashion, in that changes within the GSH system may or may not correlate with a change in cancer phenotype or cellular chemosensitivity. As outlined, the various elements can interplay, one often influencing the activity of the other (e.g., γ-GCS and MRP). As well, alterations within the GSH system are but one of a number of identified biochemical events that occur as a cell progresses through carcinogenesis. Therefore, to fully understand tumor drug resistance, we need to determine the intimate relationships that exist within the GSH system and between this system and other cellular processes. Although GSH-conjugated detoxification of antineoplastic drugs is not the sole mechanism of drug resistance, it is clear that glutathione, its related enzymes, and the GS-X pump play an important role in anticancer drug detoxification and that alteration of this system can confer chemoresistance.

REFERENCES

1. Tew K, Colvin M, Chabner B. Alkylating agents. *In*: Cancer Chemotherapy and Biotherapy: Principles and Practice, BA Chabner, DL Longo (eds.), Lippincott-Raven, Philadelphia, PA, 1996.
2. Hansson J, Lewensohn R, Ringborg U, Nilsson B. Formation and removal of DNA cross-links induced by melphalan and nitrogen mustard in relation to drug-induced cytotoxicity in human melanoma cells. Cancer Res, 47:2631-2637, 1987.
3. Pu Q, Bezwoda W. Induction of alkylator (melphalan) resistance in HL60 cells is accompanied by increased levels of topoisomerase II expression and function. Mol Pharmacol, 56:147-153, 1999.
4. Bedford P, Fichtinger-Schepman AMJ, Hill BT. Differential repair of platinum-DNA adducts in human bladder and testicular tumor continuous cell lines. Cancer Res, 48:3019-3024, 1988.
5. Redwood WR, Colvin M. Transport of melphalan by sensitive and resistant L1210 cells. Cancer Res, 40:1144-1149, 1980.

6. Richon VM, Schulte N, Eastman A. Multiple mechanisms of resistance to cis-diamminedichloroplatinum (II) in murine leukemia L1210 cells. Cancer Res, 47:2056-2061, 1987.
7. Harrison SD Jr, Brockman RW, Trader MW, *et al.* Cross resistance of drug-resistant murine leukemias to deoxyspergualin (NSC 356894) in vivo. Invest New Drugs 5:345-351, 1987.
8. Ozols RF, Masuda H, Hamilton TC. Mechanisms of cross-resistance between radiation and antineoplastic drugs. NCI Monogr, 6:159-165, 1988.
9. McGown AT, Fox BW. A proposed mechanism of resistance to cyclophosphamide and phosphoramide mustard in a Yoshida cell line in vitro. Cancer Res, 17:223-226, 1986.
10. Schecter RL, Alaoui-Jamali MA, Batist G. Glutathione S-transferase in chemotherapy resistance and in carcinogenesis. Biochem Cell Biol, 70:349-353, 1991.
11. Tew, K. Glutathione-associated enzymes in anticancer drug resistance. Cancer Res, 54:4313-4320, 1994.
12. Meister A. Metabolism and function of glutathione. *In*: Glutathione: Chemical, Biochemical and Medical Aspects, D Dolphin, A Avramovich, R Poulson (eds.), John Wiley and Sons, New York, NY, 1989.
13. Kosower NS, Kosower ES. The glutathione-glutathione disulfide system. *In*: Free Radicals in Biology, WA Pryor (ed.), Academic Press, New York, NY, 1976.
14. Kosower NS, Kosower ES. Glutathione metabolism and function. Annu Rev Biochem, 52:711-760, 1983.
15. Hanawalt PC, Cooper PK, Ganesan AK. DNA repair in bacterial and mammalian cells. Annu Rev Biochem, 48:783-836, 1979.
16. Masuda H, Ozols RF, Lai GM. Increased DNA repair as a mechanism of acquired resistance to cis-diamminedichloroplatinum (II) in human ovarian cancer cell lines. Cancer Res, 48:5713-5716, 1988.
17. Luperchio S, Tamir S, Tannenbaum SR. NO-induced oxidative stress and glutathione metabolism in rodent and human cells. Free Radic Biol Med, 21:513-519, 1996.
18. Tu Z, Anders MW. Identification of an important cysteine residue in human glutamate-cysteine ligase catalytic subunit by site-directed mutagenesis. Biochem J, 336:675-680, 1998.
19. Åslund F, Beckwith J. Bridge over troubled waters: sensing stress by disulfide bond formation. Cell, 96:751-753, 1999.
20. Zheng M, Åslund F, Storz G. Activation of the OxyR transcription factor by reversible disulfide bond formation. Science, 279:1718-1721, 1998.
21. Mulcahy RT, Wartman MA, Bailey HH, Gipp JJ. Constitutive and beta-naphthoflavone-induced expression of the human gamma-glutamylcysteine synthetase heavy subunit gene is regulated by a distal antioxidant response element/TRE sequence. J Biol Chem, 272:7445-7454, 1997.
22. Wild A, Moinova H, Mulcahy T. Regulation of γ-glutamylcysteine synthetase subunit gene expression by the transcription factor Nrf2. J Biol Chem, 274:33627-33636, 1999.
23. Wild AC, Mulcahy T. Regulation of γ-glutamylcysteine synthetase subunit gene expression: insight into transcriptional control of antioxidant defenses. Free Radic Res, 32:281-301, 2000.
24. Kondo T, Higashiyama Y, Goto S *et al.* Regulation of γ-glutamylcysteine synthetase expression in response to oxidative stress. Free Radic Res, 31:325-334, 1999.
25. Walsh AC, Li W, Rosen DR, Lawrence DA. Genetic mapping of GLCLC, the human gene encoding the catalytic subunit of γ-glutamylcysteine synthetase, to chromosome band 6p12 and characterization of a polymorphic trinucleotide repeat within its 5' untranslated region. Cytognent Cell Genet, 75:14-16, 1996.

26. Beutler E, Gelbart T, Kondo T, Matsunaga AT. The molecular basis of a case of γ-glutamylcysteine synthetase deficiency. Blood, 94:2890-2894, 1999.
27. Ristoff E, Augustson C, Geissler J *et al.* A missense mutation in the heavy subunit of γ-glutamylcysteine synthetase gene causes hemolytic anemia. Blood, 95:2193-2197, 2000.
28. Booth J, Boyland E, Sims P. An enzyme from rat liver catalysing conjugation with glutathione. Biochem J, 79:516-524, 1961.
29. Hubatsch I, Riddrestrom M, Mannervik B. Human glutathione transferase A4-4: an Alpha class enzyme with high catalytic efficiency in the conjugation of 4-hydroxynonenal and other genotoxic products of lipid peroxidation. Biochem J, 330:175-179, 1998.
30. Baez S, Segura-Aguilar J, Widersten M, *et al.* Glutathione transferases catalyse the detoxification of oxidized metabolites (o-quinones) of catecholamines and may serve as an antioxidant system preventing degenerative cellular processes. Biochem J, 324:25-28, 1997.
31. Berhane K, Widersten M, Engstrom A, *et al.* Detoxification of base propenals and other alpha, beta-unsaturated aldehyde products of radical reactions and lipid peroxidation by human glutathione transferases. Proc Natl Acad Sci. USA, 91:1480-1484, 1994.
32. Mannervik B, Alin P, Guthenberg C, *et al.* Identification of three classes of cytosolic glutathione transferase common to several mammalian species: correlation between structural data and enzymatic properties. Proc Natl Acad Sci USA, 82:7202-7206, 1995.
33. Morgenstern R, Guthenburg C, Depierre JW. Microsomal glutathione S-transferase. Purification, initial characterisation and demonstration that it is not identical to the cytosolic glutathione S-transferases A, B and C. Eur J Biochem, 128:243-248, 1982.
34. Jakobsson PJ, Mancini JA, Ford-Hutchinson AW. Identification and characterization of a novel human microsomal glutathione S-transferase with leukotriene C4 synthase activity and significant sequence identity to 5-lipoxygenase-activating protein and leukotriene C4 synthase. J Biol Chem, 271:22203-22210, 1996.
35. DeJong JL, Morgenstern R, Jornvall H, *et al.* Gene expression of rat and human microsomal glutathione S-transferases. J Biol Chem, 263:8430-8436, 1998.
36. Lam BK, Penrose JF, Freeman GJ, Austen KF. Expression cloning of a cDNA for human leukotriene C4 synthase, an integral membrane protein conjugating reduced glutathione to leukotriene A4. Proc Natl Acad Sci USA, 91:7663-7667, 1994.
37. Arca P, Hardisson C, Suarez JE. Purification of a glutathione S-transferase that mediates fosfomycin resistance in bacteria. Antimicrob Agents Chemother, 34:844-848, 1990.
38. Mannervik B, Danielson UH. Glutathione transferases-structure and catalytic activities. Crit Dev Biochem, 23:283-337, 1998.
39. Bolton MG, Colvin OM, Hilton J. Specificity of isozymes of murine hepatic glutathione S-transferase for the conjugation of glutathione with L-phenylalanine mustard. Cancer Res, 51:2410-2414, 1991.
40. Yuan Z-M, Fenselau C, Dulik DM, Martin W, *et al.* Laser desorption electron impact: application to a study of the mechanism of conjugation of glutathione and cyclophosphamide. Anal Chem, 62:868-870, 1990.
41. Ciaccio PJ, Tew KD, LaCreta FP. The spontaneous and glutathione S-transferase mediated reaction of chlorambucil with glutathione. Cancer Commun, 2:279-286, 1990.
42. Zimniak P, Nanduri B, Pikula S, *et al.* Naturally occurring human glutathione S-transferase GSTP1-1 isoforms with isoleucine and valine in position 104 differ in enzymatic properties. Eur J Biochem, 224:893-899, 1994.
43. Coles B, Ketterer B. The role of glutathione and glutathione transferases in chemical carcinogenesis. Biochem Mol Biol, 25:47-70, 1990.
44. Cole SPC, Bhardwaj G, Gerlach JH, *et al.* Overexpression of a transporter gene in a multidrug-resistant human lung cancer cell line. Science, 258:1650-1654, 1992.

45. Ishikawa T. The ATP-dependent glutathione S-conjugate export pump. Trends Biochem, 17:463-468, 1992.
46. Leier I, Jedlitschky G, Buchholz U, *et al.* ATP-dependent glutathione disulphide transport mediated by the MRP gene-encoded conjugate export pump. Biochem J, 314:433-437, 1996.
47. Jedlitschky G, Leier I, Buchholz U, *et al.* Transport of glutathione, glucuronate and sulfate conjugates by the MRP gene-encoded conjugate export pump. Cancer Res, 56:988-994, 1996.
48. Rappa G, Finch RA, Sartorelli AC, Lorico A. New insights into the biology and pharmacology of the multidrug resistance protein (MRP) from gene knockout models. Biochem Pharmacol, 58:557-562, 1999.
49. Dulik DM, Fenselau C, Hilton J. Characterization of melphalan-glutathione adducts whose formation is catalysed by glutathione S-transferases. Biochem Pharmacol, 35:3404-3409, 1986.
50. Zhang K, Wong KP. Glutathione conjugation of chlorambucil: measurement and modulation by plant polyphenols. Biochem J, 325:417-422, 1997.
51. Gamcsik MP, Hamill TG, Colvin OM. NMR studies of conjugation of mechlorethamine with glutathione. J Med Chem, 33:1009-1014, 1990.
52. Dirven HA, Megens I, Oudshoorn MJ, *et al.* Glutathione conjugation of cytostatic drug ifosfamide and the role of human glutathione S-transferases. Chem Res Toxicol, 8:979-986, 1995.
53. Zhang K, Mack P, Wong KP. Glutathione-related mechanisms in cellular resistance to anticancer drugs (review). Int J Oncol, 12:871-882, 1998.
54. Kotoh S, Naito S, Yokomizo A, *et al.* Enhanced expression of γ-glutamylcysteine synthetase and glutathione S-transferase genes in cisplatin-resistant bladder cancer cells with multidrug resistance phenotype. J Urol, 157:1054-1058, 1997.
55. Saburi Y, Nakagawa M, Ono M, *et al.* Increased expression of glutathione S-transferase gene in cis-diamminedichloroplatinum(II)-resistant variants of a Chinese hamster ovary cell line. Cancer Res, 49:7020-7025, 1989.
56. Goto S, Iida T, Oka M, *et al.* Overexpression of glutathione S-transferase π enhances the adduct formation of cisplatin with glutathione in human cancer cells. Free Radic Res, 31:549-558, 1999.
57. Ban N, Takahashi Y, Takayama T, *et al.* Transfection of glutathione S-transferase (GST)-π antisense complimentary DNA increases the sensitivity of a colon cancer cell line to adriamycin, cisplatin, melphalan and etoposide. Cancer Res, 56:3577-3582, 1996.
58. Nakagawa K, Saijo N, Tsuchida S, *et al.* Glutathione S-transferase π as a determinant of drug resistance in transfectant cell lines. J Biol Chem, 265:4296-4301, 1990.
59. Moscow JA, Townsend AJ, Cowan KH. Elevation of π class glutathione S-transferase activity in human breast cancer cells by transfection of the GSTπ gene and its effect to sensitivity to toxins. Mol Pharmacol, 36:22-28, 1989.
60. Schecter RL, Alaoui-Jamali M, Woo A, *et al.* Expression of a rat glutathione S-transferase complimentary DNA in rat mammary carcinoma cells: impact upon alkylator-induced toxicity. Cancer Res, 53:4900-4906, 1993.
61. Greenbaum M, Létourneau S, Assar H, *et al.* Retrovirus-mediated gene transfer of rat glutathione S-transferase Yc confers alkylating drug resistance in NIH 3T3 mouse fibroblasts. Cancer Res, 54:4442-4447, 1994.
62. Doroshow JH, Metz MZ, Matsumoto L, *et al.* Transduction of NIH 3T3 cells with a retrovirus carrying both human MDR1 and glutathione S-transferase π produces broad-range multidrug resistance. Cancer Res, 55:4073-4078, 1995.

63. Godwin AK, Meister A, O'Dwyer PJ *et al.* High resistance to cisplatin in human ovarian cancer cell lines is associated with marked increase of glutathione synthesis. Pro Natl Acad Sci USA, 89:3070-3074, 1992.
64. Yao XS, Godwin AK, Johnson SW *et al.* Evidence for altered regulation of γ-glutamylcysteine synthetase gene expression among cisplatin-sensitive and cisplatin-resistant human ovarian cancer cell lines. Cancer Res, 55:4367-4374, 1995.
65. Mulcahy RT, Untawale S, Gipp JJ. Transcriptional up-regulation of γ-glutamylcysteine synthetase gene expression in melphalan-resistant human prostate carcinoma cells. Mol Pharmacol, 46:909-914, 1994.
66. Iida T, Mori K, Goto S *et al.* Co-expression of gamma-glutamylcysteine synthetase sub-units in response to cisplatin and doxorubicin in human cancer cells. Int J Canc, 82:405-411, 1999.
67. Mulcahy RT, Bailey HH, Gipp JJ. Transfection of complimentary DNAs for the heavy and light subunits of human γ-glutamylcysteine synthetase results in an elevation of intracellular glutathione and resistance to melphalan. Cancer Res, 55:4771-4775, 1995.
68. Kurokawa H, Ishida T, Nishio K, *et al.* γ-glutamylcysteine synthetase gene overexpression results in increased activity of the ATP-dependent glutathione S-conjugate export pump and cisplatin resistance. Biochem Biophys Res Commun, 216:258-264, 1995.
69. Ishikawa T, Bao J-J, Yamane Y, *et al.* Coordinated induction of MRP-GS-X pump and γ-glutamylcysteine synthetase by heavy metals in human leukemia cells. J Biol Chem, 271:14981-14988, 1996.
70. Ishikawa T, Wright CD, Ishizuka H. GS-X pump is functionally overexpressed in cis-daimminechloroplatinum (II)-resistant human leukemia HL-60 cells and down-regulated by cell differentiation. J Biol Chem, 269:29085-29093, 1994.
71. Kuo MT, Bao JJ, Curley SA, *et al.* Frequent co-ordinated overexpression of the MRP/GS-X pump and γ-glutamylcysteine synthetase genes in human colorectal cancers. Cancer Res, 56:3642-3644, 1996.
72. Ogretmen B, Bahadori H, McCauley MD, *et al.* Co-ordinated over-expression of the MRP and γ-glutamylcysteine synthetase genes, but not MDR1, correlates with doxorubicin resistance in human malignant mesothelioma cell lines. Int J Cancer, 75:757-761, 1998.
73. Morrow CS, Smitherman PK, Diah SK, *et al.* Coordinated action of glutathione S-transferases (GSTs) and multidrug resistance protein 1 (MRP1) in antineoplastic drug detoxification. J Biol Chem, 273:20114-20120, 1998.
74. Zaman GJR, Lankelma J, Tellingen O, *et al.* Role of glutathione in the export of compounds from cells by the multidrug-resistance-associated protein. PNAS USA, 92:7690-7694, 1995.
75. Griffith OW. Mechanisms of action, metabolism and toxicity of butathionine sulfoximine and its higher homologues; potent inhibitors of glutathione biosynthesis. J Biol Chem, 257:13704-13708, 1982.
76. Griffith OW. Biologic and pharmacologic regulation of mammalian glutathione synthesis. Free Radic Biol Med, 27:922-935, 1999.
77. Griffith OW, Mulcahy RT. The enzymes of glutathione synthesis: γ-glutamylcysteine synthetase. *In*: Advances in Enzymology and Related Areas of Molecular Biology, Volume 73: Mechanism of Enzyme Action, Part A, D Purich (ed.), John Wiley and Sons, New York, NY, 1999.
78. Kramer RA, Greene K, Ahmad S, Vistica DT. Chemosensitization of L-phenylalanine mustard by the thiol-modulating agent buthionine sulfoximine. Cancer Res, 47:1593-1597, 1987.

79. O'Dwyer PJ, Hamilton TC, LaCreta FP, *et al.* Phase I trial of buthionine sulfoximine in combination with melphalan in patients with cancer. J Clin Oncol, 14:249-256, 1996.
80. Bailey HH, Mulcahy RT, Tutsch KD, *et al.* Phase I clinical trial of intravenous L-buthionine sulfoximine and melphalan: an attempt at modulation of glutathione. J Clin Oncol, 12:194-205, 1994.
81. Bailey HH, Ripple G, Tutsch KD *et al.* Phase I study of continuous-infusion L-S,R-buthionine sulfoximine with intravenous melphalan. J Natl Cancer Inst, 89:1789-1796, 1997.
82. O'Dwyer PJ, Hamilton TC, Young RC *et al.* Depletion of glutathione in normal and malignant human cells in vivo by butathionine sulfoximine: clinical and biochemical results. J Natl Cancer Instit, 84:264-267, 1992.
83. Hamilton TC, Lai GM, Rothenberg ML. Mechanisms of resistance to alkylating agents and cisplatin. *In*: Cancer Treatment and Research: Drug Resistance, RF Ozols (ed.), Martinus Nijhoff, Boston, MA, 1989.
84. Batist G, Schecter RL, Karp W, *et al.* Effects of BSO infusion on GSH and related proteins in patients with metastatic melanoma. Submitted.
85. Meister A. Glutathione deficiency produced by inhibition of its synthesis and its reversal; applications in research and therapy. Pharmacol Ther, 51:155-194, 1991.
86. Anderson ME, Luo J-L. Glutathione therapy: from prodrugs to genes. Sem Liver Dis, 18:415-424, 1998.
87. Russo A, Mitchell JB, McPherson SJ, Friedman N. Alteration of bleomycin cytotoxicity by glutathione depletion or elevation. Int J Radiat Oncol Biol Phys, 10:1675-1678, 1983.
88. Russo A, De Graff W, Friedman N, Mitchell JB. Selective modulation of glutathione levels in human normal versus tumor cells and subsequent differential response to chemotherapy drugs. Cancer Res, 46:2845-2848, 1986.
89. Wang T, Chen X, Schecter R, *et al.* Modulation of glutathione by a cysteine pro-drug enhances in vivo tumor response. J Pharm Exp Ther, 276:1169-1173, 1996.
90. Baruchel S, Wang T, Farah R, *et al.* In vivo selective modulation of tissue glutathione in a rat mammary carcinoma model. Biochem Pharmacol, 50:1499-1502, 1995.
91. Chen X, Batist G. Sensitization effect of L-2-oxothiazolidine-4-carboxylate on tumor cells to melphalan and the role of 5-oxo-l-prolinase in glutathione modulation in tumor cells. Biochem Pharm, 56:743-749, 1998.
92. Wellner VP, Anderson ME, Puri RN *et al.* Radioprotection by glutathione ester: transport of glutathione ester into human lymphoid cells and fibroblasts. Pro Natl Acad Sci USA, 81:4732-4735, 1984.
93. Benson AB. Oltipraz: a laboratory and clinical review. J Cell Biochem, 17F:278-291, 1993.
94. DCPC Chemoprevention Branch agents under evaluation. September 1990. Prepared under NCI contract NO1-CN-95159-03.
95. Langouët S, Machéo K, Berthou F, *et al.* Effects of administration of the chemoprotective agent oltipraz on CYP1A and CYP2B in rat liver and rat hepatocytes in culture. Carcinogenesis, 18:1343-1349, 1997.
96. Jaitovitch-Groisman I, Fotouhi-Ardakani N, Schecter R, *et al.* Modulation of glutathione s-transferase alpha by hepatitis B virus and the chemopreventive drug oltipraz. J Biol Chem, 275:33395-33403, 2000.
97. Ciaccio PJ, Shen H, Kruh GD, Tew KD. Effects of chronic ethacrynic acid exposure on glutathione conjugation and MRP expression in human colon tumor cells. Biochem Biophys Res Commun, 222:111-115, 1996.
98. Ahokas JT, Nicholls FA, Ravenscroft PJ, Emmerson PJ. Inhibition of purified rat liver glutathione S-transferase isozymes by diuretic drugs. Biochem Pharmacol, 34:2157-2161, 1990.

99. Ploemen J, van Ommen B, van Bladeren PJ. Inhibition of rat and human glutathione S-transferase isoenzymes by ethacrynic acid and its glutathione conjugate. Biochem Pharmacol, 40:1631-1635, 1990.
100. Nagourney RA, Messenger JC, Kern DH, Weisenthal LM. Enhancement of anthracycline and alkylator cytotoxicity by ethacrynic acid in primary cultures of human tissues. Cancer Chemother Pharmacol, 26:318-322, 1990.
101. Hansson J, Berhane K, Castro VM, *et al.* Sensitization of human melanoma cells to the cytotoxic effect of melphalan by the glutathione transferase inhibitor ethacrynic acid. Cancer Res, 51:94-98, 1991.
102. Xu BH, Singh SV. Effect of buthionine sulfoximine and ethacrynic acid on cytotoxic activity of mitomycin C analogues BMY 25282 and BMY 25067. Cancer Res, 52:6666-6670, 1992.
103. Tew KD, Bomber AM, Hoffman SJ. Ethacrynic acid and piripost as enhancers of cytotoxicity in drug resistant and sensitive cell lines. Cancer Res, 48:3622-3625, 1988.
104. Kuzmich S, Vanderveer LA, Walsh ES, *et al.* Increased levels of glutathione S-transferase π transcript as a mechanism of resistance to ethacrynic acid. Biochem J, 269:47-54, 1992.
105. O'Dwyer PJ, LaCreta F, Nash S, *et al.* Phase I study of thiotepa in combination with the glutathione transferase inhibitor ethacrynic acid. Cancer Res, 51:6059-6065, 1991.
106. Wijnholds J, Evers R, van Leusden MR, *et al.* Increased sensitivity to anticancer drugs and decreased inflammatory response in mice lacking the multidrug resistance-associated protein. Nat Med, 3:1275-1279, 1997.
107. Ford JM and Hait WN. Pharmacology of drugs that alter multidrug resistance in cancer. Phamacol Rev, 42:155-199, 1990.
108. Barrand MA, Rhodes T, Center MS, *et al.* Chemosensitization and drug accumulation effects of cyclosporin A, PSC 833 and verapamil in human MDR large cell lung cancer cells expressing a 190k membrance protein distinct from P-glycoprotein. Eur J Cancer, 29A:408-415, 1993.
109. Leier I, Jedlitschky G, Buchholz U *et al.* The MRP gene encodes an ATP-dependent export pump for leukotriene C_4 and structurally related compounds. J Biol Chem, 269:27807-27810, 1994.
110. Gekeler V, Ise W, Sanders KH, *et al.* The leukotriene LTD_4 receptor antagonist MK571 specifically modulates MRP associated multidrug resistance. Biochem Biophys Res Commun, 208:345-352, 1995.
111. Endo K, Maehara Y, Ichiyashi Y *et al.* Multidrug resistance-associated protein expression in clinical gastric carcinoma. Cancer, 7:1681-1687, 1996.
112. Laird DW, Fistouris P, Batist G, *et al.* Deficiency of connexin43 gap junctions is an independent marker for breast tumors. Cancer Res, 59:4104-4110, 1999.
113. Oskar S, Frankhurt D, Sugarbaker EV. Intercellular transfer of drug resistance. Cancer Res, 51:1190-1195, 1991.
114. Carystinos GD, Alaoui-Jamali MA, Phipps J, *et al.* Up-regulation of gap junctional intercellular communication and connexin 43 expression by cyclic-AMP and all-trans-retinoic acid is associated with glutathione depletion and chemosensitivity in neuroblastoma cells. Cancer Chemother Pharmacol, 47:126-132, 2001.

Chapter 5

THE ROLE OF SIGNAL TRANSDUCTION PATHWAYS IN DRUG AND RADIATION RESISTANCE

Steven Grant[1,2], Paul B. Fisher[4] and Paul Dent[1,3]
Departments of [1]Pharmacology and Toxicology, [2]Hematology/Oncology, [3]Radiation Oncology Medical College of Virginia, Virginia Commonwealth University, Richmond, Virginia, USA
[4]Department of Pathology and Urology, Columbia University College of Physicians and Surgeons, New York, New York, USA

1. THE MITOGEN ACTIVATED PROTEIN KINASE (MAPK) PATHWAY

"MAPK" was first reported by Sturgill and Ray in 1986[1]. This protein kinase was originally described as a 42-kDa insulin-stimulated protein kinase activity whose tyrosine phosphorylation increased after insulin exposure, and which phosphorylated the cytoskeletal protein MAP-2 (hence "MAP" kinase). Contemporaneous studies by Boulton and Cobb identified an additional 44-kDa isoform of MAPK, which they named ERK1 (extracellular signal regulated kinase)[2]. Since many growth factors and mitogens could activate MAPK, the acronym for this enzyme has subsequently been considered to denote mitogen-activated protein (MAP) kinase. In the following years, additional studies demonstrated that the p42/p44 MAPKs regulated another protein kinase activity ($p90^{rsk}$)[3], and that they were themselves regulated by a protein kinase activity originally designated MKK (MAPK kinase)[4,5].

MKK phosphorylates the MAPKs on tyrosine and threonine residues and became the first biochemically characterized dual specificity (threonine/tyrosine) protein kinase[4–6]. This enzyme is also often referred to as MEK (mitogen activated/extracellular regulated kinase). Shortly after the discovery of MKK1, a second isoform of this enzyme was identified (MKK1 and MKK2)[7]. MKK1/2 were also found to be regulated by reversible phosphorylation, and within 6 months of the discovery of MKK2, the protein kinase responsible for catalyzing MKK1/2 activation was discovered, the proto-oncogene Raf-1[8,9]. More recently, it has been suggested that other enzymes at the level of MKK1/2 can phosphorylate and activate p42/44 MAPK; e.g., RIP2[10]. RIP2 plays a role in TNFα-induced, but not EGF-induced, MAPK activation and may play a protective NFκ-B-activating role[10].

Raf-1 is a member of a family of serine-threonine protein kinases termed Raf-1, B-Raf, and A-Raf[11,12]. Each protein consists of an NH_2-terminal domain (termed CR1), a COOH-terminal catalytic domain (termed CR3), and a central domain that is heavily phosphorylated *in vivo* (termed CR2). All "Raf" family members can phosphorylate and activate MKK1/2, although the relative ability of each member to catalyze this reaction varies (B-Raf > Raf-1 > A-Raf)[13,14]. Raf kinases thus act at the level of a MAPK kinase kinase (MAPKKK). Several studies demonstrated that the CR1 domain of Raf-1 could reversibly interact with the Ras proto-oncogene in the plasma membrane and that the ability of Raf-1 to associate with Ras was dependent upon the Ras molecule being in the GTP-bound state[15,16]. Other findings proved that the ability of Raf-1 to be activated depended upon Raf-1 translocation to the plasma membrane[17–20]. The regulation of Raf-1 activity appears to be very complex, with several mechanisms coordinately regulating activity when in the plasma membrane environment. Stokoe and McCormick have demonstrated that association of Raf-1 with Ras is sufficient for partial stimulation of Raf-1 activity[21]. More recently, the binding of 14-3-3 proteins to phospho-serine residues (S259, S621) in Raf-1 have been suggested to play a role in Raf-1 activation[22–24]. Phosphorylation of S338 by PAK enzymes has more recently been shown to play a role in the activation process[25]. Other investigators have suggested that another lipid second messenger, ceramide, may also be able to play a role in Raf-1 activation[26,27], although this is disputed[28,29]. Data from several laboratories have suggested that protein serine/threonine and tyrosine phosphorylations play a role increasing Raf-1 activity when in the plasma membrane environment[29–31]. Other studies have also suggested that PKC (protein kinase C) isoforms can directly regulate Raf-1 activity[32,33]. Phorbol esters and the macrocyclic lactone bryostatin 1 can activate PKC, and have been shown to activate Raf-1 and the MAPK cascade in many cell types[34,35]. At the same time that Raf-1 was shown to associate with Ras, it was found that growth factors, via their plasma membrane receptors, stimulate GTP for GDP exchange in Ras using guanine nucleotide exchange factors[36,37]. Thus, over an interval of ~9 years, a "MAPK" pathway was delineated from plasma membrane growth factor receptors, through guanine nucleotide exchange factors and the Ras proto-oncogene, to the Raf-1/MKK/MAPK/p90[rsk] (Figure 1). During this period, other studies had begun to link growth factor induced MAPK and p90[rsk] activation to the ability of these mitogens to regulate transcription factor activities within the nucleus[38,39]. The relative ability of MAPK signaling to mediate increased activity of transcription factors is under intensive study because it appears that many signaling pathways, e.g., the JNK pathway, coordinately regulate transcription factor activities and gene expression along with the classical MAPK pathway[40–43].

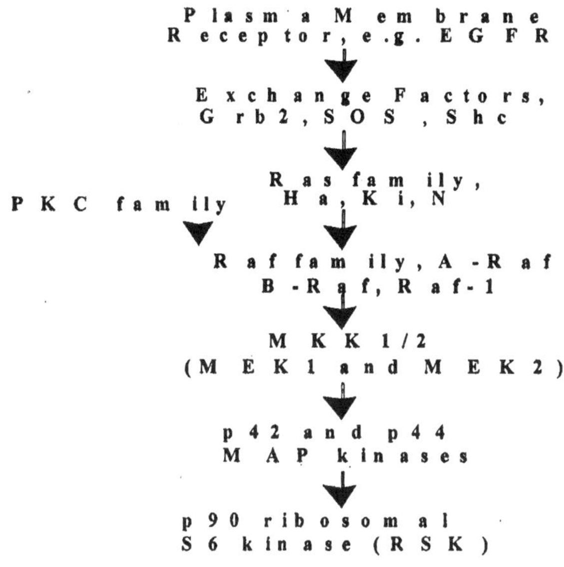

Figure 1. The MAPK pathway in mammalian cells.

2. THE C-JUN NH_2-TERMINAL KINASE (JNK)/STRESS ACTIVATED PROTEIN KINASE (SAPK) PATHWAY

The c-Jun NH_2 terminal kinase (JNK) pathway was discovered and described in the early to mid 1990's[44,45]. JNK1/2 were initially described biochemically to be a stress-induced protein kinase activity that phosphorylated the NH_2-terminus of the transcription factor c-Jun; hence the pathway is also often called the stress activated protein kinase (SAPK) pathway. Multiple stresses increase JNK1/2 activity, including UV- and γ-irradiation, cytotoxic drugs and reactive oxygen species (H_2O_2). Phosphorylation of the NH_2-terminal sites Ser63 and Ser73 in c-Jun increases its ability to transactivate AP-1 enhancer elements in the promoters of many genes[46,47]. It has been recently suggested that JNK can also phosphorylate the NH_2-terminus of c-Myc, enhancing its activity, potentially playing a role in both proliferative and apoptotic signaling[48]. In a similar manner to the previously described MAPK pathway, JNK1/2 activities were regulated by dual threonine and tyrosine phosphorylations which were found to be catalyzed by a protein kinase analogous to MKK1/2, termed stress-activated extracellular regulated kinase 1 (SEK1), also called MKK4[49]. An additional isoform of MKK4, termed MKK7, was subsequently discovered[50]. As in the case of MKK1/2, MKK4/7 were also regulated by dual serine phosphorylation. In contrast to the MAPK pathway, which appears to primarily utilize the three protein kinases of the Raf family to activate MKK1/2, at least ten protein kinases are known to phosphorylate and activate MKK4/7, including MKKK1-4, TAK-1 and Tpl-2[51]. The agonist and cell type specificity of each JNK pathway MAPKKK enzyme in the activation of this pathway is currently under intense investigation.

Upstream of the MAPKKK enzymes are another layer of JNK pathway protein kinases, e.g., Ste20-homologues and low molecular weight GTP-binding proteins of the Rho family, in particular Cdc42 and Rac1 (Figure 2)[52]. It is not clear how growth factor receptors, e.g., EGF receptor, activate the Rho family low molecular weight GTP-binding proteins; one mechanism may be via the Ras proto-oncogene, whereas others have suggested via PI_3 kinase and/or protein kinase C isoforms (Figure 2)[53,54]. In addition, other groups have shown that agonists acting through the tumor necrosis factor alpha (TNFα) receptor, *via* sphingomyelinase enzymes generating the lipid second messenger ceramide, can activate the JNK pathway by mechanism(s) which may also act through Rho family GTPases[55]. Definitive answers to all of these questions await further investigation. In the following sections, potential roles in the control of growth, proliferation, cell survival and DNA repair for the JNK and MAPK pathways are examined.

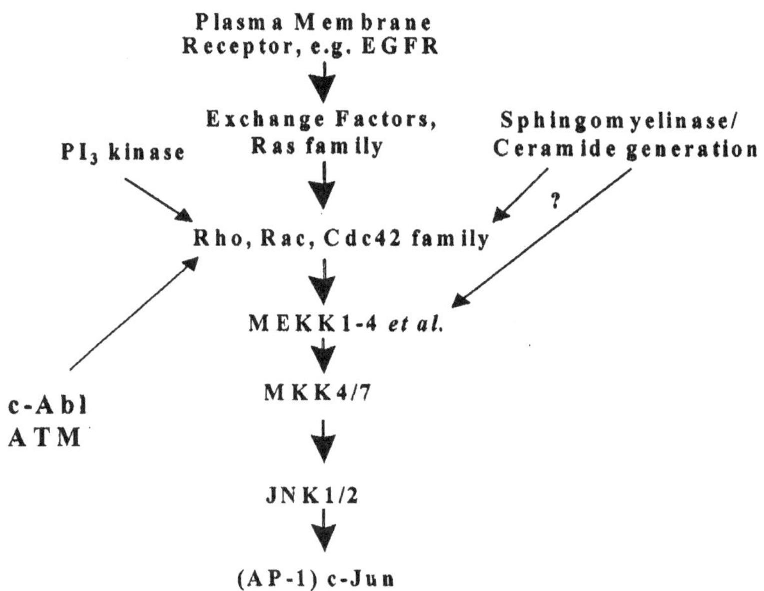

Figure 2. The JNK pathway in mammalian cells.

3. AN OVERVIEW OF THE ROLE OF THE MAPK PATHWAY IN PROLIFERATION, DIFFERENTIATION AND SURVIVAL SIGNALING

Simplistically, cell growth can be divided into five separate phases termed the cell cycle. Quiescent, non-proliferating cells are frequently termed to be in G_0 phase. Upon mitogenic stimulation, cells in G_0 enter into the first growth phase of the cell cycle, G_1. Once cell growth has reached a certain level, cells enter a new phase of the cycle as they begin to synthesize new DNA, which is termed S phase. Cells exit S phase and enter a shorter growth phase termed G_2, which is shortly followed by chromosomal alignment along the metaphase plate as cells enter into M (mitosis) phase. The chromosomes separate in M phase and two daughter cells are formed. Both the MAPK and JNK pathways have been proposed to control cell cycle progression.

Initial observations suggested that signaling by the MAPK pathway was intimately involved in the abilities of growth factors to stimulate proliferation and initially the accepted view of signaling through the pathway was that its activation promotes proliferation, and the greater the activation, the greater the proliferative response[56]. For example, in NIH 3T3 fibroblasts, transformation with either the v-Ha-Ras oncogene or the v-Raf oncogene caused constitutive activation of the MAPK cascade and increased proliferation[57,58]. In NIH 3T3 cells, expression of a constitutively active form of MKK1 also caused constitutive activation of the MAPK cascade and increased proliferation[59]. The positive role of MAPK activation in cell cycle progression may be linked to increased expression of cyclin molecules, e.g., cyclin D1[60–63]. However, more defined studies examining the extent and duration of MAPK activation are now beginning to show that a simplistic view of increased activation of MAPK equating with increased proliferation is not necessarily valid.

For example, in PC12 pheochromocytoma cells, the role of MAPK signaling appears to conflict with the conventional view linking increased activity to enhanced proliferation. It was known that exposure of PC12 cells to EGF stimulates their proliferation. In contrast, exposure of these cells to nerve growth factor (NGF) was shown to inhibit proliferation and cause a differentiation response[64,65]. Several groups then noted that whereas EGF induces an acute phasic activation of the MAPK pathway, NGF increases MAPK activity over a prolonged time period[66–68]. Other studies confirmed that prolonged signaling, via the MAPK pathway, was essential to the ability of NGF to induce differentiation. It was argued[68,69] that the ability of NGF to cause growth arrest via MAPK is dependent upon its ability to increase expression of the cyclin dependent kinase inhibitor protein (CKI) $p21^{Cip\text{-}1/MDA6/WAF1}$. Many leukemic cell types behave in a similar manner to PC12 cells when exposed to phorbol esters. For example, Whalen *et al.*[70] demonstrated that phorbol esters cause growth arrest and differentiation in megakaryocytes via activation of classical PKC isoforms. These enzymes cause prolonged activation of the MAPK pathway, leading to terminal differentiation[70]. Exposure of myeloid leukemia cells to phorbol esters can also increase $p21^{Cip-1/MDA6/WAF1}$ expression via the MAPK pathway[71].

Recently, studies performed in embryonic fibroblasts and in primary hepatocytes have demonstrated definitively that an acute phasic activation of the MAPK pathway promotes proliferation, whereas prolonged activation of the pathway promotes cell cycle arrest[72–75]. In studies by McMahon and Land, mouse embryonic fibroblasts which were p21 -/- did not arrest in response to prolonged MAPK activation, suggesting a key role for $p21^{Cip-1/MDA6/WAF1}$ in the MAPK-mediated cell cycle arrest[72,73]. In studies by Park *et al.*[75] and Tombes *et al.*[74], however, prolonged MAPK signaling was observed to increase expression of both $p21^{Cip-1/MDA6/WAF1}$ and another CKI protein, $p16^{INK4a}$, in primary hepatocytes. This suggests that MAPK can modify expression of different cassettes of CKI proteins in a cell-type specific manner, which may in turn exert cell type specific functions in mediating cell growth arrest.

However, it is notable that inhibition of PKC function in megakaryocytes promotes differentiation towards an erythroid lineage, suggesting that perturbations in PKC signaling, potentially via downstream recruitment of MAPK, can lead to a switch between specific differentiation pathways[76]. Similarly, other studies have suggested that increased or decreased MAPK signaling can influence T cell differentiation between either a CD4 or CD8 expressing cell lineage[77]. In other cell types, several groups have demonstrated that MAPK signaling can both promote and inhibit adipogenesis and myogenesis in pre-adipocytes and myoblasts, respectively, in a time and context dependent manner[78–81]. Thus in some established cell systems, *constitutive elevation* of MAPK activity can stimulate proliferation, whereas in others it triggers increased $p21^{Cip-1/MDA6/WAF1}$ levels, cell cycle arrest, and cellular maturation. In contrast, in other cell types, *prolonged inhibition* of the MAPK pathway may also promote maturation and lead to increased $p21^{Cip-1/MDA6/WAF1}$ expression. The linkage of MAPK signaling to regulation of $p21^{Cip-1/MDA6/WAF1}$ expression is potentially important from a therapeutic perspective. For example several studies have shown that p21 -/- cells or cells expressing p21 antisense have increased chemo- and radio-sensitivities[82–83], suggesting that the relative ability of a cell to express $p21^{Cip-1/MDA6/WAF1}$ will alter its responsiveness to a variety of cytotoxic cellular stresses. One implication from these studies is that a potential strategy to sensitize cells to ionizing radiation or chemotherapeutic agents may involve inhibition of the MAPK pathway. Other protective mechanisms may also exist. For example, recent studies suggest that MAPK may be involved in phosphorylation of Bcl-2 which, at least under certain conditions, may exert an anti-apoptotic effect[84]. Other groups have argued that protein levels of the anti-apoptotic protein Mcl-1 are regulated by MAPK signaling, potentially linking MAPK signaling to expression of an anti-apoptotic effector[85].

4. AN OVERVIEW OF THE ROLE OF THE JNK PATHWAY IN PROLIFERATION, DIFFERENTIATION AND APOPTOTIC SIGNALING

Since the JNK pathway was first examined as a pathway activated in response to cytotoxic insults, many of the initial studies on JNK signaling focused on the role of this pathway as either a pro-apoptotic or anti-apoptotic effector. For example, Verheij *et al.*[86] demonstrated that exposure of U937 leukemic cells to either TNFα, FAS-ligand, ceramide or γ-radiation activated the JNK pathway and that this activation was causal in an enhanced apoptotic response to these stress signals. Multiple other studies over the past 10 years, using a large variety of cytotoxic stresses, have made similar conclusions; that JNK activation is a causal effector in pro-apoptotic signaling. These conclusions were strongly supported by molecular inhibition of the JNK pathway at multiple levels by expressing dominant negative versions of MKK4/7, JNK1/2 and c-Jun[87].

However, the multiple mechanisms by which prolonged JNK signaling can cause apoptosis in response to many stimuli are still not fully elucidated. One mechanism may be by the induction of death receptors and/or their ligands, such as the APO-1/CD95/FAS-Receptor and FAS-ligand[88]. Alternatively, JNK has been proposed to phosphorylate anti-apoptotic mitochondrial proteins, e.g., Bcl-xl, causing inactivation of Bcl-xl anti-apoptotic function, thereby also promoting apoptosis[89]. Other studies have shown that while JNK signaling may play a role in apoptosis, it does not necessarily play an *initiating* role. For example, some studies have suggested that while cytotoxic drugs can activate apoptotic caspase proteases, a profound apoptotic response after drug exposure requires an additional proteolytic cleavage of MEKK enzymes followed by JNK activation[90]. In contrast, Herr *et al.*[91] demonstrated that apoptotic caspase activation did not correlate with JNK activation in cells treated with doxorubicin. In MCF-7 mammary carcinoma cells, exposure to TNFα caused JNK activation in both TNFα-sensitive and -insensitive cell lines, but only caused apoptosis in the sensitive cell line variant[92]. In part, this effect may be because the resistant cell line had a lower activation of JNK, further suggesting that the time and amplitude of pathway activation plays a key role in the cellular response to any pathway. Behrens *et al.*[93], using primary fibroblasts from transgenic mice expressing a c-Jun mutant mutated at the NH_2-terminal phosphorylation sites, found that loss of these sites impaired both proliferative and apoptotic responses of these cells. In an analogous manner to our comments surrounding MAPK signaling, these findings have shed doubt upon the concept that JNK signaling is obligatorily required for apoptosis.

Several groups have demonstrated that JNK signaling can represent an important pro-proliferative or differentiation signal in a variety of cells. As noted above a mutant c-Jun, which could no longer be phosphorylated by JNK, impaired fibroblast growth. In A549 cells loss of JNK function abolished EGF-stimulation of growth[94]; similar data have been obtained in primary hepatocytes stimulated with TNFα or hepatocyte growth factor[95]. In contrast, JNK signaling also has been linked to a differentiation response in other cells such as pre-erythrocytes and pre-T helper cells[96,97]. Thus it has been proposed that JNK signaling may either cause growth/differentiation or death in a contextual manner. For example, a short burst of high JNK activity or low sustained JNK activity may cause a growth/differentiation response whereas high sustained JNK activity, potentially after cleavage of upstream activators such as MEKK, may lead to an apoptotic response.

5. POTENTIAL DIRECT ROLES FOR MAPK AND JNK SIGNALING IN THE CONTROL OF THE CELL CYCLE AND DNA REPAIR FOLLOWING IRRADIATION AND DRUG EXPOSURE

Evidence is now emerging that the MAPK pathway can play both positive and negative roles in cell survival after treatment with various chemotherapeutic drugs and/or ionizing radiation[98–101]. More recently, other studies using cytotoxic drugs have also surprisingly suggested that enhanced JNK signaling can enhance cell survival by increasing DNA repair.

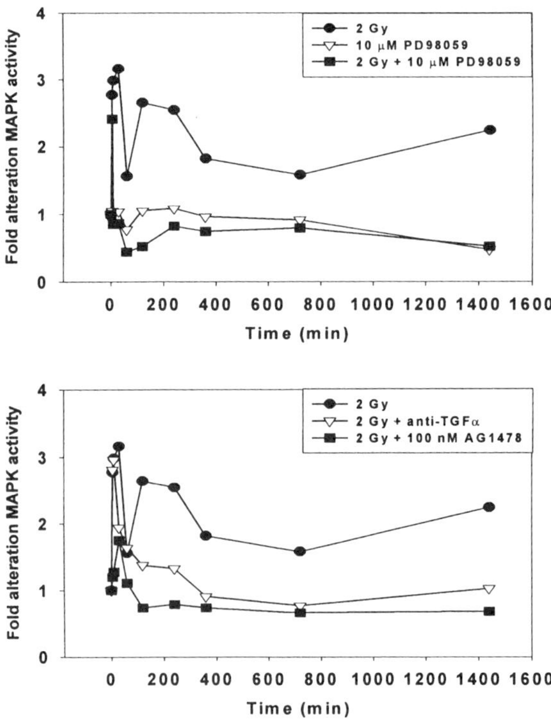

Figure 3. Ionizing radiation activates MAPK in DU145 prostate carcinoma cells via the EGFR and TGFα.

6. MAPK SIGNALING

Several studies have suggested both a radio-protective and a radio-sensitizing role for MAPK signaling. In both instances, the differential effects appear to be due to altered cell cycle progression following radiation exposure. Radiation can increase MAPK activity in a variety of cell types by causing activation of growth factor receptors in the plasma membrane[102]. One component of this activation may be operating through the actions of autocrine growth factors such as TGFα[103] (Figure 3). This may be important because tumor cells tend to express more receptors and more autocrine ligand than non-transformed cells, thus leading to higher activities and activation of protective signal transduction pathway(s) such as MAPK[104].

Previous studies have shown that activation of PKC by either phorbol esters or bryostatin 1 shortly before or after irradiation exerts cytoprotective effects toward normal human hematopoietic progenitor cells *in vitro* and in intact animals *in vivo*[105]. However, down-regulation of PKC expression by a 24 h pre-treatment with bryostatin 1 was found to sensitize cells to ionizing radiation[106]. Downstream inhibition of the MAPK pathway by the selective MEK1/2 inhibitor PD98059 also increases the radiosensitivity of cells and causes a prolonged G_2/M arrest[103,107]. Cells which are arrested in G_2/M then undergo apoptosis, and the remaining non-apoptotic cells display a loss of clonogenicity in clonogenic assays[103,107,108], in general agreement with the capacity of PKC down-regulation to exert a similar effect[106]. Thus, interruption of PKC signaling, or one of its downstream targets such as the MAPK pathway, can lower the apoptotic threshold of cells in response to ionizing radiation and certain chemotherapeutic agents.

Increased expression of Raf-1 has been shown to both radio-sensitize[109] and to enhance radio-resistance[110]. The radio-sensitizing effect of enhanced Raf-1 expression was correlated with a more rapid exit from radiation-induced G_2/M arrest and an enhanced G_1/S arrest. Other studies, however, have argued that enforced over-expression of Raf-1 is radio-protective and that ablation of Raf-1 expression by use of antisense oligonucleotides radio-sensitizes these cells[111]. In both instances it should be noted that enhanced Raf-1 protein levels may not cause a large increase in basal MAPK activity, but could enhance radiation-induced stimulation of the MAPK pathway. If enhanced Raf-1 protein levels do increase MAPK signaling, it is possible that expression of CKI molecules such as $p21^{Cip-1/WAF1/mda6}$ and $p16^{INK4a}$ may be induced, leading to a prolongation of growth arrest at both G_1/S and potentially at G_2/M phases[74,75]. Depending upon the cell type and the extent of CKI induction, it may be possible to observe these effects only at the G_1/S transition or at both G_1/S and G_2/M. This effect will in turn alter the cell cycle profile after irradiation.

In general agreement with a role for MAPK signaling in enhancing G_2/M progression, other groups have shown that inhibition of MAPK signaling can prolong radiation-induced G_2/M arrest and increase radio-sensitivity[103,107,108]. The role of the MAPK pathway in cell cycle progression at the G_2/M transition has been found to be complex, and it appears that MAPK signaling is both permissive for G_2/M entry and G_2/M exit[112,113]. These observations suggest that a certain amount of radiation-induced MAPK activity may enhance progression through G_2/M phase, increasing radio-sensitivity. In agreement with this notion, either enhanced Raf-1 expression or pre-treatment of cells with caffeine can reduce radiation-induced G_2/M arrest and radiosensitize cells. However, in studies by Abbott and Holt[107], and by Park *et al.*[108], addition of caffeine several hours after exposure abolished the prolonged portion of the G_2/M arrest caused by MAPK inhibition and was shown to be radio-protective. Thus it appears that either potentiation or inhibition of radiation-induced G_2/M arrest can decrease cell survival after exposure to ionizing radiation.

After exposure to ionizing radiation, cells arrest their growth so as to repair their DNA[114], and the time spent in growth arrest at G_2/M, DNA repair and radio-sensitivity have been correlated in several studies[115]. In the study by Abbott and Holt, no effect of MAPK inhibition was observed on DNA repair after radiation exposure[107]. However MAPK signaling has been linked to expression of at least one protein involved in nucleotide excision repair, ERCC1[116]. Under normal culture pO_2 conditions, loss of ERCC1 expression does not significantly alter radiosensitivity whereas under hypoxic conditions, loss of ERCC1 was recently found to reduce survival after irradiation[117,118] Thus MAPK signaling may be able to modify the DNA repair response of some cells under certain conditions.

Additional insights into the potential roles of MAPK in the regulation of drug-mediated lethality have arisen from studies involving the nucleoside analog ara-C. Ara-C is converted in cells to its active triphosphate derivative, ara-CTP, which is incorporated into elongating strands of DNA, resulting in interference with chain elongation and promotion of chain termination[119]. Exposure of cells to ara-C causes generation of lipid messengers that exert opposing effects on cell survival; ceramide and diglyceride. This raises the possibility that the relative extent to which these signaling molecules are generated determines the cell's ultimate fate. Furthermore, the cytoprotective effects of MAPK may exert a self-limiting effect on ara-C-mediated lethality. It would be predicted that interventions that reduce net MAPK activity would potentiate ara-C-related cytotoxicity. In agreement with this hypothesis, we and others have found that pharmacologic agents which directly inhibit PKC (e.g., staurosporine)[120], down-regulate PKC upon chronic exposure (e.g., bryostatin 1), or ablate PKC expression (e.g., PKC antisense oligonucleotides) have all been shown to enhance the lethal actions of ara-C[121–123]. Interestingly, in the latter study, ceramide exposure decreased whereas diglyceride exposure increased expression of the anti-apoptotic protein Bcl-2 in leukemic cells[123,124]. More recently, bryostatin 1 and the PKC inhibitor safingol have been shown to block ara-C-mediated MAPK activation in association with potentiation of leukemic cell apoptosis, effects which we have found to be mimicked by the MEK1 inhibitor PD98059[121,125,126]. Potentiation of ara-C-mediated lethality by inhibition of the MAPK pathway has also been observed in PC12 cells[127]. In contrast, others have shown that loss of MAPK function did not enhance ara-C cell killing[128]. Clearly, the ability of MAPK to protect cells from ara-C-induced DNA damage may be a cell-type dependent effect. Collectively, these findings raise the possibility that interruption of the PKC/MAPK pathway facilitates apoptosis, perhaps by preventing one or more cytoprotective responses.

Finally, attention has also been focused on alternate downstream MAPK cytoprotective effectors. These include the transcription factors NFκB[129] and CREB[130], which have recently been shown to protect cells from growth factor deprivation-induced apoptosis in cells of a neural origin. Whether these effectors contribute to the cytoprotective effects of the MAPK cascade in cells exposed to radiation or drugs remains to be determined.

7. JNK SIGNALING

As previously discussed, inhibition of PKC and/or MAPK function radiosensitizes fibroblast and epithelial cell types, and conversely, PKC activation has been shown to attenuate ionizing radiation-mediated lethality[131,132]. The lethal effects of ionizing radiation in some cell types, e.g., in peripheral lymphoblasts from individuals with Neimann-Pick disease, has been directly attributed to the cytotoxic actions of ceramide[133]. The ability of radiation to activate the JNK pathway has been investigated in leukemia cells and demonstrated to be dependent upon activation of sphingomyelinase enzymes[134]. These data suggest that sphingomyelinase enzymes, via the JNK pathway, play key roles in mediating radiation-induced cytotoxic signals.

However, based on studies using growth factors and non-lymphoid cell types, many other stimuli could play a role in JNK activation following irradiation. For example, in carcinoma cells radiation-induced signaling from TGFα and the EGFR, and the TNFα receptor, can play a role in JNK activation[103]. Of note, many ligands utilize signaling through the cytoprotective PI_3 kinase pathway to activate JNK, suggesting that JNK signaling under certain circumstances may be protective[53]. Other studies have argued that radiation-induced DNA damage may play a role in JNK activation by protein kinases such as ATM (mutated in ataxia telangiectasia) and c-Abl[135]. These observations raise the intriguing possibility that stress-induced JNK pathway activation may be under the control of multiple factors; receptor ligands; growth factor receptors; sphingomyelinase enzymes and ceramide; and DNA damage-activated protein kinases such as ATM and c-Abl.

Multiple studies have documented the cytotoxic effects of prolonged JNK signaling in a variety of cell types[93]. It is also clear that increased JNK signaling does not always correlate with increased apoptosis after exposure to a cytotoxic stress. For example, Reardon *et al.*[136] demonstrated that radiation-induced activation of JNK was not causal in the apoptotic response of MDA-MB-231 mammary carcinoma cells. This observation may be in part due to the fact that a parallel balanced activation of both JNK and MAPK signaling occurs in response to this stimulus.

It is also becoming evident that JNK signaling may play an important cytoprotective effector in the response of cells to DNA damage. For example, Potapova *et al.*[137] demonstrated that cells exposed to cisplatin were more sensitive to drug-induced apoptosis if their JNK signaling pathway was inhibited. In addition, in cells which were DNA repair deficient, Nehme *et al.*[138] showed that no activation of c-Abl or JNK took place, leading to a more cisplatin-sensitive phenotype. Exposure of cells to UV radiation causes DNA damage and several investigators have argued that JNK pathway signaling is involved in the repair of UV-damaged DNA. Engelberg *et al.*[139] and Schreiber *et al.*[140] have both shown data arguing that the AP-1 (c-Jun:c-Fos) transcription factor complex is an essential component in the protective response of cells exposed to UV radiation. Since c-Fos expression, which is under control of the transcription factor Elk-1, is dependent upon both MAPK and JNK signaling, it is likely that both JNK and MAPK signaling play roles in the protective response to UV radiation.

In the previous section examining MAPK signaling and DNA repair, it was proposed that MAPK regulates the ERCC1 promoter[116]. Other groups have shown that phorbol esters can increase ERCC1 promoter activity through an AP-1 responsive element, suggesting that signaling by the JNK pathway may also enhance ERCC1 expression[141,142]. Exposure of cells to nitrosoureas has been shown to induce cytotoxic DNA lesions by alkylation of guanine residues, and these lesions are repaired by O^6-methylguanine-DNA methyltransferase (MGMT) enzymes. The MGMT promoter contains two AP-1 binding sites and its activity increased after exposure to phorbol esters, suggesting a role for JNK/c-Jun signaling in this process[143]. Thus it is probable that both JNK and MAPK signaling will impact on c-Jun and c-Fos protein levels, respectively, and ultimately the function of the AP-1 complex leading to enhanced expression of multiple proteins involved in DNA repair processes.

CONCLUSION

From the previous sections it can be deduced that signaling by the MAPK and JNK pathways can control many of the responses of cells following exposure to toxic agents. Signaling by the MAPK pathway has been largely associated with cytoprotective responses whereas signaling by the JNK pathway has been associated with cytotoxic responses. However, although evidence in some cell systems indicates that JNK signaling can protect cells from death, in others it appears that JNK/AP-1 function is essential for the expression of certain DNA repair enzymes. Thus it seems likely that moderate levels of JNK activity may be required for protective responses of cells to DNA damage. In other systems, increased MAPK activity may enhance expression of cytotoxic ligands potentially leading to cell death, whereas in others it could enhance expression of anti-apoptotic proteins, leading to a protective response. The overall balance of protective and toxic signals generated by each pathway will ultimately depend upon the cell type examined and the culture conditions used. Currently, relatively little is known about the mechanism(s) by which signaling pathways control the expression and function of DNA repair genes. Further studies will thus be required to link enhanced signal transduction pathway function with enhanced DNA repair following exposure to DNA damaging agents.

ACKNOWLEDGMENTS

This work was funded; to PD from PHS grants as P.I. (R01DK52825) and Co-P.I. (P01CA72955) and (R01CA65896), and the Department of Defense (BC980148). To PBF from PHS grants (R01CA35675; R01CA74468) and the Chernow Endowment. To SG from PHS awards (P01-CA72955; R01-CA63753; R01-CA77141) and a Leukemia Society of America grant 6405-97.

REFERENCES

1. Sturgill, TW, Ray LB. Muscle proteins related to microtubule associated protein-2 are substrates for an insulin-stimulatable kinase. Biochem Biophys Res Commun, 134:565-571, 1986.
2. Boulton TG, Cobb MH. Identification of multiple extracellular signal-regulated kinases (ERKs) with antipeptide antibodies. Cell Regul, 2:357-371, 1991.
3. Sturgill TW, Ray LB, Erikson E, *et al.* Insulin-stimulated MAP-2 kinase phosphorylates and activates ribosomal protein S6 kinase II. Nature, 334:715-718, 1988.
4. Wu J, Michel H, Rossomando A, *et al.* Renaturation and partial peptide sequencing of mitogen-activated protein kinase (MAP kinase) activator from rabbit skeletal muscle. Biochem J, 285:701-705, 1992.
5. Haystead CM, Wu J, Gregory P, *et al.* Functional expression of a MAP kinase-kinase in COS cells and recognition by an anti-STE7/byr1 antibody. FEBS Lett, 317:12-16, 1993.
6. Robbins DJ, Zhen E, Owaki H, *et al.* Regulation and properties of extracellular signal-regulated protein kinases 1 and 2 in vitro. J Biol Chem, 268:5097-5106, 1993.
7. Wu J, Harrison JK, Dent P, *et al.* Identification and characterization of a new mammalian mitogen-activated protein kinase kinase, MKK2. Mol Cell Biol, 13:4539-4548, 1993.
8. Kyriakis JM, App H, Zhang XF, *et al.* Raf-1 activates MAP kinase-kinase. Nature, 358:417-421, 1992.
9. Dent P, Haser W, Haystead TA, *et al.* Activation of mitogen-activated protein kinase kinase by v-Raf in NIH 3T3 cells and in vitro. Science, 257:1404-1407, 1992.
10. Navas TA, Baldwin DT, Stewart TA. RIP2 is a Raf1-activated mitogen-activated protein kinase kinase. J Biol Chem, 274:33684-33690, 1999.
11. Morrison DK, Cutler RE. The complexity of Raf-1 regulation. Curr Opin Cell Biol, 9:174-179, 1997.
12. Chow YH, Pumiglia K, Jun TH, *et al.* Functional mapping of the N-terminal regulatory domain in the human Raf-1 protein kinase. J Biol Chem, 270:14100-14106, 1995.
13. Bosch E, Cherwinski H, Peterson D, McMahon M. Mutations of critical amino acids affect the biological and biochemical properties of oncogenic A-Raf and Raf-1. Oncogene, 15:1021-1033, 1997.
14. Marais R, Light Y, Paterson HF, *et al.* Differential regulation of Raf-1, A-Raf, and B-Raf by oncogenic ras and tyrosine kinases. J Biol Chem, 272:4378-4383, 1997.
15. Moodie SA, Willumsen BM, Weber MJ, Wolfman A. Complexes of Ras.GTP with Raf-1 and mitogen-activated protein kinase kinase. Science, 260:1658-1661, 1993.
16. Van Aelst L, Barr M, Marcus S, *et al.* Complex formation between RAS and RAF and other protein kinases. Proc Natl Acad Sci USA, 90:6213-6217, 1993.

17. Leevers SJ, Paterson HF, Marshall CJ. Requirement for Ras in Raf activation is overcome by targeting Raf to the plasma membrane. Nature, 369:411-414. 1994.
18. Stokoe D, Macdonald SG, Cadwallader K, *et al.* Activation of Raf as a result of recruitment to the plasma membrane. Science, 264:1463-1467, 1994.
19. Dent P, Sturgill TW. Activation of $(His)_6$-Raf-1 in vitro by partially purified plasma membranes from v-Ras-transformed and serum stimulated fibroblasts. Proc Natl Acad Sci USA, 91:9544-9548, 1994.
20. Mason CS, Springer CJ, Cooper RG, *et al.* Serine and tyrosine phosphorylations cooperate in Raf-1, but not B-Raf, activation. EMBO J, 18:2137-2148, 1999.
21. Stokoe D, McCormick F. Activation of c-Raf-1 by Ras and Src through different mechanisms: activation in vivo and in vitro. EMBO J, 16:2384-2396, 1997.
22. Tzivion G, Luo Z, Avruch J. A dimeric 14-3-3 protein is an essential cofactor for Raf kinase activity. Nature, 394:88-92, 1998.
23. Thorson JA, Yu LWK, Hsu AL, *et al.* 14-3-3 proteins are required for maintenance of Raf-1 phosphorylation and kinase activity. Mol Cell Biol, 18:5229-5238, 1998.
24. McPherson RA, Harding A, Roy S, *et al.* Interactions of c-Raf-1 with phosphatidylserine and 14-3-3. Oncogene, 18:3862-3869, 1999.
25. Sun H, King AJ, Diaz HB, Marshall MS. Regulation of the protein kinase Raf-1 by oncogenic Ras through phosphatidylinositol 3-kinase, Cdc42/Rac and Pak. Curr Biol, 10:281-284, 2000.
26. Zhang Y, Yao B, Delikat S, *et al.* Kinase suppressor of Ras is ceramide-activated protein kinase. Cell, 89:63-72, 1997.
27. Muller G, Storz P, Bourteele S, *et al.* Regulation of Raf-1 kinase by TNF via its second messenger ceramide and cross-talk with mitogenic signalling. EMBO J, 17:732-742, 1998.
28. Joneson T, Fulton JA, Volle DJ, *et al.* Kinase suppressor of Ras inhibits the activation of extracellular ligand-regulated (ERK) mitogen-activated protein (MAP) kinase by growth factors, activated Ras, and Ras effectors. J Biol Chem, 273:7743-7748, 1998.
29. Fabian JR, Daar IO, Morrison DK. Critical tyrosine residues regulate the enzymatic and biological activity of Raf-1 kinase. Mol Cell Biol, 13:7170-7179, 1993.
30. Dent P, Jelinek T, Morrison DK, *et al.* Reversal of Raf-1 activation by purified and membrane associated protein phosphatases. Science, 268:1902-1906, 1995.
31. Marais R, Light Y, Paterson HF, Marshall CJ. Ras recruits Raf-1 to the plasma membrane for activation by tyrosine phosphorylation. EMBO J, 14:3136-3145, 1995.
32. Schonwasser DC, Marais RM, Marshall CJ, Parker PJ. Activation of the mitogen-activated protein kinase/extracellular signal-regulated kinase pathway by conventional, novel, and atypical protein kinase C isotypes. Mol Cell Biol, 18:790-798, 1998.
33. Cai H, Smola U, Wixler V, *et al.* Role of diacylglycerol-regulated protein kinase C isotypes in growth factor activation of the Raf-1 protein kinase. Mol Cell Biol, 17:732-741, 1997.
34. Marais R, Light Y, Mason C, *et al.* Requirement of Ras-GTP-Raf complexes for activation of Raf-1 by protein kinase C. Science, 280:109-112, 1998.
35. Siddhanti SR, Hartle JE 2nd, Quarles LD. Forskolin inhibits protein kinase C-induced mitogen activated protein kinase activity in MC3T3-E1 osteoblasts. Endocrinology, 136:4834-4841, 1995.
36. Li N, Batzer A, Daly R, *et al.* Guanine-nucleotide-releasing factor hSos1 binds to Grb2 and links receptor tyrosine kinases to Ras signalling. Nature, 363:85-88, 1993.
37. Olivier JP, Raabe T, Henkemeyer M, *et al.* A Drosophila SH2-SH3 adaptor protein implicated in coupling the sevenless tyrosine kinase to an activator of Ras guanine nucleotide exchange, Sos. Cell, 73:179-191, 1993.

38. Yang SH, Whitmarsh AJ, Davis RJ, Sharrocks AD. Differential targeting of MAP kinases to the ETS-domain transcription factor Elk-1. EMBO J, 17:1740-1749, 1998.
39. Chung KC, Gomes I, Wang D, *et al.* Raf and fibroblast growth factor phosphorylate Elk1 and activate the serum response element of the immediate early gene pip92 by mitogen-activated protein kinase-independent as well as -dependent signaling pathways. Mol Cell Biol, 18:2272-2281, 1998.
40. Johnson CM, Hill CS, Chawla S, *et al.* Calcium controls gene expression via three distinct pathways that can function independently of the Ras/mitogen-activated protein kinases (ERKs) signaling cascade. J Neurosci, 17:6189-6202, 1997.
41. Whitmarsh AJ, Yang SH, Su MS, *et al.* Role of p38 and JNK mitogen-activated protein kinases in the activation of ternary complex factors. Mol Cell Biol, 17:2360-2371, 1997.
42. Cuenda A, Cohen P, Buee-Scherrer V, Goedert M. Activation of stress-activated protein kinase-3 (SAPK3) by cytokines and cellular stresses is mediated via SAPKK3 (MKK6); comparison of the specificities of SAPK3 and SAPK2 (RK/p38). EMBO J, 16:295-305, 1997.
43. Price MA, Cruzalegui FH, Treisman R. The p38 and ERK MAP kinase pathways cooperate to activate ternary complex factors and c-fos transcription in response to UV light. EMBO J, 15:6552-6563, 1996.
44. Hibi M, Lin A, Smeal T, *et al.* Identification of an oncoprotein- and UV-responsive protein kinase that binds and potentiates the c-Jun activation domain. Genes Dev, 7:2135-2148, 1993.
45. Derijard B, Hibi M, Wu IH, *et al.* JNK1: a protein kinase stimulated by UV light and Ha-Ras that binds and phosphorylates the c-Jun activation domain. Cell, 76:1025-1037, 1994.
46. Davis RJ. Signal transduction by the c-Jun N-terminal kinase. Biochem Soc Symp, 64:1-12, 1999.
47. Yang SH, Whitmarsh AJ, Davis RJ, Sharrocks AD. Differential targeting of MAP kinases to the ETS-domain transcription factor Elk-1. EMBO J, 17:1740-1749, 1998.
48. Noguchi K, Kitanaka C, Yamana H, *et al.* Regulation of c-Myc through phosphorylation at Ser-62 and Ser-71 by c-Jun N-terminal kinase. J Biol Chem, 274:32580-32587, 1999.
49. Derijard B, Raingeaud J, Barrett T, *et al.* Independent human MAP-kinase signal transduction pathways defined by MEK and MKK isoforms. Science, 267:682-685, 1995.
50. Tournier C, Whitmarsh AJ, Cavanagh J, *et al.* The MKK7 gene encodes a group of c-Jun NH2-terminal kinase kinases. Mol Cell Biol, 19:1569-1581, 1999.
51. Schlesinger TK, Fanger GR, Yujiri T, Johnson GL. The TAO of MEKK. Front Biosci, 3:D1181-1186, 1998.
52. Yustein JT, Li D, Robinson D, Kung HJ. KFC, a Ste20-like kinase with mitogenic potential and capability to activate the SAPK/JNK pathway. Oncogene, 19:710-718, 2000.
53. Timokhina I, Kissel H, Stella G, Besmer P. Kit signaling through PI 3-kinase and Src kinase pathways: an essential role for Rac1 and JNK activation in mast cell proliferation. EMBO J, 17:6250-6262, 1998.
54. Assefa Z, Valius M, Vantus T, *et al.* JNK/SAPK activation by platelet-derived growth factor in A431 cells requires both the phospholipase C-gamma and the phosphatidylinositol 3-kinase signaling pathways of the receptor. Biochem Biophys Res Commun, 261:641-645, 1999.
55. Lu Y, Settleman J. The Drosophila Pkn protein kinase is a Rho/Rac effector target required for dorsal closure during embryogenesis. Genes Dev, 13:1168-1180, 1999.

56. Mansour SJ, Matten WT, Hermann AS, *et al.* Transformation of mammalian cells by constitutively active MAP kinase kinase. Science, 265:966-970, 1994.
57. Dlugosz AA, Hansen L, Cheng C, *et al.* Targeted disruption of the epidermal growth factor receptor impairs growth of squamous papillomas expressing the v-ras(Ha) oncogene but does not block in vitro keratinocyte responses to oncogenic Ras. Cancer Res, 57:3180-3188, 1997.
58. Cleveland JL, Troppmair J, Packham G, *et al.* v-raf suppresses apoptosis and promotes growth of interleukin-3-dependent myeloid cells. Oncogene, 9:2217-2226, 1994.
59. Mansour SJ, Candia JM, Gloor KK, Ahn NG. Constitutively active mitogen-activated protein kinase kinase 1 (MAPKK1) and MAPKK2 mediate similar transcriptional and morphological responses. Cell Growth Differ, 7:243-250, 1996.
60. Aktas H, Cai H, Cooper GM. Ras links growth factor signaling to the cell cycle machinery via regulation of cyclin D1 and the Cdk inhibitor p27KIP1. Mol Cell Biol, 17:3850-3857, 1997.
61. Cheng M, Sexl V, Sherr CJ, Roussel MF. Assembly of cyclin D-dependent kinase and titration of p27Kip1 regulated by mitogen activated protein kinase kinase (MEK1). Proc Natl Acad Sci USA, 95:1091-1096, 1998.
62. Okuda K, Sanghera JS, Pelech SL, *et al.* Granulocyte-macrophage colony-stimulating factor, interleukin-3, and steel factor induce rapid tyrosine phosphorylation of p42 and p44 MAP kinase. Blood, 79:2880-2887, 1992.
63. Towatari, M, Iida H, Tanimoto M, *et al.* Consititutive activation of mitogen activated protein kinase pathway in acute leukemia cells. Leukemia, 11:479-484, 1997.
64. Wood KW, Sarnecki C, Roberts TM, Blenis J. Ras mediates nerve growth factor receptor modulation of three signal-transducing protein kinases: MAP kinase, Raf-1, and RSK. Cell, 68:1041-1050, 1992.
65. Jaiswal RK, Weissinger E, Kolch W, Landreth GE. Nerve growth factor-mediated activation of the mitogen-activated protein (MAP) kinase cascade involves a signaling complex containing B-Raf and HSP90. J Biol Chem, 271:23626-23629, 1996.
66. Traverse S, Gomez N, Paterson H, *et al.* Sustained activation of the mitogen-activated protein (MAP) kinase cascade may be required for differentiation of PC12 cells. Comparison of the effects of nerve growth factor and epidermal growth factor. Biochem J, 288:351-355, 1992.
67. Cowley S, Paterson H, Kemp P, Marshall CJ. Activation of MAP kinase kinase is necessary and sufficient for PC12 differentiation and for transformation of NIH 3T3 cells. Cell, 77:841-852, 1994.
68. Pumiglia KM, Decker SJ. Cell cycle arrest mediated by the MEK/mitogen-activated protein kinase pathway. Proc Natl Acad Sci USA, 94:448-452, 1997.
69. Decker SJ. Nerve growth factor-induced growth arrest and induction of p21Cip1/WAF1 in NIH-3T3 cells expressing TrkA. J Biol Chem, 270:30841-30844, 1995.
70. Whalen AM, Galasinski SC, Shapiro PS, *et al.* Megakaryocytic differentiation induced by constitutive activation of mitogen-activated protein kinase kinase. Mol Cell Biol, 17:1947-1958, 1997.
71. Kharbanda S, Saleem A, Emoto Y, *et al.* Activation of Raf-1 and mitogen-activated protein kinases during monocytic differentiation of human myeloid leukemia cells. J Biol Chem, 269:872-878, 1994.
72. Woods D, Parry D, Cherwinski H, *et al.* Raf-induced proliferation or cell cycle arrest is determined by the level of Raf activity with arrest mediated by p21Cip1. Mol Cell Biol, 17:5598-5611, 1997.
73. Sewing A, Wiseman B, Lloyd AC, Land H. High-intensity Raf signal causes cell cycle arrest mediated by p21Cip1. Mol Cell Biol, 17:5588-5597, 1997.

74. Tombes R, Auer KL, Brenz-Verca S, *et al.* The Mitogen-Activated Protein (MAP) kinase cascade can either stimulate or inhibit DNA synthesis in primary cultures of rat hepatocytes depending upon whether its activation is acute/phasic or chronic. Biochem J, 330:1451-1460, 1998.
75. Park JS, Boyer S, Mitchell K, *et al.* Expression of human papilloma virus E7 protein causes apoptosis and inhibits DNA synthesis in primary hepatocytes via increased expression of p21(Cip-1/WAF1/MDA6). J Biol Chem, 275:18-28, 2000.
76. Hong Y, Martin JF, Vainchenker W, Erusalimsky JD. Inhibition of protein kinase C suppresses megakaryocytic differentiation and stimulates erythroid differentiation in HEL cells. Blood, 87:123-131, 1996.
77. Sharp LL, Schwarz DA, Bott CM, *et al.* The influence of the MAPK pathway on T cell lineage commitment. Immunity, 7:609-618, 1997.
78. Hu E, Kim JB, Sarraf P, Spiegelman BM. Inhibition of adipogenesis through MAP kinase-mediated phosphorylation of PPARgamma. Science, 274:2100-2103, 1996.
79. Lacasa D, Garcia E, Agli B, Giudicelli Y. Control of rat preadipocyte adipose conversion by ovarian status: regional specificity and possible involvement of the mitogen-activated protein kinase-dependent and c-fos signaling pathways. Endocrinology, 138:2729-2734, 1997.
80. Ramocki MB, Johnson SE, White MA, *et al.* Signaling through mitogen-activated protein kinase and Rac/Rho does not duplicate the effects of activated Ras on skeletal myogenesis. Mol Cell Biol, 17:3547-3555, 1997.
81. Bennett AM, Tonks NK. Regulation of distinct stages of skeletal muscle differentiation by mitogen-activated protein kinases. Science, 278:1288-1291, 1997.
82. Barboule N, Chadebech P, Baldinm V, *et al.* Involvement of p21 in mitotic exit after paclitaxel treatment in MCF-7 breast adenocarcinoma cell line. Oncogene, 15:2867-2875, 1997.
83. Deng C, Zhang P, Harper JW, *et al.* Mice lacking p21 Cip-1/WAF-1 undergo normal development, but are defective in G1 checkpoint control. Cell, 82:675-684, 1995.
84. Deng X, Ruvolo P, Carr B, *et al.* Survival function of ERK1/2 as IL-3-activated, staurosporine-resistant Bcl2 kinases. Proc Natl Acad Sci USA, 97:1578-1583, 2000.
85. Leu CM, Chang C, Hu C. Epidermal growth factor (EGF) suppresses staurosporine-induced apoptosis by inducing mcl-1 via the mitogen-activated protein kinase pathway. Oncogene, 19:1665-1675, 2000.
86. Verheij M, Bose. R, Lin X.H, *et al.* Requirement for ceramide-initiated SAPK/JNK signalling in stress-induced apoptosis. Nature, 380:75-79, 1996.
87. Leppa S, Bohmann D. Diverse functions of JNK signaling and c-Jun in stress response and apoptosis. Oncogene, 18:6158-6162, 1999.
88. Zhang J, Gao JX, Salojin K, *et al.* Regulation of fas ligand expression during activation-induced cell death in T cells by p38 mitogen-activated protein kinase and c-Jun NH2-terminal kinase. J Exp Med, 191:1017-1030, 2000.
89. Kharbanda S, Saxena S, Yoshida K, *et al.* Translocation of SAPK/JNK to mitochondria and interaction with Bcl-x(L) in response to DNA damage. J Biol Chem, 275:322-327, 2000.
90. Gebauer G, Mirakhur B, Nguyen Q, *et al.* Cisplatin-resistance involves the defective processing of MEKK1 in human ovarian adenocarcinoma 2008/C13 cells. Int J Oncol, 16:321-325, 2000.
91. Herr I, Wilhelm D, Bohler T, *et al.* JNK/SAPK activity is not sufficient for anticancer therapy-induced apoptosis involving CD95-L, TRAIL and TNF-alpha. Int J Cancer, 80:417-424, 1999.

92. Doman RK, Perez M, Donato NJ. JNK and p53 stress signaling cascades are altered in MCF-7 cells resistant to tumor necrosis factor-mediated apoptosis. J Interferon Cytokine Res, 19:261-269, 1999.
93. Behrens A, Sibilia M, Wagner EF. Amino-terminal phosphorylation of c-Jun regulates stress-induced apoptosis and cellular proliferation. Nat Genet, 21:326-329, 1999.
94. Bost F, McKay R, Bost M, *et al.* The Jun kinase 2 isoform is preferentially required for epidermal growth factor-induced transformation of human A549 lung carcinoma cells. Mol Cell Biol, 19:1938-1949, 1999.
95. Auer KL, Contessa J, Brenz-Verca S, *et al.* The Ras/Rac1/Cdc42/SEK/JNK/c-Jun cascade is a key pathway by which agonists stimulate DNA synthesis in primary cultures of rat hepatocytes. Mol Biol Cell, 9:561-573, 1998.
96. Nagata Y, Takahashi N, Davis RJ, *et al.* Activation of p38 MAP kinase and JNK but not ERK is required for erythropoietin-induced erythroid differentiation. Blood, 92:1859-1869, 1998.
97. Yang DD, Conze D, Whitmarsh AJ, *et al.* Differentiation of CD4+ T cells to Th1 cells requires MAP kinase JNK2. Immunity, 9:575-585, 1998.
98. Xia Z, Dickens M, Raingeaud J, Davis RJ, Greenberg ME. Opposing effects of ERK and JNK-p38 MAP kinases on apoptosis. Science, 270:1326-1331, 1995.
99. Lotem J, Sachs L. Control of apoptosis in hematopoiesis and leukemia by cytokines, tumor suppressor and oncogenes. Leukemia, 10:925-931, 1996.
100. Chmura SJ, Nodzenski E, Weichselbaum RR, *et al.* Protein kinase C inhibition induces apoptosis and ceramide production through activation of a neutral sphingomyelinase. Cancer Res, 56:2711-2714, 1996.
101. Vrana J, Grant S, Dent P. Inhibition of the MAPK pathway abrogates Bcl-2 -mediated leukemic cell survival after exposure of HL60 cells to ionizing radiation. Radiat Res, 151:559-569, 1999.
102. Balaban N, Moni J, Shannon M, *et al.* The effect of ionizing radiation on signal transduction: antibodies to EGF receptor sensitize A431 cells to radiation. Biochim Biophys Acta, 1314:147-156, 1996.
103. Dent P, Reardon DB, Park JS, *et al.* Radiation-induced release of transforming growth factor alpha activates the epidermal growth factor receptor and mitogen-activated protein kinase pathway in carcinoma cells, leading to increased proliferation and protection from radiation-induced cell death. Mol Biol Cell, 10:2493-2506, 1999.
104. Sebolt-Leopold JS, Dudley DT, Herrera R, *et al.* Blockade of the MAP kinase pathway suppresses growth of colon tumors in vivo. Nature Med, 5:810-816, 1999.
105. Grant S, Traylor R, Pettit GR, Lin PS. The macrocyclic lactone protein kinase C activator, bryostatin 1, either alone, or in conjunction with recombinant murine granulocyte-macrophage colony-stimulating factor, protects Balb/c and C3H/HeN mice from the lethal in vivo effects of ionizing radiation. Blood, 83:663-667, 1994.
106. Watson, NC, Jarvis WD, Orr MS, *et al.* Radiosensitization of HL-60 human leukemia cells by bryostatin-1 in the absence of increased DNA fragmentation or apoptotic cell death. Int J Radiat Biol, 69:183-192, 1996.
107. Abbott DW, Holt JT. Mitogen-activated protein kinase kinase 2 activation is essential for progression through the G2/M checkpoint arrest in cells exposed to ionizing radiation. J Biol Chem, 274:2732-2742, 1999.
108. Park JS, Carter S, Reardon DB, *et al.* Roles for basal and stimulated p21(Cip-1/WAF1/MDA6) expression and mitogen-activated protein kinase signaling in radiation-induced cell cycle checkpoint control in carcinoma cells. Mol Biol Cell, 10:4231-4246, 1996.

109. Warenius HM, Jones MD, Thompson CC. Exit from G2 phase after 2 Gy gamma irradiation is faster in radiosensitive human cells with high expression of the RAF1 proto-oncogene. Radiat Res, 146:485-493, 1996.
110. Kasid U, Pfeifer A, Brennan T, *et al.* Effect of antisense c-raf-1 on tumorigenicity and radiation sensitivity of a human squamous carcinoma. Science, 243:1354-1356, 1989.
111. Gokhale PC, McRae D, Monia BP, *et al.* Antisense raf oligodeoxyribonucleotide is a radiosensitizer in vivo. Antisense Nucleic Acid Drug Dev, 9:191-201, 1999.
112. Tamemoto H, Kadowaki T, Tobe K, *et al.* Biphasic activation of two mitogen-activated protein kinases during the cell cycle in mammalian cells. J Biol Chem, 267:20293-20297, 1992.
113. Wright JH, Munar E, Jameson DR, *et al.* Mitogen-activated protein kinase kinase activity is required for the G(2)/M transition of the cell cycle in mammalian fibroblasts. Proc Natl Acad Sci USA, 96:11335-11340, 1999.
114. O'Connor PM, Fan S. DNA damage checkpoints: implications for cancer therapy. Prog Cell Cycle Res, 2:165-173, 1996.
115. Zhou BB, Chaturvedi P, Spring K, *et al.* Caffeine abolishes the mammalian G(2)/M DNA damage checkpoint by inhibiting ataxia-telangiectasia-mutated kinase activity. J Biol Chem, 275:10342-10348, 2000.
116. Lee-Kwon W, Park D, Bernier M. Involvement of the Ras/extracellular signal-regulated kinase signalling pathway in the regulation of ERCC-1 mRNA levels by insulin. Biochem J, 331:591-597, 1998.
117. Murray D, Macann A, Hanson J, Rosenberg E. ERCC1/ERCC4 5'-endonuclease activity as a determinant of hypoxic cell radiosensitivity. Int J Radiat Biol, 69:319-327, 1996.
118. Murray D, Rosenberg E. The importance of the ERCC1/ERCC4[XPF] complex for hypoxic-cell radioresistance does not appear to derive from its participation in the nucleotide excision repair pathway. Mutat Res, 364:217-226, 1996.
119. Mikita T, Beardsley GP. Functional consequences of the arabinosylcytosine structural lesion in DNA. Biochem, 27:4698-4705, 1998.
120. Grant S, Turner AJ, Bartimole TM, *et al.* Modulation of 1-[beta-D arabinofuranosyl] cytosine-induced apoptosis in human myeloid leukemia cells by staurosporine and other pharmacological inhibitors of protein kinase C. Oncol Res, 6:87-99, 1994.
121. Jarvis WD, Fornari FA, Auer KL, *et al.* Differential involvement of stress-activated protein kinases in the apoptotic actions of ceramide and sphingosine. Mol Pharm, 52:935-947, 1997.
122. Grant S. Ara-C: cellular and molecular pharmacology. Adv Cancer Res, 72:197-233, 1998.
123. Whitman SP, Civoli F, Daniel LW. Protein kinase CbetaII activation by 1-beta-D-arabinofuranosylcytosine is antagonistic to stimulation of apoptosis and Bcl-2alpha down-regulation. J Biol Chem, 272:23481-23484, 1997
124. Strum JC, Small GW, Pauig SB, Daniel LW. 1-beta-D-Arabinofuranosylcytosine stimulates ceramide and diglyceride formation in HL-60 cells. J Biol Chem, 269:15493-15497, 1994.
125. Jarvis WD, Fornari FA, Traylor RS, *et al.* Induction of apoptosis and potentiation of ceramide-mediated cytotoxicity by sphingoid bases in human myeloid leukemia cells. J Biol Chem, 271:8275-8284, 1996.
126. Jarvis WD, Fornari FA, Tombes RM, *et al.* Evidence for involvement of MAPK, rather than SAPK, in potentiation of 1-beta-D-arabinofuranosylcytosine-induced apoptosis by interruption of PKC signaling. Mol Pharm, 54:844-856, 1998.

127. Anderson CNG, Tolkovsky AM. A role for MAPK/ERK in sympathetic neuron survival: protection against a p53-dependent, JNK-independent induction of apoptosis by cytosine arabinoside. J Neurosci, 19:664-673, 1999.
128. Stadheim TA, Saluta GR, Kucera GL. Role of c-Jun N-terminal kinase/p38 stress signaling in 1-beta-D-arabinofuranosylcytosine-induced apoptosis. Biochem Pharmacol, 59:407-418, 2000.
129. Troppmair J, Hartkamp J, Rapp UR. Activation of NF-kappa B by oncogenic Raf in HEK 293 cells occurs through autocrine recruitment of the stress kinase cascade. Oncogene, 17:685-690, 1998.
130. Bonni A, Brunet A, West AE, *et al.* Cell survival promoted by the Ras-MAPK signaling pathway by transcription-dependent and -independent mechanisms. Science, 286:1358-1362, 1999.
131. Fuks Z, Haimovitz-Friedman A, Kolesnick RN. The role of the sphingomyelin pathway and protein kinase C in radiation-induced cell kill. Important Adv Oncol, 10:19-31, 1995.
132. Haimovitz-Friedman A, Balaban N, McLoughlin M, *et al.* Protein kinase C mediates basic fibroblast growth factor protection of endothelial cells against radiation-induced apoptosis. Cancer Res, 54:2591-2597, 1994.
133. Haimovitz-Friedman A, Kan CC, Ehleiter D, *et al.* Ionizing radiation acts on cellular membranes to generate ceramide and initiate apoptosis. J Exp Med, 180:525-535, 1994.
134. Santana P, Pena LA, Haimovitz-Friedman A, *et al.* Acid sphingomyelinase-deficient human lymphoblasts and mice are defective in radiation-induced apoptosis. Cell, 86:189-199, 1996.
135. Kharbanda S, Yuan ZM, Weichselbaum R, Kufe D. Determination of cell fate by c-Abl activation in the response to DNA damage. Oncogene, 17:3309-3318, 1998.
136. Reardon DB, Contessa JN, Mikkelsen RB, *et al.* Dominant negative EGFR-CD533 and inhibition of MAPK modify JNK1 activation and enhance radiation toxicity of human mammary carcinoma cells. Oncogene, 18:4756-4766, 1999.
137. Potapova O, Haghighi A, Bost F, *et al.* The Jun kinase/stress-activated protein kinase pathway functions to regulate DNA repair and inhibition of the pathway sensitizes tumor cells to cisplatin. J Biol Chem, 272:14041-14044, 1997.
138. Nehme A, Baskaran R, Aebi S, *et al.* Differential induction of c-Jun NH2-terminal kinase and c-Abl kinase in DNA mismatch repair-proficient and -deficient cells exposed to cisplatin. Cancer Res, 57: 3253-3257, 1997.
139. Engelberg D, Klein C, Martinetto H, *et al.* The UV response involving the Ras signaling pathway and AP-1 transcription factors is conserved between yeast and mammals. Cell, 77:381-390, 1994.
140. Schreiber M, Baumann B, Cotten M, *et al.* Fos is an essential component of the mammalian UV response. EMBO J, 14:5338-5349, 1995.
141. Li Q, Zhang L, Tsang B, *et al.* Phorbol ester exposure activates an AP-1-mediated increase in ERCC-1 messenger RNA expression in human ovarian tumor cells. Cell Mol Life Sci, 55:456-466, 1999.
142. Li Q, Tsang B, Bostick-Bruton F, Reed E. Modulation of excision repair cross complementation group 1 (ERCC-1) mRNA expression by pharmacological agents in human ovarian carcinoma cells. Biochem Pharmacol, 57:347-353, 1999.
143. Boldogh I, Ramana CV, Chen Z, *et al.* Regulation of expression of the DNA repair gene O6-methylguanine-DNA methyltransferase via protein kinase C-mediated signaling. Cancer Res, 58:3950-3956, 1998.

Chapter 6

MECHANISMS OF REPAIR OF INTERSTRAND CROSSLINKS IN DNA

Randy J. Legerski and Christopher Richie
Department of Molecular Genetics, The University of Texas MD Anderson Cancer Center, Houston, Texas, USA

1. INTRODUCTION

The chemotherapeutic use of the early forms of DNA interstrand crosslinking agents, such as mustard gas and nitrogen mustard, predates the Second World War, making these agents among the oldest, and yet still most effective, anticancer drugs available in the clinic. The alkylation chemistry of these drugs was elucidated shortly after the War, and their cellular pharmacology was studied extensively during the 1970s and 1980s[1]. In contemporary chemotherapy treatment, interstrand crosslinking agents such as cyclophosphamide, melphalan, and cisplatin are among the most potent antitumor agents. Despite this lengthy history of clinical usage and pharmacologic investigation, the mechanisms of repair of the lesions produced in DNA by interstrand crosslinking agents have not been extensively studied. This relative neglect of investigation into the biochemical pathways of interstrand crosslink (ICL) repair is to be contrasted with the striking advances that have been accomplished in the past decade in other DNA damage processing pathways, such as nucleotide excision repair (NER), double-strand break (DSB) repair, and mismatch repair[2].

Resolving the mechanisms by which the lesions created by these drugs are repaired is an important adjunct to the overall understanding of the efficacy of these chemotherapeutic agents. An additional important aspect is to characterize the mechanisms by which recurrent tumors acquire resistance to these agents. There are any number of modes by which cells can acquire resistance to chemotherapeutic agents, including membrane alterations that reduce drug uptake, increased drug removal from the cell effected by multidrug resistance genes, increased metabolic degradation of the drug, loss of the apoptotic response, and enhanced repair of drug-induced lesions. In regard to the final possibility, a number of studies have demonstrated increased DNA repair capability in cell lines resistant to cisplatin[3]. Similarly, an enhanced removal of ICLs was observed in lymphocytes from patients with melphalan-resistant chronic lymphocytic leukemia[4] and in a melphalan-resistant human breast cancer cell line[5].

2. REPAIR OF ICLs IN *E. COLI*

Current evidence indicates that the error-free repair of both ICLs and DSBs involves a recombinational mechanism in which an undamaged donor chromosome provides a homologous copy for the repair of the damaged template. Both of these lesions are highly deleterious, and it has been shown in certain yeast genetic backgrounds, in which particular DNA repair pathways have been abolished, that a single occurrence of either lesion in the genome has proven to be lethal[6,7]. The most extensive studies of ICL repair have been carried out in *E. coli*. Cole and his coworkers[8,9] were the first to show that the repair of ICL damage in *E. coli* depends upon the products of the *uvrA*, *uvrB*, *uvrC*, *uvrD*, *recA*, and *polA* genes. The products of the *uvrA*, *B*, and *C* genes comprise the (A)BC exinuclease, which is a component of the NER pathway, and which initiates damage recognition and incision at sites of lesions. These findings indicated that components of both the NER and recombination pathways of *E. coli* were required for ICL repair. Cole[8] was unable to find evidence for a double-strand break intermediate, and therefore proposed a model for the removal of ICLs in *E. coli* (Figure 1) in which repair is initiated by dual incisions in one strand on either side of the ICL. The resulting gap is then repaired by a *recA*-mediated recombination process using a donor template. The remaining monoadduct is repaired by a second round of incision by the NER apparatus, and the resulting gap is filled in by the product of the *polA* gene (DNA polymerase I). Elements of this model, as well as additional insights into this pathway, have been elucidated by subsequent investigators. Sancar, Hearst, and their colleagues[10] used photoactivated psoralen as a model crosslinking agent and showed that the uvr (A)BC exinuclease initially cleaved only at the furan side of a psoralen ICL, and that the sites of the double incision differed from those previously determined for a cyclobutane pyrimidine dimer (CPD). CPDs evoke a dual incision by the (A)BC exinuclease seven nucleotides 5' and four or five nucleotides 3' to the lesion; however, psoralen ICLs were incised nine nucleotides 5' and three nucleotides 3' on the furan side of the lesion. In a further extension of this work, it was shown that the (A)BC exinuclease will cleave a triple-stranded crosslinked substrate on the pyrone side of the ICL[11]. This structure mimics the proposed repair intermediate that occurs after the recombination step as shown in Figure 1. This group also showed that a triple-stranded crosslinked substrate, formed in a plasmid by the invasion of a RecA-coated oligonucleotide, was also a substrate for cleavage on the pyrone side of the ICL by the (A)BC exinuclease[12]. Sladek *et al.*[13] showed that a substrate with dual incisions on either side of the ICL did not stimulate strand exchange by RecA. However, if the nick is processed into a gap, RecA-mediated strand exchange is stimulated, suggesting that an exonucleolytic step is required prior to recombination. This group postulated that the 5'-3' exonuclease activity of DNA polymerase I might extend the gap *in vivo* since it has been shown to be required for repair of ICLs. Taken together, these findings strongly support a recombinational mode of ICL repair, which is consistent with Cole's model; however, an *in vitro* reconstitution of this pathway has not yet been reported.

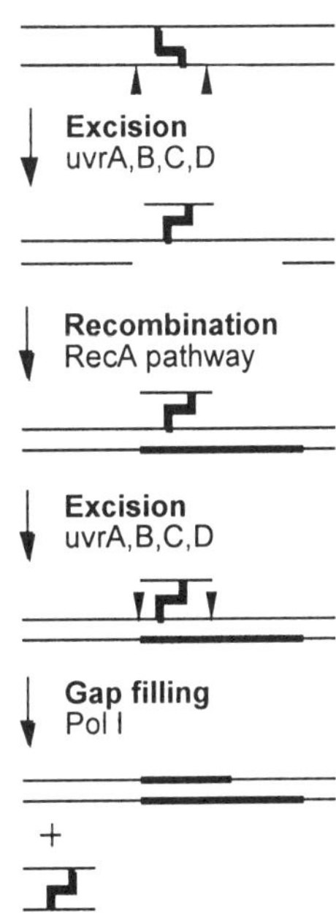

Figure 1. The Cole model of the recombination-dependent repair of ICLs in *E. coli.*

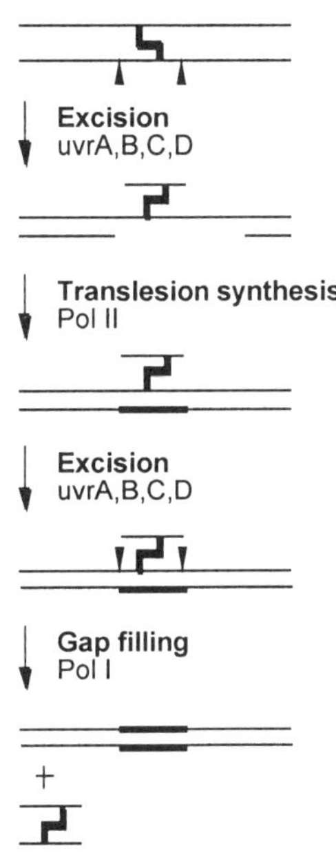

Figure 2. The Loechler model of the recombination-independent repair of ICLs in *E. coli.*

More recently, Loechler and his colleagues[14,15] have defined a pathway of ICL repair in *E. coli* that is recombination independent. Like the mechanism described by Cole and colleagues[8,9], this pathway also requires the incision components of NER, and in addition the product of the *polB* gene, DNA polymerase II. The lack of a requirement for recombination elements, and the involvement of DNA polymerase II, suggested a model (Figure 2) in which the NER components initiate repair by dual incisions on either side of the ICL, and the resulting gap is repaired by translesion synthesis as opposed to recombination. It is highly probable that the translesion synthesis pathway is more error-prone than the recombination pathway, and is, therefore, likely to be a minor pathway of ICL removal. Indeed, survival of *E. coli* cells exposed to nitrogen mustard indicate that *polB* mutants are only moderately more sensitive than wild type cells, whereas, *recA* or *uvrA* mutants are extremely sensitive[15].

3. RECOMBINATION IN EUCARYOTES

The genetics of recombinational repair in the yeast *S. cerevisiae* have been extensively studied. There are three major DNA repair epistasis groups in yeast which are termed *RAD3*, *RAD6*, and *RAD52* which represent distinct pathways of lesion processing. The *RAD3* and *RAD6* epistasis groups primarily mediate repair by the NER and postreplication repair pathways, respectively, while the *RAD52* epistasis group represents recombinational repair pathways. Many of the members of the *RAD52* group are also required for both mitotic and meiotic recombination. Similar to the situation in *E. coli*, the biochemistry of recombinational repair in yeast is not as advanced as for the NER pathway, but recent findings indicate that rapid progress can be expected. The underlying recombinational nature of the repair process performed by the *RAD52* group is indicated by the observation that haploid G_2 cells and diploid G_1 cells, where a second homolog is present, are highly resistant to ionizing radiation (IR) compared to haploid G_1 cells[16].

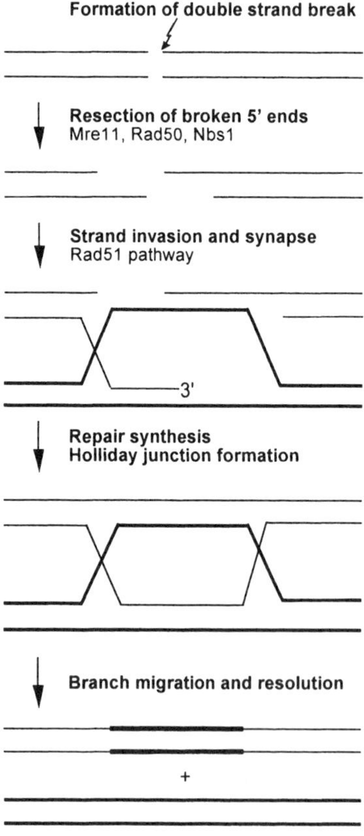

Figure 3. The eukaryotic mechanism for double-strand break repair by homologous recombination (HR) requires collaboration between the Rad50 complex and the Rad51 pathway.

There are essentially four distinct pathways of recombinational repair that have been identified in eucaryotic cells largely as a result of studies conducted in yeast on the repair of DSBs in DNA[17]. These include homologous recombination (HR), non-homologous end joining (NHEJ), single-strand annealing (SSA), and break-induced replication (BIR). Both HR and BIR require a donor template containing regions of DNA sequence that are highly homologous with the damaged chromosome. These segments of homology allow the initiation of a strand transfer reaction from the broken chromosome into the undamaged chromosome.

In the case of HR this initial strand invasion, often referred to as D-loop formation, is converted into a Holliday junction which can extensively branch migrate through regions of homology (Figure 3); in contrast, BIR requires no further homology because the resulting D-loop is extended by DNA synthesis (Figure 4). SSA is utilized to repair DSBs by extensive resection of the ends which produces long single-stranded tails, which allows regions of homology on either side of the break to anneal, creating a restored chromosome with an intervening deletion (Figure 5). In contrast to the other three pathways, which require significant homology, NHEJ catalyzes the direct rejoining of broken ends in a process that requires as little as one base pair of homology (Figure 6).

4. MEDIATORS OF RECOMBINATION

Early studies indicated that mutational inactivation of the *RAD51* gene results in defects in both meiotic and mitotic recombination as well as increased sensitivity to both IR and crosslinking agents[18,19]. Cloning of the *RAD51* gene showed that the encoded protein had significant homology to the RecA protein of *E. coli*[20–22]. This homology is contained in the middle portion of the two proteins encompassing approximately 220 amino acids which share an identity of about 30%. Like RecA, in the presence of ATP, Rad51 forms a helical filament with both single-stranded and double-stranded DNA[23,24]; however, only the filament with single-stranded DNA is functionally relevant[25]. It was also shown that formation of the filament on single-stranded DNA, and strand transfer reactions, are greatly stimulated by the single-strand binding protein, replication protein A (Rpa), when it is added subsequent to Rad51. Addition of Rpa simultaneously was found to be inhibitory. In addition to *RAD51*, two other members of the *RAD52* epistasis group, *RAD55* and *RAD57*, also have significant homology to *RecA*[26,27]. However, mutants of *RAD55* and *RAD57* are differentiated from *RAD51* mutants by the observation that their sensitivity to IR is only observed at low temperatures. In addition, over-expression of *RAD51* can suppress the phenotype of *RAD55* or *RAD57* mutants[28,29]. Recently, it has also been shown that the Rad55-Rad57 heterodimer overcomes the inhibitory effect of Rpa when it is added simultaneously with Rad51[30]. It has also been shown through the use of the two-hybrid system that Rad51 interacts with Rad52 and Rad55, and that Rad55 interacts with Rad57[28,29,31], suggesting the existence of a large recombination complex, or recombinasome, in yeast.

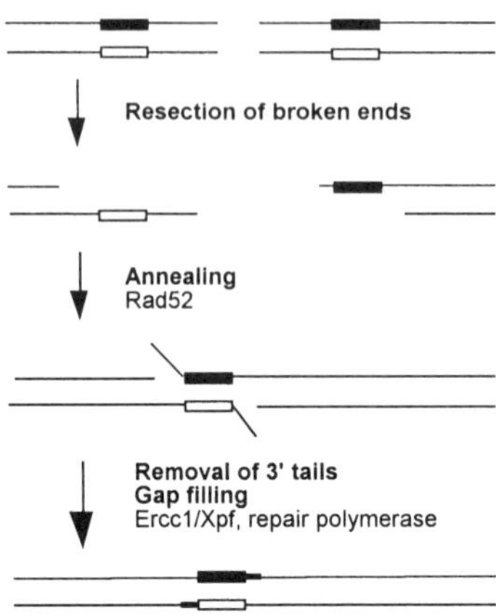

Figure 4. Break-induced replication (BIR) utilizes a Rad52-mediated mechanism to prime new DNA synthesis using a donor template.

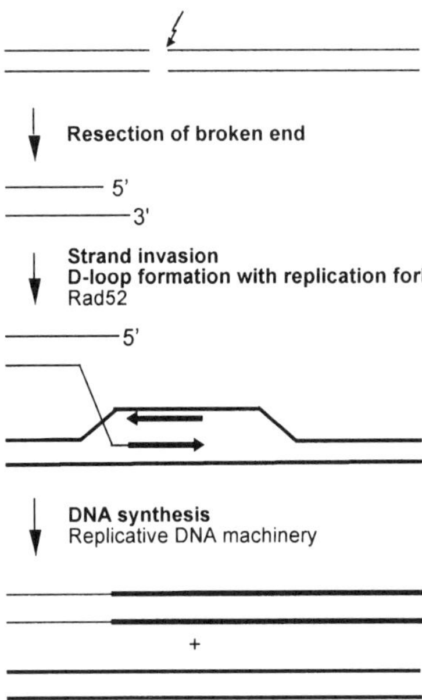

Figure 5. Single-strand annealing (SSA) uses a Rad52-mediated mechanism to join broken DNA ends via small regions of homology with deletion of intervening sequences.

Mammalian cells have been shown to contain at least six homologs of the *RAD51* family, which includes *RAD51*, *RAD51B*, *RAD51C*, *RAD51D*, *XRCC2*, and *XRCC3*. Like its yeast counterpart, mammalian Rad51 has also been shown to mediate strand transfer reactions in the presence of Rpa[32]. However, unlike its yeast counterpart, mammalian *RAD51* has been shown to be an essential gene in that its disruption by gene targeting techniques in the mouse has resulted in an embryonic lethal phenotype[33,34]. A similar lethal phenotype has also been obtained by disruption of the *RAD51B*[35], *RAD51D*[36], and *XRCC2*[37] genes in the mouse. Disruption of *RAD51* in chicken DT40 cells also resulted in lethality[38]; however, disruption of *RAD51B* in these cells resulted in viable cells that were mildly sensitive to IR, highly sensitive to mitomycin C (MMC) and cisplatin, and defective in generalized homologous recombinational repair[39]. Cellular localization studies of Rad51 have shown that this protein typically has a diffuse nuclear staining; however, upon entrance into S phase of the cell cycle, or after exposure to DNA damaging agents such as IR, it is partitioned into distinct nuclear foci or dots[40,41]. While the function or role of these foci is still not entirely clear, a likely possibility is that they represent DNA repair factories localized to sites of damage. In fact, it has been shown that these foci contain a large multifactorial complex of recombination proteins, which in addition to the Rad51 homologs[42], also include two proteins involved in hereditary breast cancer susceptibility, Brca1[43] and Brca2[44,45]. Interactions among the components of this complex have been identified by various methods, and an illustration of the currently described composition and structure of this complex is shown in Figure 7. This complex is clearly the primary mediator of the HR pathway in mammalian cells.

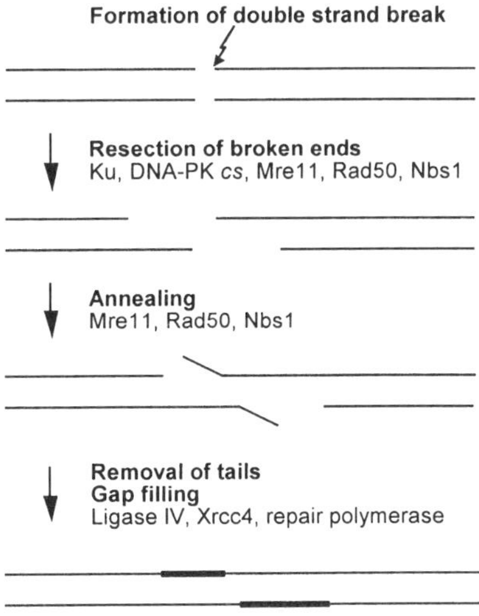

Figure 6. Nonhomologous end-joining (NHEJ) uses sequence microhomology to ligate two broken DNA ends in a Ku-dependent manner.

Yeast *RAD52* mutants are quite similar to *RAD51* mutants in their phenotype, having a general defect in both meiotic and mitotic recombination, and in DSB repair[46]. As indicated above the Rad52 protein interacts with Rad51[28,29], and it has been shown in yeast and mammals that Rad52 stimulates homologous pairing and strand exchange by Rad51. Yeast and mammalian Rad52 has been shown to form a heptameric ring structure that directly binds broken ends of DNA[47,48]. In yeast, Rad52 appears to be one of the most important recombination proteins since it is not only required for the HR pathway, but also for the SSA and BIR pathways of recombination. Rad51 is not required for either the SSA or BIR pathways. It was, thus, surprising that disruption of the mouse homolog of *RAD52* did not result in hypersensitivity to either IR or MMC, but only in a mild homologous recombination defect[49]. This finding suggests the possibility that there is a functional redundancy for the activity of Rad52 in mammalian cells. In fact, the yeast *RAD59* gene does share some homology with *RAD52*[50], and Rad59 has been shown, like Rad52, to be involved in both the HR and SSA recombination mechanisms, although, Rad59 cannot substitute for Rad52 in these pathways.

Yeast *RAD54* mutants have a severe defect in DSB repair; however, meiotic recombination is much less affected[51]. The *RAD54* gene encodes a protein that is a member of the SNF2 gene superfamily, members of which contain canonical ATPase and helicase domains, although helicase activity has not been demonstrated for any of these proteins *in vitro*[52]. At least some members of this family are involved in altering protein-DNA interactions in chromatin during cellular processes such as transcription and DNA repair. Rad54 protein possesses a double-stranded DNA-dependent ATPase activity, and has been shown to interact with Rad51, and to stimulate the rate of pairing between homologous single-stranded and double-stranded DNA[53].

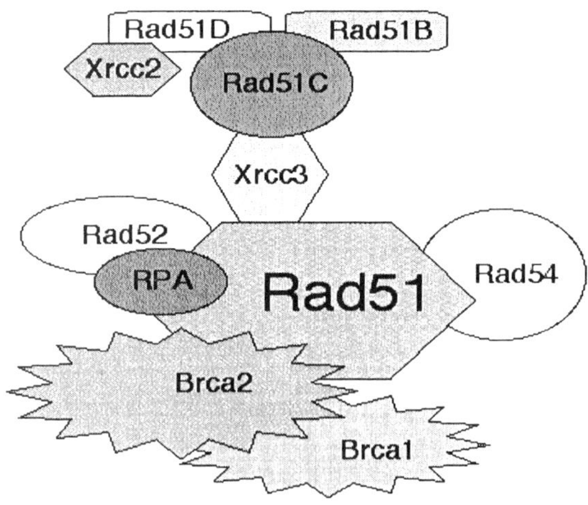

Figure 7. The Rad51 protein complex. Components of the Rad51 recombination complex that have been identified by two- and three-hybrid analyses and/or coimmunoprecipitation experiments are indicated.

Disruption of *RAD54* in the mouse has led to a viable phenotype with sensitivity to IR, MMC, and methylmethane sulfonate (MMS), and a deficiency in homologous recombination[54], indicating that as in yeast, mammalian *RAD54* plays a major role in recombinational repair.

RAD50 mutants of *S. cerevisiae* have been shown to be highly sensitive to IR and crosslinking agents, severely defective in meiotic recombination, but not in homologous integration of linearized plasmids[55,56]. The *RAD50* gene encodes a 153 kDa protein containing a nucleotide binding motif and a predicted coiled coil domain[57]. Rad50 forms a highly stable complex with the products of the *MRE11* and *XRS2* genes, and mutants in these latter genes have a similar phenotype to *RAD50* mutants[58]. This complex appears to play a role in a variety of processes of DNA metabolism including HR, NHEJ, telomere maintenance, and meiotic recombination. Genetic evidence indicates that the defect in HR is in a reduction in the cell's ability to resect the 5' strand at broken ends, which creates 3' single-stranded tails necessary for the initiation of the strand invasion step of HR[59]. Surprisingly, biochemical findings with purified proteins indicate that this complex actually possesses a 3'-5' exonuclease encompassed in the Mre11 protein, and not the expected 5'-3' activity[58]. It has been suggested that this complex could mediate 5' resection by clipping off a single-stranded 5' tail that had been created by the unwinding activity of a DNA helicase, although mutations in Mre11 that disrupt its nuclease activity are not deficient in HR[60].

Homologs of *RAD50*, and *MRE11*, have also been identified in mammalian cells, and a functional homolog of *XRS2* with little sequence similarity has been identified as defective in the Nijmegen breakage syndrome and has been termed *NBS1*[61,62]. It has also been found that *MRE11* is mutated in a human syndrome that is highly similar in phenotype to ataxia telangiectasia that is mutated in the *ATM* gene. The newly identified syndrome is referred to as the ataxia telangiectasia-like disorder (ATLD)[63]. However, disruption of either *MRE11* or *RAD50* in embryonic stem cells creating a homozygous null genotype results in a lethal phenotype indicating the essential nature of these genes[64,65]. The role of the Mre11/Rad50/Nbs1 complex in NHEJ has been better clarified in mammalian cells since this pathway plays a far greater role in the repair of DSBs due to IR than does the HR pathway. This relative importance of these pathways is opposite to that found in yeast where NHEJ appears to be a minor pathway. *In vitro*, Mre11 is able to resect broken ends in a 3'-5' direction, and in the presence of DNA ligase can directly rejoin these ends through regions of microhomology encompassing as little as one base pair[66]. This process is stimulated by Rad50, and the addition of Nbs1 adds new activities to the complex including partial unwinding of a DNA duplex, and efficient cleavage of fully paired hairpins[67]. The Mre11/Rad50/Nbs1 complex has been shown to form damage inducible foci in the nucleus which are distinct from those formed by the Rad51 complex[68], and which appear to migrate to sites of damage induced by IR[69]. Mre11 has also been found to interact with Ku70, a protein required for NHEJ, and in the absence of Ku70 the Mre11 damage inducible foci do not form suggesting that Ku70 may direct the Mre11 complex into the NHEJ pathway[70]. Regulation of the Mre11/Rad50/Nbs1 complex is also achieved by damage-induced phosphorylation. IR results in the phosphorylation of Nbs1 mediated by the ATM kinase[71], and in the phosphorylation of Mre11 in a process that requires Nbs1[72].

As indicated above, the products of the familial breast cancer genes *BRCA1* and *BRCA2* are also components of the mammalian Rad51 multifactorial complex. Brca2 has been shown to interact directly with both Rad51 and Brca1[43–45,73]. Inactivation of either Brca1 or Brca2 results in loss of damage-induced Rad51 foci formation, and Brca2 has been shown to have an essential function in suppressing gross chromosomal rearrangements such as translocations after chromosome breakage[74]. This essential function is emphasized by the finding that disruption of either gene in the mouse results in an embryonic lethal phenotype[44,75,76]. Thus, current evidence indicates that Brca1 and Brca2 participate in a common DNA damage response pathway associated with the activation of homologous recombination, and the repair of DSBs and ICLs[77]. Brca1 may, in fact, not only be required for homologous recombination, but may also act to suppress mutagenic nonhomologous repair processes[78]. Indeed, Brca1 has been shown to interact with Rad50, and is required for the formation of damage-induced Mre11/Rad50/Nbs1 foci[79]. Coimmunoprecipitation experiments performed with Brca1 have indicated the presence of a large number of additional proteins in this complex (referred to as the Brca1 associated surveillance complex or BASC) including the mismatch repair proteins Msh2, Msh6, and Mlh1, the checkpoint kinase Atm, the product of the Bloom's syndrome gene Blm, and replication factor C[80] (Figure 8). Brca1 has also been shown to be a substrate of the Atm kinase, and becomes phosphorylated upon exposure of cells to IR[81], possibly providing a mechanistic explanation of the role of Atm in breast cancer. In addition, Brca1 has also been shown to interact with a component of a Swi/Snf-related complex, which suggests that Brca1 may also mediate transcriptional control through modulation of chromatin structure[82]. Brca1 has also been shown to be involved in DNA repair pathways that are independent of recombination, such as transcription-coupled repair of oxidative damage[83].

In contrast to yeast, NHEJ is considered the primary pathway of DSB repair in mammalian cells. Recently, much progress has been made on the analysis of this pathway with the identification, cloning and characterization of the Ku70/80 heterodimer, its associated DNA-dependent protein kinase (DNA-PK$_{cs}$), and the products of the *XRCC4* and *Ligase IV* (L-IV) genes[84]. Mutation of any of these genes leads to extreme sensitivity to IR, but not to agents which induce ICLs. The Ku heterodimer binds to the free ends of double-stranded DNA, and recruits DNA-PK$_{cs}$, and the Xrcc4/L-IV heterodimer, both of which directly interact with Ku[85]. *In vitro*, the Xrcc4/L-IV heterodimer has been shown to be sufficient to mediate rejoining of DNA DSBs, and this activity is greatly stimulated by Ku, DNA-PK$_{cs}$, and inositol hexakisphosphate[86]. Additionally, these proteins are also involved in V(D)J recombination, a process required for the immunological diversity that is achieved in T and B lymphocytes. In the yeast, although homologs for *XRCC4*, *Ligase IV*, and the Ku genes have been identified, this pathway represents only a minor mechanism for the repair of DSBs. A homolog for DNA-PK$_{cs}$ has not been identified in the sequenced genome of *S. cerevisiae*.

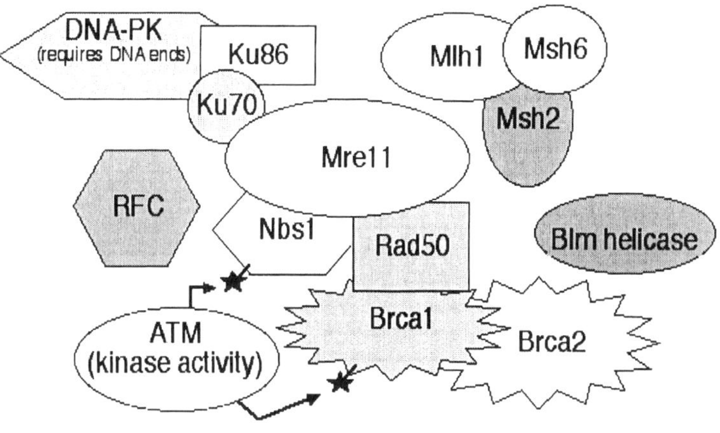

Figure 8. The Rad50 protein complex. Components of the Rad50 repair complex that have been identified by two-hybrid analyses and/or coimmunoprecipitation experiments are indicated.

Mutant hamster cell lines that are defective in the *ERCC1* or *XPF* genes have been shown to exhibit extreme sensitivity to interstrand crosslinking agents and UV without a corresponding sensitivity to IR[2]. The homologs of these genes in yeast, *RAD10* and *RAD1*, respectively, were originally identified as components of NER; however, subsequently, mutants in these genes were also found to be defective in some aspects of mitotic, but not meiotic, recombination. This role in recombination is unique to these genes since other components of the NER pathway are not required. Ercc1 and Xpf, and their yeast counterparts, form a stable heterodimer, and an examination of the role of these proteins in NER revealed that the complex is an endonuclease that specifically cleaves at junctions between single-stranded and double-stranded DNA that form as an intermediate during the excision repair process. This activity of the complex may also function in recombination since Rad1 and Rad10, in conjunction with Msh2 and Msh3, are involved in removing regions of nonhomology during both the SSA and HR pathways of DSB repair[17]. A similar involvement in recombination has also recently been reported for the mammalian proteins[87]. Rad1 and Rad10 have also been implicated in some pathways of mismatch repair in yeast[88].

5. PROCESSING OF INTERSTRAND CROSSLINKS IN DNA

The early stages of recognition and processing of ICLs in mammalian cells remain to a large extent unresolved. In yeast, current evidence indicates that ICL repair proceeds by a mechanism somewhat similar to the model proposed by Cole for ICL repair in *E. coli*, in that it requires a combination of the NER and the *RAD51*-mediated recombination pathways[89]. However, differences apparently exist in these mechanisms since DSBs have been shown to occur during processing of ICLs in yeast[90], but not in *E. coli*. The origin of these DSBs is unclear since mutants defective in either NER or recombination are not deficient in their formation. The initial stages of ICL repair in mammalian cells appear to be far more complex than those found in either *E. coli* or yeast. The first distinct difference is that an intact NER pathway does not seem to play a major role in the removal of these lesions since most mutants in this pathway exhibit only slight to moderate sensitivity to bifunctional alkylating agents[91]. However, *in vitro* findings using reconstituted NER components have shown that ICLs induce specific incisions, both of which occur 5' to the site of the lesion[92]. A subsequent report from this same laboratory, however, postulated that these incisions lead to a futile cycle of incision and gap filling that does not result in the removal of the ICL[93]. However, recent results obtained from reactivation studies of plasmids crosslinked with psoralen adducts, and transfected into mammalian cells, indicates that their repair requires an intact NER pathway, but not an intact homologous recombinational pathway[94]. Taken together, these results suggest that NER is probably involved in a minor pathway of ICL repair that is recombination independent, and which may require the activity of a translesion polymerase somewhat similar to the secondary pathway of ICL repair in *E. coli* discussed above.

Although most NER mutants are not highly sensitive to ICL-inducing agents, mutations in either *ERCC1* or *XPF* lead to extreme sensitivity to these agents of up to 90-fold above that observed in wild-type cells. The exact role of Ercc1 and Xpf in ICL repair is still somewhat unclear since, as indicated above, these proteins are known to play a role in some aspects of recombination. However, current evidence suggests that they are likely involved in the initial stages of recognition and incision of ICLs. Li *et al.*[95] have shown in an *in vitro* assay using mammalian cell extracts that site-specific psoralen adducts in plasmid DNAs stimulate DNA synthesis at or near these lesions. Extracts from hamster mutant cell lines defective in either Ercc1 or Xpf were found to be deficient in this assay, suggesting that these proteins are involved in the early stages of ICL repair. Interestingly, extracts from XPF patient cells, while deficient in NER *in vitro*, were found to be proficient in ICL-induced DNA synthesis, suggesting that the activities of Xpf in NER and ICL repair are separable[96]. Mu *et al.*[93] have shown that Ercc1 and Xpf can, in the presence of Rpa, degrade one strand of a linear duplex fragment containing an ICL in the 3'-5' direction. This degradation can proceed past the ICL resulting in a single-stranded fragment crosslinked to a single nucleotide residue. In addition, Kobertz *et al.*[97] have shown that a Y DNA structure with an ICL at the junction between the single- and double-stranded DNA can be incised in the duplex portion just 5' to the ICL. These findings all suggest a role for the Ercc1-Xpf heterodimer in the early stages of ICL repair; however, it remains possible that this complex also functions in the subsequent recombination stages as well.

In addition to the laboratory-derived hamster cell mutants, there is also a series of human cell lines derived from patients with the highly cancer-prone syndrome Fanconi anemia (FA). FA is an autosomal recessive disorder characterized by a diversity of clinical symptoms including skeletal abnormalities, progressive bone marrow failure, and a marked predisposition to acute myeloid leukemia. Cells from FA patients exhibit a variable, but marked, hypersensitivity to bifunctional alkylating agents, but not to other treatments such as IR, UV, or monofunctional alkylating agents. There are seven identified complementation groups of FA termed A through G, and five of these genes, representing groups A, C, E, F, and G, have been cloned[98–103]. Interestingly, all five of the proteins encoded by these genes are novel, and are not represented in the genomes of either *S. cerevisiae* or *C. elegans*. The hypersensitivity of FA cell lines to ICL-inducing agents has suggested that FA represents a disease defective in a DNA repair pathway; however, there is little direct evidence to date that FA proteins play a role in lesion removal, and the pleiotropic nature of the disorder suggests a more complex etiology. Initial immunohistochemical analysis of the Fancc protein indicated that it is localized entirely in the cytoplasm[104,105]. Furthermore, the cytoplasmic location of Fancc is essential for its function since when it is targeted to the nucleus it fails to correct the defect in FAC cells[106]. These results and others suggested that FA proteins may be involved in a cytoplasmic defense mechanism, such as prevention of oxidative damage induced by alkylating agents[107], rather than having a direct role in DNA repair processing. However, later findings have contradicted these results, and indicated an interaction between Fanca and Fancc that results in translocation of the complex into the nucleus[108]. Additional studies have shown that the Fancg protein is a component of this complex, and that its presence is required to stabilize the interaction between Fanca and Fancc[109]. These findings are consistent with a role in DNA repair, but other studies have suggested an involvement of FA proteins in regulating apoptosis and/or the cell cycle after exposure to crosslinking agents, or in a pathway of feedback control of DNA replication during S phase of the cell cycle[110].

Similar to the human FA mutants, mutants of the *SNM1* (sensitivity to nitrogen mustard) gene of *S. cerevisiae* are specifically sensitive to all bi- or polyfunctional alkylating agents that induce substantial levels of ICLs[111]. *SNM1* is allelic to the *PSO2* gene which was identified by selecting for mutants sensitive to psoralen plus UVA. Biochemical analysis of the function of Snm1 indicated that incision at the sites of ICLs proceeded normally in these mutants, but that a later step involving reconstitution of high molecular weight DNA from low molecular weight DNA was defective. Thus, Snm1 may function specifically in ICL repair to couple the initial stages of damage recognition and incision to the later states of recombinational repair. Interestingly, however, *SNM1* mutants have been reported to be proficient in the preferential incision of ICLs at the active *MATα* locus, but not at the silent *HMLa* locus, suggesting a role for Snm1 in the early stages of ICL repair. Recently, three homologs of *SNM1* have been identified in mammalian cells. All Snm1 family proteins, including homologs from *S. cerevisiae* and C. *elegans*, contain a conserved region of approximately 300 amino acids, but differ outside of this domain. A disruption of one of the three mammalian homologs in the mouse resulted in a definite but not dramatic sensitivity of the mice and cultured epithelial stem cells to MMC[112]. Future studies should help to determine whether all three mammalian *SNM1* homologs are involved in the repair processing of ICLs in DNA.

There are several other additional mammalian mutants, all of which are derived from hamster cell lines, that exhibit extreme sensitivity to agents that induce ICLs[113]. The *XRCC2* and *XRCC3* genes defective in two of these mutants, referred to as *irs1* and *irs1SF*, respectively, have been cloned, and found to be members of the *RecA/RAD51* gene family[114]. The proteins expressed by these genes have been shown to be components of the Rad51 foci-forming complex (Figure 7), and both mutants have been shown to be defective in the repair of DSBs mediated by HR[115,116]. Despite this demonstrated defect in the repair of DSBs, these mutants exhibit only a 2-3 fold increase in sensitivity to IR, while exhibiting a 60-100 fold increase in sensitivity to bifunctional alkylating agents. Interestingly, mutations in genes that mediate NHEJ, such as Ku or DNA-PK_{cs}, confer a high degree of sensitivity to IR, but little sensitivity to agents that induce ICLs. These findings appear to indicate that NHEJ, and perhaps SSA and BIR, have only a minor, if any, role in the repair of ICLs, and that repair of these lesions normally proceeds through the HR pathway. This lack of a major redundant pathway for ICL repair accounts for the extreme sensitivity of mutants, such as *irs1* and *irs1SF*. There are also additional hamster cell mutants, such as *V-C8* and *V-H4*, which also exhibit extreme sensitivity to bifunctional alkylating agents. In fact, *V-C8* is the most sensitive mutant yet identified with an approximate 110-fold decrease in resistance to these agents compared to wild-type cells[117]. The genes defective in either the *V-C8* or *V-H4* mutant have not yet been identified.

CONCLUSION

One can envision that the ICL is perhaps the most formidable lesion that a cell has to resolve in order to maintain genomic stability. DSBs, which are also extremely lethal, are repaired by a variety of mechanisms, the simplest of which is a direct rejoining of the broken molecules through the annealing of a few base pairs of microhomology by NHEJ. ICLs, however, appear to be largely shunted into the more complex homologous recombination pathway, and rapid progress is being made in the understanding of the intricacies of this mechanism in both yeast and mammalian cells. However, the early stages of ICL repair in mammalian cells have lagged behind the progress made in the elucidation of the other major pathways of DNA repair, and this part of the pathway remains to be clearly defined. It is apparent, though, that unlike *E. coli* and perhaps yeast, NER is not the major pathway of initiation of ICL repair in mammalian cells. The Ercc1-Xpf heterodimer appears to be a required component, but the other elements involved in the recognition and incision processes remain to be identified. In addition, there may also be a requirement for a coupling of the incision stages of ICL processing to the later stages of recombination. Possible candidates for this step are the Snm1 proteins, which in yeast have been shown to be required for restoring high molecular weight after the initial incision events. Finally, the possibility remains that the FA proteins are involved in some stage of ICL repair, and with the cloning of the remaining FA genes rapid progress can also be expected on elucidating their role in mediating resistance to ICL-inducing agents.

REFERENCES

1. Kohn KW. Beyond DNA cross-linking: history and prospects of DNA-targeted cancer treatment. Fifteenth Bruck F Can Memorial Award Lecture. Cancer Res, 56:5533-5546, 1996.
2. Friedberg EC, Walker GC, Siede W. DNA Repair and Mutagenesis. ASM Press, Washington, DC, 1995.
3. Calsou P, Salles B. Role of DNA repair in the mechanisms of cell resistance to alkylating agents and cisplatin. Cancer Chemother Pharmacol, 32:85-95, 1993.
4. Panasci L, Henderson D, Torres-Garcia SJ, *et al.* Transport, metabolism, and DNA interaction of melphalan in lymphocytes from patients with chronic lymphocytic leukemia. Cancer Res, 48:1972-1979, 1988.
5. Batist G, Torres-Garcia S, Demuys J-M, *et al.* Enhanced DNA cross-link removal: the apparent mechanisms of resistance in a clinically relevant melphalan-resistant human breast cancer cell line. Mol Pharmacol, 36:224-230, 1989.
6. Frankenburg DM, Frankenburg-Schwager M, Blocher D, Harbich R. Evidence for DNA double-strand breaks as the critical lesions in yeast cells irradiated with sparsely or densely ionizing radiation under oxic and anoxic conditions. Radiat Res, 88:524-532, 1989.
7. Magana-Schwencke N, Henriques JA, Chanet R, Moustacchi E. The fate of 8-methoxypsoralen photoinduced crosslinks in nuclear and mitochondrial yeast DNA: comparison of wild-type and repair-deficient strains. Proc Natl Acad Sci USA, 79:1722-1726, 1982.
8. Cole RS. Repair of DNA containing interstrand crosslinks in Escherichia coli: sequential excision and recombination. Proc Natl Acad Sci USA, 70:1064-1068, 1973.
9. Cole RS, Levitan D, Sinden RR. Removal of psoralen interstrand cross-links from DNA of Escherichia coli: mechanism and genetic control. J Mol Biol, 103:39-59, 1976.
10. Van Houten B, Gamper H, Holbrook SR, *et al.* Action mechanism of ABC excision nuclease on a DNA substrate containing a psoralen crosslink at a defined position. Proc Natl Acad Sci USA, 83:8077-8081, 1986.
11. Cheng S, van Houten B, Gamper HB, *et al.* Use of psoralen-modified oligonucleotides to trap three-stranded RecA-DNA complexes and repair of these cross-linked complexes by ABC exinuclease. J Biol Chem, 263:15110-15117, 1988.
12. Cheng S, Sancar A, Hearst JE. RecA-dependent incision of psoralen-crosslinked DNA by (A)BC exinuclease. Nucleic Acids Res, 19:657-663, 1989.
13. Sladek FM, Munn MM, Rupp WD, Howard-Flanders P. In vitro repair of psoralen-DNA cross-links by RecA, UvrABC, and the 5'-exonuclease of DNA polymerase I. J Biol Chem, 264:6755-6765, 1989.
14. Berardini M, Mackay W, Loechler EL. Evidence for a recombination-independent pathway for the repair of DNA interstrand cross-links based on a site-specific study with nitrogen mustard. Biochem, 36:3506-3513, 1997.
15. Berardini M, Foster PL, Loechler EL. DNA polymerase II (polB) is involved in a new DNA repair pathway for DNA interstrand cross-links in *Escherichia coli.* J Bacteriol, 181:2878-2882, 1999.

16. Game JC. DNA double-strand breaks and the RAD50-RAD57 genes in Saccharomyces. Semin Cancer Biol, 4:73-83, 1993.
17. Paques F, Haber JE. Multiple pathways of recombination induced by double-strand breaks in Saccharomyces cerevisiae. Microbiol Mol Biol Rev, 63:349-404, 1999.
18. Contopoulou CR, Cook VE, Mortimer RK. Analysis of DNA double-strand breakage and repair using orthogonal field alternation gel electrophoresis. Yeast, 3:71-76, 1987.
19. Petes TD, Malone RE, Symington LS. Recombination in yeast. *In*: The Molecular and Cellular Biology of the Yeast Saccharomyces: Genome Dynamics, Protein Synthesis, and Energetics, JR Broach, JR Pringle, EW Jones (eds.), Cold Spring Harbor Laboratory Press, Cold Spring Harbor, NY, 1991.
20. Aboussekhra A, Chanet R, Adjiri A, Fabre F. Semi-dominant suppressors of Srs2 helicase mutations of Saccharomyces cerevisiae map in the RAD51 gene, whose sequence predicts a protein with similarities to procaryotic RecA proteins. Mol Cell Biol, 12:3224-3234, 1992.
21. Basile G, Aker M, Mortimer RK. Nucleotide sequence and transcriptional regulation of the yeast recombinational repair gene RAD51. Mol Cell Biol, 12:3235-3246, 1992.
22. Shinohara A, Ogawa H, Ogawa T. RAD51 protein involved in repair and recombination in S. cerevisiae is a RecA-like protein. Cell, 69:457-470, 1992.
23. Ogawa T, Yu X, Shinohara A, Egelman EH. Similarity of the yeast RAD51 filament to the bacterial RecA filament. Science, 259:1896-1899, 1993.
24. Sung P. Catalysis of ATP-dependent homologous DNA pairing and strand exchange by yeast RAD51 protein. Science, 265:1241-1243, 1994.
25. Sung P, Robberson DL. DNA strand exchange mediated by a RAD51-ssDNA nucleoprotein filament with polarity opposite to that of RecA. Cell, 82:453-461, 1995.
26. Kans JA, Mortimer RK. Nucleotide sequence of the RAD57 gene of Saccharomyces cerevisiae. Gene, 105:139-140, 1991.
27. Lovett ST. Sequence of the RAD55 gene of Saccharomyces cerevisiae: similarity of RAD55 to prokaryotic RecA and other RecA-like proteins. Gene, 142:103-106, 1994.
28. Johnson RD, Symington LS. Functional differences and interactions among the putative RecA homologs Rad51, Rad55, and Rad57. Mol Cell Biol, 15:4843-4850, 1995.
29. Hays SL, Firmenich AA, Berg P. Complex formation in yeast double-stranded break repair: participation of Rad51, Rad52, Rad55, and Rad57. Proc Natl Acad Sci USA, 92:6925-6929, 1995.
30. Sung P. Yeast Rad55 and Rad57 proteins form a heterodimer that functions with replication protein A to promote DNA strand exchange by Rad51 recombinase. Genes Dev, 11:1111-1121, 1997.
31. Milne GT, Weaver DT. Dominant negative alleles of RAD52 reveal a DNA repair/recombination complex including Rad51 and Rad52. Genes Dev, 7:1755-1765, 1993.
32. Baumann P, Benson FE, West SC. Human Rad51 protein promotes ATP-dependent homologous pairing and strand transfer reactions in vitro. Cell, 87:757-766, 1996.
33. Tsuzuki T, Fujii Y, Sakumi K, *et al.* Targeted disruption of the Rad51 gene leads to lethality in embryonic mice. Proc Natl Acad Sci USA, 93:6236-6240, 1996.
34. Lim DS, Hasty P. A mutation in mouse rad51 results in an early embryonic lethal that is suppressed by a mutation in p53. Mol Cell Biol, 16:7133-7143, 1996.
35. Shu Z, Smith S, Wang L, *et al.* Disruption of muREC2/RAD51L1 in mice results in early embryonic lethality which can be partially rescued in a p53(-/-) background. Mol Cell Biol, 19:8686-8693, 1999.
36. Pittman, DL, Schimenti JC. Midgestation lethality in mice deficient for the RecA-related gene, Rad51d/Rad51l3. Genesis, 26:167-173, 2000.

37. Thacker J. American Society for Microbiology. DNA Repair and Mutagenesis. Hilton Head, SC, 1999.
38. Sonoda E, Sasaki MS, Buerstedde JM, *et al.* Rad51-deficient vertebrate cells accumulate chromosomal breaks prior to cell death. EMBO J, 17:598-608, 1998.
39. Takata M, Sasaki MS, Sonoda E, *et al.* The Rad51 paralog Rad51B promotes homologous recombinational repair. Mol Cell Biol, 20:6476-6482, 2000.
40. Haaf T, Golub EI, Reddy G, *et al.* Nuclear foci of mammalian Rad51 recombination protein in somatic cells after DNA damage and its localization in synaptonemal complexes. Proc Natl Acad. Sci USA, 92:2298-2302, 1998.
41. Tashiro S, Kotomura N, Shinohara A, *et al.* S phase specific formation of the human Rad51 protein nuclear foci in lymphocytes. Oncogene, 12:2165-2170, 1996.
42. Schild D, Lio Y, Collins DW, *et al.* Evidence for simultaneous protein interactions between human Rad51 paralogs. J Biol Chem, 275:16443-16449, 2000.
43. Scully R, Chen J, Plug A, *et al.* Association of BRCA1 with Rad51 in mitotic and meiotic cells. Cell, 88:265-275, 1997.
44. Sharan SK, Morimatsu M, Albrecht U, *et al.* Embryonic lethality and radiation hypersensitivity mediated by Rad51 in mice lacking Brca2. Nature, 386:804-810, 1997.
45. Mizuta R, LaSalle JM, Cheng HL, *et al.* RAB22 and RAB163/mouse BRCA2: proteins that specifically interact with the RAD51 protein. Proc Natl Acad Sci USA, 94:6927-6932, 1997.
46. Game JC, Zamb TJ, Braun RJ, *et al.* The role of radiation (rad) genes in meiotic recombination in yeast. Genetics, 94:51-68, 1980.
47. Van Dyck E, Stasiak AZ, Stasiak A, West SC. Binding of double-strand breaks in DNA by human Rad52 protein. Nature, 398:728-731, 1999.
48. Stasiak AZ, Larquet E, Stasiak A, *et al.* The human Rad52 protein exists as a heptameric ring. Current Biol, 10:337-340, 2000.
49. Rijkers T, Van Den Ouweland J, Morolli B, *et al.* Targeted inactivation of mouse RAD52 reduces homologous recombination but not resistance to ionizing radiation. Mol Cell Biol, 18:6423-6429, 1998.
50. Bai Y, Symington, LS. A *RAD52* homologue is required for *RAD51*-independent mitotic recombination in Saccharomyces cerevisiae. Genes Dev, 10:2025-2037, 1996.
51. Game JC. DNA double-strand breaks and the RAD50-RAD57 genes in Saccharomyces. Semin Cancer Biol, 4:73-83, 1993.
52. Emery HS, Schild D, Kellogg DE, *et al.* Sequence of RAD54, a Saccharomyces cerevisiae gene involved in recombination and repair. Gene, 104:103-106, 1991.
53. Petukhova G, Stratton S, Sung P. Catalysis of homologous DNA pairing by yeast Rad51 and Rad54 proteins. Nature, 393:91-94, 1998.
54. Essers J, Hendriks RW, Swagemakers SM, *et al.* Disruption of mouse RAD54 reduces ionizing radiation resistance and homologous recombination. Cell, 89:195-204, 1997.
55. Alani E, Padmore R, Kleckner N. Analysis of wild-type and rad50 mutants of yeast suggests an intimate relationship between meiotic chromosome synapsis and recombination. Cell, 61:419-436, 1990.
56. Game JC, Mortimer RK. A genetic study of X-ray sensitive mutants in yeast. Mutat Res, 24:281-292, 1974.
57. Alani E, Subbiah S, Kleckner N. The yeast RAD50 gene encodes a predicted 153-Kd protein containing a purine-nucleotide binding domain and two large heptad-repeat regions. Genetics, 122:47-57, 1989.
58. Usui T, Ohta T, Oshumi H, *et al.* Complex formation and functional versatility of Mre11 of budding yeast in recombination. Cell, 95:705-716, 1998.

59. Ivanov EL, Sugawara N, White CI, *et al.* Mutations in XRS2 and RAD50 delay but do not prevent mating-type switching in Saccharomyces cerevisiae. Mol Cell Biol, 14:3414-3425, 1994.
60. Bressan DA, Baxter BK, Petrini JH. The Mre11-Rad50-Xrs2 protein complex facilitates homologous recombination-based double-strand break repair in Saccharomyces cerevisiae. Mol Cell Biol, 19:7681-7687, 1999.
61. Le Beau M, Yates JR, Hays L, *et al.* The hMre11/hRad50 protein complex and Nijmegen breakage syndrome: linkage of double-strand break repair to the cellular DNA damage response. Cell, 93:477-486, 1998.
62. Matsuura S, Tauchi H, Nakamura A, *et al.* Positional cloning of the gene for Nijmegen breakage syndrome. Nature Genet, 19:179-181, 1998.
63. Stewart GS, Maser RS, Stankovic T, *et al.* The DNA double-strand break repair gene hMRE11 is mutated in individuals with an ataxia-telangiectasia-like disorder. Cell, 99:577-587,1999.
64. Luo G, Yao MS Bender CF, *et al.* Disruption of mRad50 causes embryonic stem cell lethality, abnormal embryonic development, and sensitivity to ionizing radiation. Proc Natl Acad Sci USA, 96:7376-7381, 1999.
65. Xiao Y, Weaver DT. Conditional gene targeted deletion by Cre recombinase demonstrates the requirement for the double-strand break repair Mre11 protein in murine embryonic stem cells. Nucleic Acids Res, 25:2985-2991, 1999.
66. Paull TT, Gellert M. The 3' to 5' exonuclease activity of Mre11 facilitates repair of DNA double-strand breaks. Mol Cell, 1:969-980, 1998.
67. Paull TT, Gellert M. Nbs1 potentiates ATP-driven DNA unwinding and endonuclease cleavage by the Mre11/Rad50 complex. Genes Dev, 13:1276-1288, 1999.
68. Maser RS, Monsen KJ, Nelms BE, Petrini JH. hMre11 and hRad50 nuclear foci are induced during the normal cellular response to DNA double-strand breaks. Mol Cell Biol, 17:6087-6096, 1998.
69. Nelms BE, Maser RS, MacKay JF, *et al.* In situ visualization of DNA double-strand break repair in human fibroblasts. Science, 280:590-592, 1998.
70. Goedecke W, Eijpe M, Offenberg HH, *et al.* Mre11 and Ku70 interact in somatic cells, but are differentially expressed in early meiosis. Nature Genet, 23:194-198, 1999.
71. Gatei M, Young D, Cerosaletti KM, *et al.* ATM-dependent phosphorylation of nibrin in response to radiation exposure. Nature Genet, 25:115-119, 2000.
72. Dong Z, Zhong Q, Chen PL. The Nijmegen breakage syndrome protein is essential for Mre11 phosphorylation upon DNA damage. J Biol Chem, 274:19513-19516, 1999.
73. Chen J, Silver DP, Walpita D, *et al.* Stable interaction between the products of the BRCA1 and BRCA2 tumor suppressor genes in mitotic and meiotic cells. Mol Cell, 2:317-328, 1998.
74. Yu VP, Koehler M, Steinlein C, *et al.* Gross chromosomal rearrangements and genetic exchange between nonhomologous chromosomes following BRCA2 inactivation. Genes Dev, 14:1400-1406, 2000.
75. Gowen LC, Johnson BL, Latour AM, *et al.* Brca1 deficiency results in early embryonic lethality characterized by neuroepithelial abnormalities. Nature Genet, 12:191-194, 1996.
76. Liu CY, Flesken-Nikitin A, Li S, *et al.* Inactivation of the mouse Brca1 gene leads to failure in the morphogenesis of the egg cylinder in early postimplantation development. Genes Dev, 10:1835-1843, 1996.
77. Chen JJ, Silver D, Cantor S, *et al.* BRCA1, BRCA2, and Rad51 operate in a common DNA damage response pathway. Cancer Res, 59:1752s-1756s, 1999.
78. Moynahan ME, Chiu JW, Koller BH, Jasin M. Brca1 controls homology-directed DNA repair. Mol Cell, 4:511-518, 1999.

79. Zhong Q, Chen CF, Li S, *et al.* Association of BRCA1 with the hRad50-hMre11-p95 complex and the DNA damage response. Science, 285:747-750, 1999.
80. Wang Y, Cortez D, Yazdi P, *et al.* Basc, a super complex of BRCA1-associated proteins involved in the recognition and repair of aberrant DNA structures. Genes Dev, 14:927-939, 2000.
81. Cortez D, Wang Y, Qin J, Elledge SJ. Requirement of ATM-dependent phosphorylation of BRCA1 in the DNA damage response to double-strand breaks. Science, 286:1162-1166, 1999.
82. Bochar DA, Wang L, Beniya, H, *et al.* BRCA1 is associated with a human SWI/SNF-related complex: linking chromatin remodeling to breast cancer. Cell, 102:257-265, 2000.
83. Gowen LC, Avrutskaya AV, Latour AM, *et al.* BRCA1 required for transcription-coupled repair of oxidative DNA damage. Science, 281:1009-1012, 1998.
84. Jeggo PA, Taccioli GE, Jackson SP. Menage a trois: double strand break repair, V(D)J recombination and DNA-PK. Bioessays, 17:949-957, 1995.
85. McElhinny SAN, Snowden CM, McCarville J, Ramsden DA. Ku recruits the XRCC4-Ligase complex to DNA ends. Mol Cell Biol, 20:2996-3003, 2000.
86. Hanakahi LA, Bartlett-Jones M, Chappell C, *et al.* Binding of inositol phosphate to DNA-PK and stimulation of double-strand break repair. Cell, 102:721-729, 2000.
87. Adair GM, Rolig RL, Moore-Faver D, *et al.* Role of ERCC1 in removal of nonhomologous tails during targeted homologous recombination in mammalian cells. EMBO J, 19:5552-5561, 2000.
88. Kirkpatrick DT, Petes TD. Repair of DNA loops involves DNA-mismatch and nucleotide-excision repair proteins. Nature, 387:929-931, 1997.
89. Jachymczyk WJ, von Borstel RC, Mowat MRA, Hastings PJ. Repair of interstrand crosslinks in DNA of Saccharomyces cerevisiae requires two systems for DNA repair: the RAD3 system and the RAD51 system. Mol General Genet, 182:196-205, 1991.
90. McHugh PJ, Gill RD, Waters R, Hartley JA. Excision repair of nitrogen mustard-DNA adducts in Saccharomyces cerevisiae. Nucleic Acids Res, 27: 3259-3266, 1999.
91. Andersson BS, Sadeghi T, Sicilano MJ, *et al.* Nucleotide excision repair genes as determinants of cellular sensitivity to cyclophosphamide analogs. Cancer Chemother and Pharmacol, 38:406-416, 1996.
92. Bessho T, Mu D, Sancar A. Initiation of DNA interstrand crosslink repair in humans: the nucleotide excision repair system makes dual incisions 5' to the crosslinked base and removes a 22- to 28 nucleotide-long damage-free strand. Mol Cell Biol, 17:6822-6830, 1997.
93. Mu D, Bessho T, Nechev LV, *et al.* DNA interstrand cross-links induce futile repair synthesis in mammalian cell extracts. Mol Cell Biol, 20:2446-2454, 2000.
94. Wang X, Peterson CA, Zheng H, *et al.* Involvement of nucleotide excision repair in a recombination-independent and error-prone pathway of DNA interstrand cross-link repair. Mol Cell Biol, 21:713-20, 2001.
95. Li L, Peterson CA, Lu X, *et al.* Interstrand crosslinks induce DNA synthesis in damaged and undamaged plasmids in mammalian cell-free extracts. Mol Cell Biol, 19:5619-5630, 1999.
96. Zhang N, Zhang X, Peterson C, *et al.* Differential processing of UV mimetic and interstrand crosslink damage by XPF cell extracts. Nucleic Acids Res, 28:4800-4804, 2000.
97. Kobertz WR, Ariza RR, Biggerstaff M, *et al.* Repair of an interstrand DNA cross-link initiated by ERCC1-XPF repair/recombination nuclease. J Biol Chem, 275:26632-26636, 2000.

98. Strathdee CA, Gavish H, Shannon WR, Buchwald M. Cloning of cDNAs for Fanconi's anaemia by functional complementation. Nature, 358:434-436, 1992.
99. Lo Ten Foe JR, Rooimans MA, Bosnoyan-Collins L, *et al.* Expression cloning of a cDNA for the major Fanconi anaemia gene, FAA. Nature Genet, 14:320-323, 1996.
100. Consortium TFABC. Positional cloning of the Fanconi anaemia group A gene. Nature Genet, 14:324-328, 1996.
101. de Winter JP, Waisfisz Q, Rooimans MA, *et al.* The Fanconi anaemia group G gene FANCG is identical with XRCC9. Nature Genet, 20:281-283, 1998.
102. de Winter JP, Rooimans MA, van Der Weel L, *et al.* The Fanconi anaemia gene FANCF encodes a novel protein with homology to ROM. Nature Genet, 24:15-16, 2000.
103. de Winter JP, Leveille F, van Berkel CGM, *et al.* Isolation of a cDNA representing the Fanconi Anemia complementation group E gene. Am J Hum Genet, 67:1306-1308, 2000.
104. Yamashita T, Barber DL, Zhu Y, *et al.* The Fanconi anaemia polypeptide FACC is localized to the cytoplasm. Proc Natl Acad Sci USA, 91:6712-6716, 1994.
105. Youssoufian H. Localization of Fanconi anaemia C protein to the cytoplasm of mammalian cells. Proc Natl Acad Sci USA, 91:7975-7979, 1994.
106. Youssoufian H. Cytoplasmic localization of FAC is essential for the correction of a prerepair defect in Fanconi anaemia group C cells. J Clin Invest, 97:2003-2010, 1996.
107. Pagano G. Mitomycin C and diepoxybutane action mechanisms and FANCC protein functions: further insights into the role for oxidative stress in Fanconi's anaemia phenotype. Carcinogenesis, 21:1067-1068, 2000.
108. Kupfer GM, Naf D, Suliman A, *et al.* The Fanconi anaemia proteins, FAA and FAC, interact to form a nuclear complex. Nature Genet. 17:487-490, 1997.
109. Garcia-Higuera I, Kuang Y, Naf D, *et al.* Fanconi anemia proteins FANCA, FANCC, and FANCG/XRCC9 interact in a functional nuclear complex. Mol Cell Biol, 19:4866-4873, 1999.
110. Buchwald M, Moustacchi E. Is Fanconi anaemia caused by a defect in the processing of DNA damage? Mutat Res, 408:75-90, 1998.
111. Henriques JAP, Brozmanova J, Brendel M. Role of PSO genes in the repair of photoinduced interstrand crosslinks and photooxidative damage in the DNA of the yeast *Saccharomyces cerevisiae*. J Photochem Photobiol B Biol, 39:185-196, 1999.
112. Dronkert MLG, de Wit J, Boeve M, *et al.* Disruption of mouse SNM1 causes increased sensitivity to the DNA interstrand cross-linking agent mitomycin C. Mol Cell Biol, 20:4553-4560, 2000.
113. Collins AR. Mutant rodent cell lines sensitive to ultraviolet light, ionizing radiation and cross-linking agents: a comprehensive survey of genetic and biochemical characteristics. Mutat Res, 293:99-118, 1993.
114. Liu N, Lamerdin JE, Tebbs RS, *et al.* XRCC2 and XRCC3, new human Rad51-family members, promote chromosome stability and protect against DNA cross-links and other damages. Mol Cell 1, 783-793, 1998.
115. Johnson RD, Liu N, Jasin M. Mammalian XRCC2 promotes the repair of DNA double-strand breaks by homologous recombination. Nature, 401:397-399, 1999.
116. Pierce AJ, Johnson RD, Thompson LH, Jasin M. XRCC3 promotes homology-directed repair of DNA damage in mammalian cells. Genes Dev, 13:2633-2638, 1999.
117. Zdzienicka MZ, Simons JWI. Mutagen-sensitive lines are obtained with a high frequency in V79 Chinese hamster cells. Mutat Res, 178:235-244, 1987.

Chapter 7

DNA REPAIR IN RESISTANCE TO BIFUNCTIONAL ALKYLATING AND PLATINATING AGENTS

David Murray
Department of Oncology, University of Alberta, Edmonton, Alberta, Canada, and Department of Experimental Oncology, Cross Cancer Institute, Edmonton, Alberta, Canada

1. INTRODUCTION

Identifying and exploiting metabolic and genetic differences between normal and tumor cells is an important aspect of the development of cancer therapeutic agents. This rationale naturally extends to understanding the properties of tumor cells that make them responsive versus resistant to anticancer drugs. Many factors can contribute to the drug-resistant phenotype of individual tumor cells, and indeed, clinically relevant resistance in a given tumor or cell line often involves more than one mechanism. However, with a specific anticancer drug, one or more mechanisms may dominate. Thus, cyclophosphamide-resistant tumor cells display a high incidence of elevation of aldehyde dehydrogenase (ALDH), an enzyme that eliminates the active metabolite of the drug before it can react with and damage the cells' DNA[1] (see chapter 8 in this volume by Dr. N. Sladek). Similarly, tumor cells that are resistant to bis-chloroethyl nitrosourea (BCNU) display a high incidence of increased activity of the protein O^6-alkylguanine DNA alkyltransferase (AGT) which removes mono-alkylated adducts from the O^6 position of guanine (section 7). With cisplatin and melphalan, the ability of the tumor cells to repair drug-DNA adducts is a frequent contributor to the drug-resistant phenotype[2–5]. It is the latter mechanism that is the subject of this chapter.

We will focus on resistance to a group of commonly-used anticancer drugs, namely the bifunctional alkylating and platinating agents. The major classes of chemotherapeutic alkylating agents are: (i) the nitrogen mustards (e.g., mechlorethamine, melphalan, cyclophosphamide); (ii) the chloroethyl nitrosoureas (e.g., BCNU); and (iii) the methane sulfonic acid esters (e.g., busulfan). The platinating agents include cisplatin and its analogs (see chapter 13 in this volume by Dr. Z. Siddik). These electrophilic drugs share the common feature of inducing the type of DNA lesion referred to as the DNA interstrand crosslink (ISC), although they also cause other types of lesions (such as mono-adducts, intrastrand crosslinks, DNA-protein crosslinks and strand breaks). The proportion of the different classes of DNA lesion, and hence the nature of the DNA repair response invoked by the cell, varies with the drug[6]. For cisplatin, the majority of the induced lesions locally involve only one strand of the DNA and are thus substrates for the nucleotide excision repair (NER) pathway (section 2.1); however, the drug also induces a small proportion of ISCs (between 0.1 and 5% of the total lesions)[2,7,8] that can not be repaired by NER *per se* (section 2.2). Even low levels of ISCs may be important for cytotoxicity (and thus anti-tumor effect) because of the difficulty which these lesions present to the cell with respect to their impact on DNA metabolism and to their repair[9].

Because of the obvious value in distinguishing cancer patients who may not benefit from initial therapy involving a particular drug (intrinsic resistance), or whose tumors may develop resistance to that drug during treatment (acquired resistance), numerous molecular techniques have been developed with the purpose of rapidly identifying such individuals. As will be discussed in sections 3-5, assays for the ability of tumor cells to repair DNA damage caused by antitumor drugs fall into 3 groups: (i) direct assays of genomic DNA damage following treatment of the tumor cells with a genotoxic agent; (ii) surrogate assays where an exogenous DNA sequence is damaged and reactivated/repaired by the tumor (host) cells or by cell extracts; and (iii) assays of pre-treatment levels of DNA repair gene transcripts or their encoded proteins. First, we will briefly review the most relevant DNA repair processes for chemotherapy.

2. DNA REPAIR PATHWAYS

Mammalian cells possess several partially overlapping DNA repair pathways that enable them to circumvent the potentially harmful effects of a variety of genotoxic agents. Here we will focus on those that have a significant impact on the response of mammalian cells to the antitumor alkylating and platinating agents.

2.1 The NER Pathway

NER is the major pathway for the repair of bulky lesions that locally involve only one strand of the DNA, such as UV-induced cyclopyrimidine dimers or cisplatin-induced intrastrand crosslinks[10,11]. The proteins involved in the rate-limiting incision step of NER were identified using both rodent mutant cell lines (the so-called excision repair cross complementing or "ERCC" proteins) and human cells obtained from individuals afflicted with the hereditary NER-deficiency disorders xeroderma pigmentosum (XP) and Cockayne's syndrome (CS). The *XP/CS* genes are homologous to the rodent *ERCC* genes, although there is not always a corresponding mutant. For example, there is no known human syndrome associated with mutation of the *ERCC1* gene. For the remainder of this chapter (other than for *ERCC1*) we will follow the convention of using the XP or CS designations for these genes or proteins.

About 25 repair factors are required to complete NER[10,11]. XPA (in combination with replication protein A, RPA) appears to be involved in the initial damage recognition step of NER, where it serves as a nucleation factor for damage excision; this complex subsequently forms an association with ERCC1. The ERCC1/XPF heterodimer is an endonuclease that incises the DNA 5' to the bulky lesion. XPD and XPB are DNA helicases associated with local unwinding of the DNA at the damaged site. XPG is an endonuclease associated with the 3' incision step. CSB is involved in the coupling of NER to transcription (section 3.4). The lesion is removed along with an ~28 bp single-stranded DNA fragment. DNA polymerase and ligase activities complete the sealing of the repair patch, using the undamaged strand as a template.

2.2 The Repair of Interstrand Crosslinks

Several commonly used anticancer agents exert a significant proportion of their cytotoxic effects via the induction of ISCs. However, the mechanism of ISC repair is poorly understood (see chapter 6 in this volume by Drs. R. Legerski and C. Richie). The repair of ISCs utilizes some of the components of NER, specifically the ERCC1 and XPF proteins. This is apparent from the consistent finding that mutation of the *ERCC1* and *XPF* genes (but not of other NER genes) imparts a dramatic (~50 fold) sensitivity to antitumor agents such as cyclophosphamide analogs and cisplatin that induce ISCs[12–15].

The role of the ERCC1 and XPF proteins in NER and ISC repair may involve different mechanisms, and in particular different modes of endonuclease activity[16–19]. Clearly, an ISC can not be repaired by NER alone. Because an ISC involves local damage to both strands of the DNA, and thus leaves no intact template for the repair polymerase, some type of homologous recombination event must be involved for its correct repair[20]. This pathway is the subject of very active research. It was recently shown that proliferating cell nuclear antigen (PCNA) and RPA are important factors for the repair of ISCs in a cell-free plasmid assay[21]. A variety of additional proteins, such as XRCC2 and XRCC3, have been implicated in the repair of ISCs induced by drugs such as mitomycin C, cisplatin[22] and cyclophosphamide analogs[23]. The XRCC2 and XRCC3 proteins, which are homologs of RAD51, are presumed to catalyze recombination, possibly involving a break-induced replication event[18] (see chapter 6 by Drs. Legerski and Richie). There may be more than one pathway for repairing ISCs[20], and different types of ISCs may have different repair-factor requirements[18,24].

2.3 AGT

The AGT protein (it is not strictly an enzyme because it is inactivated by the transfer of an alkyl group from DNA)[10,25,26] protects cells from certain genotoxic agents by removing single alkylation products from the O^6 position of guanine. Its importance in cancer therapeutics results primarily from the fact that some methylating and chloroethylating agents produce such O^6-guanine adducts[27]. An important example is BCNU, a chloroethylnitrosourea widely used for the treatment of brain tumors. These mono-adducts can thus be removed by AGT before they react further to generate a more complex lesion, such as an ISC. The involvement of AGT in resistance to bifunctional alkylating agents such as cyclophosphamide analogs will be discussed in section 7.

2.4 Mismatch Repair (MMR)

The MMR pathway is best known (and named) for its role in correcting replicative mismatches that escape DNA polymerase proof-reading. DNA mismatches or unpaired short heterologies are recognized by hMSH2/GTBP, followed by binding of the hMLH1–hPMS1 heterodimer. The resulting DNA-bound ternary complex probably recruits additional repair factors, such as helicases and exonucleases. As will be discussed in section 6, MMR proteins can be an important factor in tumor-cell resistance to some anticancer drugs[28–30]. Rather than repairing damage caused by these drugs, however, the MMR complex appears to recognize and process such DNA lesions in a way that promotes cytotoxicity. Thus, the ***lack*** of MMR activity has been widely associated with drug resistance.

2.5 The Base Excision Repair (BER) Pathway

Many types of base damage induced by environmental mutagens and anticancer drugs are substrates for the BER pathway[10,31–34]. BER involves the sequential action of a damage-specific DNA glycosylase (which cleaves the N-glycosylic bond between the damaged base and the deoxyribose), an AP endonuclease (which cleaves 5' to the abasic site) or AP lyase (which cleaves 3' to the abasic site, an activity associated with most DNA glycosylases), a 5'-phosphodiesterase (which removes the remaining deoxyribose phosphate), polymerase β (which fills in the gap), and DNA ligase (which seals the resulting break). Several additional proteins appear to be involved in this process, including XRCC1, which associates with DNA ligase III. Although BER is most commonly identified with the cellular response to ionizing radiation and monofunctional alkylating agents, it can be important in the response to bifunctional alkylating and platinating agents under some circumstances. Among the most commonly studied BER enzymes in this regard is 3-methyladenine DNA glycosylase, also known as alkyl adenine glycosylase or N-methylpurine-DNA glycosylase (MPG), which can release several altered bases, including 3-methyladenine and N-7-alkylations of guanine[10,35].

3. DIRECT MEASUREMENT OF THE REPAIR OF DNA LESIONS IN GENOMIC DNA FOLLOWING TREATMENT OF TUMOR CELLS WITH ANTICANCER AGENTS

Many studies implicating a role for DNA repair in drug resistance have used techniques that are sensitive to alterations in the physical properties of the DNA from drug-treated cells. Techniques used for measuring ISCs, strand breaks and DNA adducts include alkaline filter elution[36], alkaline unwinding/ethidium bromide fluorescence[37,38], and the comet assay[39,40]. Assays based on gel electrophoresis[41] or PCR[42,43] are particularly useful because they permit the characterization of repair in specific genomic sequences (section 3.4). Other studies evaluate the persistence of total DNA adducts. For example, for cisplatin, techniques such as atomic absorption spectrometry (AAS) can readily detect total platinations. Immunochemical methods involving antibodies to some type of DNA adduct, e.g., for cisplatin[44] and melphalan[45], have also been devcloped. Many of these types of study compared a parental tumor line with a resistant line derived in the laboratory by repeated exposure of the parental cells to the drug. Some compared unrelated tumor cell lines with differing intrinsic sensitivity to a drug. Others focused on clinical material, both before and after treatment of patients with chemotherapy, or compared clinically responsive and refractory tumor types. We will consider these studies by drug.

3.1 Cisplatin

Although cellular resistance to cisplatin is clearly multifactorial[46], increased DNA repair activity has been identified as a major factor in a variety of human tumor models. These include testicular teratoma cell lines established from chemotherapy-naïve patients[47,48] and teratoma cells with resistance to cisplatin resulting from *in vitro* exposure to X rays[49]. Independent sub-lines established from primary teratomas from previously untreated patients that expressed clinically relevant levels of cisplatin resistance (~3 fold) were also more proficient in repairing cisplatin adducts (both intrastrand adducts and ISCs) than the sensitive lines[50]. Advanced testicular germ cell tumors are very sensitive to cisplatin-based chemotherapy, and cell lines derived from these tumors are deficient in the repair of Pt-DNA adducts[51]. Lung cancer cell lines with intrinsic resistance to cisplatin are also characterized by increased repair of Pt-DNA adducts[52].

Similar approaches have been applied to ovarian cancer, where drug resistance is a major obstacle to treatment. Although these tumors initially respond well to cisplatin or carboplatin-based chemotherapy, relapse is frequent and subsequent chemotherapy is largely ineffective. Several investigators have studied ovarian cancer cell lines with laboratory-induced (acquired) resistance to cisplatin[53,54]. One such cell line removed ISCs more efficiently than the parental line, as well as showing increased repair of individual Pt-DNA adducts as determined by HPLC/AAS[55]. Among a series of such lines, not only were total cisplatin-DNA adducts removed more rapidly by resistant cells, but this differential was particularly great for the removal of ISCs from an actively transcribed gene[56]. Similarly, Zhen *et al.*[57] described human ovarian cancer lines with acquired resistance to cisplatin that did not have an altered ability to repair ISCs or intrastrand adducts in their overall genome but which showed more efficient gene-specific removal of ISCs from the *DHFR*, *MDR1* and *δ-globin* genes than parental cells.

Thus, studies with human ovarian cancer cells with artificially induced drug resistance indicate a major role for DNA repair. However, in this disease, subsequent studies have underscored the importance of using clinical material for evaluating factors identified using *in vitro* models. Specifically, tolerance to Pt-DNA adducts (rather than enhanced repair) appears to be the major resistance mechanism occurring in tumor cells from clinically drug-resistant patients[58,59]. Such resistance may arise from the inactivation of pathways involved in recognizing and processing cisplatin-DNA adducts and which ordinarily activate pro-apoptotic pathways.

3.2 Melphalan

Several human tumor cell lines with laboratory-induced resistance to melphalan have increased levels of DNA repair. For example, a breast cancer cell line with ~3 fold resistance to melphalan and cross-resistance to other alkylating agents[38] and a melphalan-resistant ovarian carcinoma cell line[60] showed enhanced removal of drug-induced ISCs. Similar observations have been reported in clinical material, e.g., where lymphocytes from previously-treated patients with melphalan-resistant chronic lymphocytic leukemia (CLL) exhibited an increased rate of removal of melphalan-induced ISCs compared with lymphocytes from untreated patients[61]. Similarly, the melphalan resistant WSU-CLL human B lymphoid cell line showed faster removal of ISCs than melphalan-sensitive WIL2 cells[62].

3.3 Cyclophosphamide Analogs

Dong *et al.*[41] studied the repair of 4-hydroperoxycyclophosphamide (4HC)-induced ISCs in parental versus 4HC-resistant human medulloblastoma cell lines. The 4HC-resistant D283 Med (4-HCR) line exhibits multifactorial resistance involving at least three mechanisms[63]; (i) increased ALDH activity, (ii) elevated glutathione levels, and (iii) enhanced DNA repair, as illustrated by the more efficient removal of 4HC-induced ISCs from the c-*myc* gene[41]. A similar multifactorial resistance to 4HC was apparent in an *in vitro* model for acquired resistance to cyclophosphamide analogs in human chronic myeloid leukemia (CML)[64,65] (see chapter 11 of this volume by Drs. B. Andersson and D. Murray). These studies compared the parental KBM7/B5 CML cell line with its derivative 4HC-resistant line, B5-180[3]. A major component of the B5-180[3] phenotype derived from ALDH elevation. The second major component of 4HC resistance in these cells appeared to reflect the differential processing of DNA damage by sensitive and resistant cells, i.e., to increased repair or tolerance[64].

Subsequent measurements indicated that B5-180[3] cells may indeed repair drug-induced global ISCs somewhat faster than the parental cells[65].

3.4 Gene-specific Repair

The gene-specific or transcription-coupled repair (TCR) of DNA damage may be an important determinant of tumor-cell resistance to chemotherapeutic drugs that might not be detected by "global" (i.e., genome-wide) repair measurements. For example, human ovarian cancer cells with acquired resistance to cisplatin performed gene-specific repair of ISCs more efficiently than parental cells while showing either no[57] or modest[56] alteration in their ability to repair global DNA damage. Similarly, two cisplatin-resistant murine leukemia lines displayed no difference in global repair of ISCs while showing enhanced repair of ISCs in the *DHFR* gene as compared with the parental cells[66]. Similar data have been reported with alkylating agents such as 4HC[41] (section 3.3) and with new-generation platinating agents. For example, the ability to remove drug-DNA adducts from the N-*ras* gene induced by JM216, an oral platinating agent entering Phase III clinical trials, was greater in ovarian carcinoma cells with acquired or intrinsic drug resistance than in drug-sensitive cells[67]. Not surprisingly, given the multifactorial nature of drug resistance, not all cisplatin-resistant cells show significant alterations in the repair of DNA damage in non-transcribed or transcribed genes[68].

Accounting for gene-specific repair is also important when comparing cell lines derived from tumors of different histological types. Thus, testicular tumor lines showed much reduced repair of cisplatin-DNA adducts in the global genome, in the actively transcribed N-*ras* gene, and in the inactive $CD3\delta$ gene, when compared with bladder cancer lines[69]. These data support the suggestion[51] that inefficient DNA repair may contribute to the drug sensitivity of testicular tumor cells.

3.5 Caveats

"Direct" measurements of the repair of DNA lesions in drug-treated cells can be difficult to interpret unequivocally because the populations of parental and resistant cells are inevitably differentially compromised in terms of their survival and other biological responses. For example, if the drug concentrations are selected to produce similar levels of cell killing in the two cell types, the resistant line will have greater initial levels of DNA damage to contend with. Conversely, if the drug concentrations are selected to be iso-effective for DNA damage induction, this will result in greater cytotoxicity towards the parental cells. An excellent discussion of such factors can be found elsewhere[56]. Such data must therefore be viewed with some caution in the absence of supporting evidence using other approaches.

4. SURROGATE ASSAYS WHERE AN EXOGENOUS DNA SEQUENCE IS DAMAGED AND REACTIVATED BY A HOST (TUMOR) CELL

Viral and plasmid probes have been widely used to characterize the DNA repair proficiency of human cells. Such assays led to the discovery that some human tumor cell lines lack the ability to effect the AGT-mediated repair of O^6-methylguanine[70], the first demonstration of a tumor-specific repair defect. A major advantage of such host-cell reactivation (HCR) assays is that the human (host) cells are not exposed directly to the drug, thereby circumventing the above-mentioned problems associated with different levels of dying/degrading cells that are inherent to assays measuring DNA damage *per se*. This does not preclude direct exposure of the host cell to the drug if information on the activation of cellular responses is desired[71]. Another important feature of HCR assays is that the various host cells contend with an equal amount of DNA damage. A potential limitation is that not all repair factors may operate efficiently on non-genomic DNA lesions.

In HCR assays, the probe molecule is treated with an agent that produces DNA damage that is removed by the particular repair pathway under investigation. For example, infectious adenovirus can be treated with UV light to produce "bulky" DNA lesions, with psoralen plus near-UV light to produce ISCs, or with monofunctional alkylating agents to produce methylated bases. The damaged virus is then assayed for its ability to form plaques on cultures of various host cell types. Because the virus depends entirely on the host cell for repair factors, host cells that are defective in a specific repair factor tend to poorly support the plaquing of adenovirus treated with an agent that produces lesions that require that factor for their repair.

4.1 UV-irradiated Virus or Plasmid Probes for NER

To assess their functional NER capability, cells can be assayed for their ability to reactivate UV-irradiated adenovirus (UV-Ad)[72,73]. An example of the use of this assay to detect defects in NER is shown in Figure 1 for members of a panel of human malignant glioma cell lines. Of the 24 glioma lines studied, 23 had repair characteristics that were indistinguishable from normal fibroblasts. Only one glioma line, M085K1, showed an impaired ability to reactivate UV-Ad. M085K1 cells were also unusual in that they exhibited a 2-component reactivation curve. A similar 2-component curve was observed when UV-Ad was plaqued on three human colon tumor lines, LOVO, DLD-1 and SW620[74]. Two of these lines, LOVO and DLD-1, are defective in MMR; SW620 is proficient in MMR but lacks the AGT protein. These 2-component viral inactivation curves may reflect a defect in the TCR of UV-induced DNA damage that is also characteristic of CS cells[75].

Interestingly, the M085K1 glioma line does appear to lack MMR activity (R. Day and D. Murray, unpublished data).

UV-Ad reactivation assays have been developed that do not depend on plaque formation. For example, adenovirus containing either a *CAT* (chloramphenicol acetyltransferase) or *SEAP* (secreted alkaline phosphatase) reporter gene under the control of a strong constitutive promoter can be used to measure DNA repair in human cells[76]. HCR activity in cells that do not support plaque formation can be monitored by quantitating viral replication[77] or using an adenovirus containing the *lacZ* gene inserted in place of the viral *E1* gene[71]. An alternative to adenovirus is to use a UV-irradiated plasmid that can be expressed in mammalian cells[78].

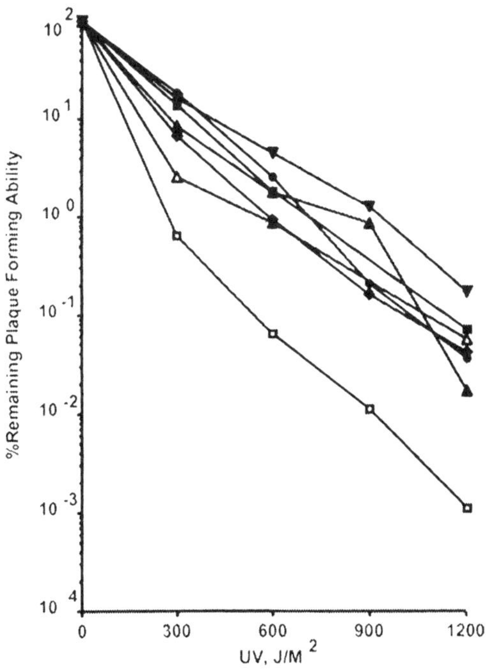

Figure 1. NER capability of selected members of a panel of human malignant glioma cell lines derived by Allalunis-Turner and colleagues[192] as indicated by their ability to reactivate UV-irradiated adenovirus. Of 24 glioma lines studied only one, M085K1 (□), showed an impaired NER capability (R. Day, J. Meservy and D. Murray, unpublished data).

4.2 Reactivation or Repair of DNA Probes Treated With Cisplatin

One of the attractions of using UV-irradiated probes is that they report exclusively on NER activity. The downside of this simplicity is that few anticancer agents exert their cytotoxicity exclusively via NER-repairable lesions. Rather, most of the drugs of interest here also cause ISCs, lesions that require different enzymatic factors for their repair (section 2.2). Some investigators have therefore used anticancer drugs themselves, most commonly cisplatin, to damage the probe molecule. Mammalian cells can indeed reactivate cisplatin-treated viruses or plasmids. The interpretation of such data is, however, complicated by the inevitability that the assay will report on *all* lesions that can contribute to probe inactivation and that can be reactivated by the host cell. The extent of probe reactivation may therefore be skewed towards repair responses such as NER. This is clearly illustrated in studies by Sheibani and colleagues[79], who used the pRSVcat plasmid treated with cisplatin to demonstrate a partial role for increased DNA repair capability in the *in vitro*-induced cisplatin resistance of murine leukemia L1210 cells. Rodent cells with mutations the *ERCC1*, *XPD* and *XPF* genes were uniformly ~8 fold sensitive in this HCR assay; however, in terms of cell killing, rodent *XPD* mutants exhibit only modest sensitivity to cisplatin, whereas the *ERCC1* and *XPF* mutants are *extremely* sensitive. This suggests that NER-repairable lesions such as intrastrand crosslinks are responsible for most of the inhibition of *CAT* expression and its subsequent reactivation. A similar conclusion was reached in a study of the reactivation of cisplatin-treated pSVgpt plasmid by cisplatin-sensitive and -resistant rodent cells[80]. The observation that the reactivation of cisplatin-Ad was reduced in *ERCC1*-deficient UV20 hamster cells, but only by ~2 fold, further suggests that HCR assays are relatively insensitive to differences in ISC repair capability[71].

With respect to human tumor cells, HeLa cells with laboratory-induced resistance to cisplatin showed an ~3 fold increased ability to reactivate a cisplatin-damaged plasmid containing *CAT* reporter sequences[81,82]. These cells also displayed an increased initial rate of repair of cisplatin-DNA adducts when measured by AAS or immunoassays[83,84]. Parker and colleagues[85] studied the human ovarian cancer cell line A2780 and its ~13 fold resistant A2780/CP70 variant, which was developed by continuous stepwise exposure to cisplatin. (This was felt to reasonably approximate the clinical problem caused by repeated drug exposure). Increased DNA repair appeared to be an important mechanism of resistance in A2780/CP70 cells; not only did the resistant cells effect the global genomic repair of Pt-DNA adducts more efficiently (~2 fold as indicated by AAS) but they also showed ~2 fold increased HCR of cisplatin-treated pRSVcat plasmid. The clinical unresponsiveness of non-small cell lung cancer to chemotherapy (relative to small cell lung cancer) has also been associated with elevated DNA repair capacity, based on the ability of primary tumor cultures and established cell lines to reactivate cisplatin-treated pRSV-CAT plasmid[86]. Given the multifactorial nature of resistance to platinating and alkylating agents, however, it is not surprising that some studies show conflicting results. Thus, overall DNA repair capability among a panel of eight human cancer cell lines as determined by HCR of cisplatin-treated pGL2 (luciferase) plasmid did not correlate with the sensitivity of these cells to either cisplatin or melphalan[87]. Similarly, there was no alteration of DNA repair activity in human melanoma (MeWo) sub-lines selected *in vitro* for resistance to cisplatin and fotemustine, based on HCR of pRSVcat plasmid exposed to either UV, fotemustine, or cisplatin[88].

Another type of plasmid-based assay applicable to clinical material involves incubating a UV- or cisplatin-treated plasmid with cellular protein extracts and monitoring the level of repair re-synthesis in the plasmid[89,90]. For example, marked (~10 fold) differences in the ability to repair cisplatin-treated pBluescript KS$^+$ plasmid DNA were observed among protein extracts of biopsy material from chemotherapy-naïve human ovarian tumors[91]. Repair in fresh malignant lymphocytes from CLL patients (7 untreated, 11 who had received chemotherapy) was similarly monitored using cisplatin-treated pBS plasmid[92]. The only extracts that exhibited measurable repair activity were obtained from treated patients, suggesting that chemotherapy might increase the NER status of tumor cells. This assay was also used to examine extracts from human testicular germ cell tumors which, as noted in section 3.1, are very sensitive to cisplatin and repair Pt-DNA adducts poorly. Consistent with this phenotype, such extracts displayed a limited ability to carry out the incision steps of NER[51]. Extracts from cisplatin-resistant human ovarian cancer cells exhibited ~3 fold greater ability to repair a plasmid substrate containing a site-specific cisplatin adduct than extracts from parental A2780 cells[93].

Several investigators have studied the repair of cisplatin-treated adenovirus (cisplatin-Ad) by human cells. Parsons *et al.*[94] observed no difference among a panel of human tumor cell lines of varying cisplatin sensitivity with respect to their ability to reactivate cisplatin-Ad. Similarly, Maynard and colleagues[95] found that only some DNA repair defects could be detected by HCR of cisplatin-Ad. Whereas XP fibroblasts and cisplatin-sensitive ovarian tumor cells were deficient in reactivating cisplatin-Ad, a teratoma cell line known to be deficient in the repair of both intrastrand crosslinks and ISCs (section 3.1) showed no defect in cisplatin-Ad reactivation. Parental (2008) and cisplatin-resistant (C13*) human ovarian carcinoma cells also reactivated cisplatin-Ad with similar efficiency[71].

4.3 HCR of DNA Probes Treated with Other Agents that Induce ISCs

Assessing the ISC-repair competency of tumor cells by their ability to reactivate DNA probes that have been reacted with drugs such as melphalan, mechlorethamine or cyclophosphamide analogs (which induce a significant number of ISCs) is an attractive concept. Unfortunately, it is nowhere near as straightforward as for UV-HCR assays for NER. For example, Dean *et al.*[96] examined the ability of human cell lines to reactivate the pCMVcat plasmid treated with mechlorethamine. As in an earlier study of the reactivation by human fibroblasts of adenovirus treated with psoralen plus near-UV light[97], it was concluded that there was little or no reactivation of

ISCs and that non-ISC lesions such as intrastrand crosslinks were responsible for the observed probe reactivation.

Consideration of these data and those described above for cisplatin suggests that HCR assays can not generally discriminate differences in ISC repair among cell lines. There are a number of potential reasons for this. First, the machinery involved in ISC repair might not assemble on the probe sequence, perhaps because there are damage recognition/verification factors that are specific for chromatin. Second, lesions other than ISCs can contribute to inactivation/reactivation of the probe. A third factor is the multiplicity of infection with the probe molecule. Intuitively, for proper ISC repair to occur, the multiplicity must be sufficiently high to allow genetic recombination between viral genomes[71,96,98]. The available data in this regard are contradictory. Thus, a high multiplicity of probe infection appeared to be necessary for the reactivation of psoralen/UV-induced ISCs in SV40 DNA by human fibroblasts[99,100], whereas the reactivation of mechlorethamine-treated HSV-I by human cells did not depend on the multiplicity of infection[101].

Regardless of whether or not ISCs in non-integrated probe molecules are repaired by the host cell, it is apparent that such assays can not systematically discriminate differences in ISC repair. This conclusion is consistent with reports such as the lack of a difference among human tumor cell lines with respect to their ability to reactivate adenovirus treated with the cyclophosphamide analog mafosfamide[94]. Although one study reported that a melphalan-resistant human breast cancer cell line known to have enhanced ISC repair capability compared to the parental cells[38] showed an increased ability to reactivate melphalan-treated pRSV-CAT plasmid[102], it is possible that this reflects the HCR of NER-repairable lesions[103] rather than of ISCs. Assays involving recombination between different probe molecules[21] may ultimately prove to be useful for the examination of ISC repair in clinical material.

5. LEVELS OF DNA REPAIR GENE TRANSCRIPTS OR PROTEINS IN TUMOR CELLS

The successful cloning of a number of DNA repair genes since the mid-1980s generated molecular probes that were rapidly applied to the study of laboratory and clinical models of drug resistance. Because of their simplicity and applicability to biopsy material (because the material does not need to be viable), slot/Northern blotting and RT-PCR are widely used approaches to measuring levels of repair gene transcripts. Because many useful anticancer agents induce DNA damage that is repaired (at least in part) by the NER pathway, and because *ERCC1* was the first NER gene to be cloned[104], *ERCC1* expression has been extensively studied in the context of drug resistance in a variety of tumor types, and especially those which are commonly treated with drugs such as cisplatin and melphalan.

5.1 Cisplatin

High pre-treatment levels of *ERCC1* mRNA in freshly-obtained malignant tissue from chemotherapy-naïve ovarian cancer patients have been associated with a poor response to cisplatin/carboplatin-based chemotherapy[105,106]. Mean pre-treatment *ERCC1* mRNA levels in tumor cells from 26 patients were ~2.6 fold higher in non-responders than in responders[105]. Mean tumor *XPD* mRNA levels, on the other hand, were comparable in the two groups of patients. One patient who developed clinical drug resistance showed an increase in *ERCC1* mRNA in their leukocytes (5 fold) and tumor cells (10 fold) following 6 cycles of chemotherapy as compared with pre-treatment levels. In a subsequent study, pre-treatment *XPA* and *ERCC1* mRNA levels in fresh ovarian cancer tissue from 28 patients were negatively correlated with tumor response to chemotherapy[106]. Tumors that responded to treatment had low *XPA* expression regardless of their *ERCC1* level, whereas clinically-resistant tumors showed concurrent high expression of both *XPA* and *ERCC1*.

Such data led Reed[107] to propose a model in which disruption of the normal coordination of NER is an important etiological factor in the development and malignant progression of ovarian cancer. One feature of this disruption is highly variable splicing of the *ERCC1* transcript[107,108]. Alterations in NER gene copy number are rare[109]. Reed has further proposed that the primary mechanism of tumor-cell resistance in ovarian cancer is increased NER capability[107]. Specifically, resistant tumors are suggested to re-establish the coordinated expression of their NER genes that is characteristic of normal tissues.

In contrast to the above-mentioned data, Codegoni and colleagues[110] reported a weak ***positive*** correlation between *ERCC1* mRNA expression and outcome (survival) following cisplatin-based chemotherapy among 33 previously untreated ovarian cancer patients. Thus, high *ERCC1* mRNA levels do not universally predict for poor responsiveness to platinating agents in this disease. Potential reasons for this discrepancy will be discussed in section 5.5. These authors also found no correlation between response to chemotherapy and the expression of two other DNA repair genes, *AGT* and *MPG*[110]. Although ectopic expression of the BER enzyme MPG *can* result in resistance to alkylating agents such as chloroethylnitrosoureas[111] and methyl methane sulfonate (MMS)[112], its importance in the clinically relevant response of tumor cells to drugs such as cisplatin and melphalan is questionable[113].

As in the studies of Reed and colleagues[105–107] with ovarian tumors, a high pre-treatment *ERCC1* mRNA titer in primary gastric adenocarcinoma-derived biopsy material was also associated with a poor patient response to cisplatin/5-fluorouracil chemotherapy[114] and remained predictive after correcting for the expression of thymidylate synthase, a known independent predictor of response to 5-fluorouracil-containing regimens.

Another perspective on the importance of repair factors in drug resistance has been to study cells derived from tumor types that differ in their clinical response to chemotherapy. For example, as was noted in sections 3.1 and 4.2, testicular germ cell tumors are clinically very responsive to cisplatin-based combination chemotherapy, and individual tumor cells repair Pt-DNA adducts poorly and display a deficiency in performing the incision step of NER in a cell-free assay[51]. Testicular tumor cells were found to contain normal levels of most NER proteins (compared with known repair-proficient cells) but to have low levels of the XPA and ERCC1-XPF proteins[51]. Low XPA levels could explain the poor repair capability of these tumors, as well as their sensitivity to cisplatin. Similarly, parental and cisplatin-resistant cells derived from an ovarian carcinoma line (SKOV-3 and SKOV-3/DXR10) expressed much higher levels of *ERCC1* mRNA (up to 50 fold) than testicular teratoma cells (SuSa and SuSa/DXR10)[115]. *XPB* mRNA expression was similar in all four cell types. The drug-resistant teratoma (but not ovarian cancer) cells showed ~2 fold increased titers of *ERCC1* mRNA relative to the parental cells.

Still another avenue has been to study panels of tumor cell lines derived from either a single histological tumor type or from unrelated tumor types. Thus, *ERCC1* mRNA levels in a panel of fifteen early-passage cervical tumor cell lines were positively correlated with the cells' resistance to cisplatin [116], whereas *ERCC1* mRNA levels were ***not*** predictive of *in vitro* resistance to cisplatin among a panel of eight unrelated human tumor cell lines[87]. It is of interest to note that the mRNA levels of *ERCC1* (and indeed other NER genes) in the latter study did not correlate with the cells' DNA repair capability as determined by HCR of a cisplatin-treated plasmid[87]; similarly, among selected members of the above-mentioned panel of cervical carcinoma cell lines there was no obvious relationship between *ERCC1* mRNA levels[116] and the cells' NER capability as evidenced by HCR of UV-Ad (D. Murray and R. A. Britten, unpublished data). Elevated constitutive *ERCC1* mRNA levels were also significantly associated with cisplatin resistance in the A2780/C-series human ovarian cancer model system[93] that had previously been shown to exhibit a number of manifestations of elevated DNA repair capability[55]. Although these cell lines, which were established by exposing A2780 cells to incrementally increasing concentrations of cisplatin, represent an exaggerated model of drug resistance, they have proven highly instructive with respect to potential mechanisms that might be operating clinically. Thus, several NER gene transcripts (e.g., *ERCC1* (~3 fold), *XPA*, *XPB*, *XPC*, and *XPG* (all ~1.4 fold)) were constitutively over-expressed in the most resistant line, C200, compared with parental A2780 cells[93]; constitutive mRNA levels of *RPA* and *XPD* were not elevated.

5.2 Melphalan and Mechlorethamine

An initial study of five CLL patients who developed clinical resistance to melphalan (following treatment with chlorambucil and/or cyclophosphamide) indicated 2-3 fold higher levels of the 1.1-kb *ERCC1* transcript in their lymphocytes than did five melphalan-responsive patients[117]. As was noted above for ovarian tumors, these CLL cells exhibited marked alternative splicing of the *ERCC1* transcript. The activity of MPG, when corrected for cell proliferation, did not differ between the lymphocytes from the two groups of patients. It is apparent in this study, however, that 1 of the 5 resistant patients had unusually high *ERCC1* mRNA levels that might have been largely responsible for the observed overall significance of the data set. In fact, when this study was later expanded to include lymphocytes from 11 untreated and 12 treated/resistant CLL patients, it was apparent that resistance to melphalan was ***not*** significantly associated with altered expression of *ERCC1*, *XPD* or polymerase β mRNAs[118]. Furthermore, there was no difference in the levels of ERCC1 protein between melphalan-sensitive and -resistant CLL B-lymphocytes. It should be noted, however, that repair-gene transcript levels in two of the resistant patients were markedly elevated, suggesting that a sub-group of these patients may indeed have a drug-resistant phenotype caused by elevated expression of repair genes. The importance of DNA repair in the response of CLL cells to alkylating agents was recently summarized[119].

Studies using established human tumor cell lines also indicate an inconsistent relationship between NER gene expression and melphalan resistance. For example, a melphalan-resistant ovarian carcinoma line that exhibited an increased rate of removal of drug-induced ISCs also displayed increased levels of *ERCC1* and *XPD* mRNA[60]. In contrast, *ERCC1* mRNA levels were not altered in melphalan-resistant breast cancer cells that showed enhanced ISC repair capability[38] and ability to reactivate melphalan-treated pRSV-CAT plasmid[102] compared to the parental cells. The two breast cancer lines also had similar levels of *ERCC1*, *XPD*, *XPB*, and polymerase β mRNA and of ERCC1, AP endonuclease, poly(ADP-ribose) polymerase (PARP), and MPG protein[102]. Similarly, *ERCC1* (and indeed *XPA*, *XPB*, *XPC*, *XPD* and *XPF*) mRNA levels were not predictive of *in vitro* resistance to melphalan among a panel of human tumor lines[87].

5.3 Cyclophosphamide and its Analogs

Dong and colleagues[120] looked for possible genetic alterations that might underlie the preferential repair of ISCs by the 4HC-resistant D-283 Med (4-HCR) medulloblastoma cell line (section 3.3). *XPF* mRNA and PARP levels were similar in the two cell lines, whereas *ERCC1* mRNA levels were ~2 fold ***lower*** in the resistant cells. Thus, while there are differences between the parental and resistant lines, they do not readily explain the enhanced ISC repair observed in the latter cells. In fact, the most obvious difference between these cell lines was that AGT levels in the resistant line were ~6 fold elevated compared with the parental line. However, as noted in section 7, AGT should have little impact on 4HC-induced ISCs. AGT may in fact be a factor in resistance to cyclophosphamide analogs such as 4HC, but because of its effect on acrolein-induced DNA adducts rather than on ISCs[121]. In another laboratory model of cyclophosphamide resistance associated with an enhanced ability to tolerate 4HC-induced ISCs, namely the 4HC-resistant B5-180[3] CML cell line[64,65], *ERCC1* mRNA levels were only modestly increased compared with the parental B5 line.

5.4 Chemotherapeutic Nitrosoureas

Abnormal *ERCC1* and *XPD* gene copy numbers were observed in 11 of 24 brain tumor specimens obtained from patients prior to treatment; however, these abnormalities were not predictive of the subsequent response to chemotherapy (primarily nitrosourea-based, although another alkylating agent, procarbazine, as well as the vinca alkaloid vincristine, was also given)[122]. Such findings, combined with reports that malignant brain tissues show disregulated expression of NER genes compared with non-malignant tissues[123,124], have led to the suggestion that, like ovarian cancers, the disruption of NER may be an early event in the evolution of some brain tumors[107]. Such a predisposing NER deficit is not apparent in the data shown in Figure 1, however, where 23 of 24 human malignant glioma cell lines had normal ability to reactivate UV-Ad.

5.5 Caveats

The fact that studies with established tumor cell lines even from the same tumor type and treated with the same drug show contributions from DNA repair to resistance that range from minimal to total is not surprising, given the number of potential mechanisms involved and the multifactorial nature of resistance[46]. Thus, each individual drug-resistant cell line will have its own "signature" of molecular alterations. What is perhaps surprising is the variability among data reported for clinical material of the same tumor type obtained from patients undergoing similar treatment protocols, notably ovarian cancers treated with platinating agent-based combination chemotherapy[105,110]. What should be being sampled in such studies is a cross-section of all resistance mechanisms that might contribute in that particular disease, which to a first approximation should be similar in each cohort of patients. Obvious factors to consider include potential differences in: (i) genetic/etiologic factors in the different patient groups; (ii) the exact combination chemotherapy protocol used; and (iii) the end-points used to assess patient response. For example, in a study of gastric cancer tissue[114], it was unclear whether the poor clinical response of patients whose tumors had high *ERCC1* mRNA levels resulted from tumor-cell resistance to the chemotherapy or from a more aggressive tumor biology. In fact, as noted above, a relationship between the loss of DNA repair capability and malignant progression has been suggested for ovarian and brain cancers[107]. The increased mutation rate in MMR-deficient tumors has also been suggested to contribute to the clinical aggressiveness of primary tumors and their metastases[30] as well as to drug resistance (section 6).

Significantly, many studies that report on mRNA expression lack direct measurements of repair proteins or of the functional DNA repair capability of the tumor cells. It is not guaranteed that such mRNA levels will always have a direct connection to the tumor cells' actual ability to repair DNA damage. Indeed, among eight members of the panel of cervical carcinoma cell lines discussed in section 5.1, there was no clear relationship between *ERCC1* mRNA and ERCC1 protein levels[116], nor was there a major difference in the ability of cisplatin-resistant versus -sensitive cells to perform NER as evidenced by HCR of UV-Ad (D. Murray and R. A. Britten, unpublished data).

Finally, it should be noted that the studies referred to above generally relate to the constitutive pre-treatment expression of DNA repair genes/proteins. A number of studies indicate that the expression of some NER genes/proteins can be induced by drugs such as cisplatin *in vitro*[107,125–127]. The consequences of such events remain to be established.

6. MISMATCH REPAIR

The MMR proteins, in addition to correcting replicative mismatches, recognize and bind to some types of DNA adducts induced by chemotherapy agents such as cisplatin and carboplatin[29]. Rather than repairing such adducts, however, the MMR complex appears to act as a DNA damage sensor (recognizing either the damaged bases themselves or the mismatch that results from attempted replication across the lesion), followed by events (which are poorly understood) that generate a pro-apoptotic signal. Paradoxically, the ***loss*** of MMR can therefore result in tumor-cell ***resistance*** to some chemotherapy agents because the apoptotic machinery is not activated.

Curiously, it has been reported that MMR-proficient and -deficient clones of the HCT116 human colorectal adenocarcinoma cell line removed global Pt-DNA adducts at equal rates, although the deficient cells showed superior HCR of a cisplatin-damaged plasmid carrying the luciferase gene[128].

Information with respect to other antitumor alkylating agents is scant. Some MMR-deficient cells display resistance to procarbazine and busulfan[29,129]. However, the evidence to date indicates that melphalan and the cyclophosphamide analog perfosfamide are not differentially cytotoxic to MMR-proficient and -deficient tumor cells[29,130], suggesting that the major DNA adducts produced by these agents are not recognized by the MMR complex. It has been suggested that the MMR proteins may recognize ISCs induced by some drugs[29], but this needs to be clearly established. It should be noted that the parental and 4HC-resistant medulloblastoma cell lines referred to in sections 3.3 and 5.3 were ***both*** deficient in the MMR protein MutLα[120], suggesting that alterations in MMR did not contribute to cyclophosphamide resistance in that particular model.

7. AGT

AGT is an important determinant of tumor-cell response to certain alkylating agents that produce O^6-alkyl guanine adducts and to some extent O^4-alkyl thymine. AGT also repairs 2-chloroethyl-, benzyl- and pyridyloxobutyl-adducts[26]. Many studies have examined the impact of AGT levels on the chemotherapeutic nitrosoureas such as BCNU, which is widely used for the treatment of gliomas. AGT protects against BCNU-induced cytotoxicity by removing the O^6-alkyl guanine mono-adducts before these can react with a nucleophilic group on the opposite strand to form an ISC[23]. Once an ISC is formed, AGT plays no further role. The alkylated AGT protein is rapidly degraded by the ubiquitin/proteasome system[26].

A large body of evidence has implicated AGT in tumor-cell resistance to chemotherapeutic nitrosoureas and alkylating agents in a variety of model systems, and especially brain tumors[26,27,70,131–139]. Clinical studies also support a role for AGT in the response of brain tumors to BCNU[140,141]. Studies with clinical biopsy material likewise suggest that high AGT levels may contribute to the resistance of ovarian cancers to nitrosourea chemotherapy[142].

Several investigators have examined the role of AGT in the cytotoxicity of other classes of anticancer drugs, although there is no clear consensus in this regard[23]. Thus, AGT levels in tumor tissues from 20 ovarian cancer patients were negatively correlated with response to postoperative cisplatin-cyclophosphamide combination chemotherapy in one study[143], whereas another study reported no correlation between AGT expression and the response of ovarian cancer patients to platinating agent-based chemotherapy with or without doxorubicin and cyclophosphamide[110]. As noted elsewhere[23], these studies were confounded by the use of multiple (alkylating) agent therapy. Equally conflicting results have been reported using human tumor xenografts[144,145]. AGT does appear to be involved in resistance to cyclophosphamide, but this effect is related to the acrolein metabolite of cyclophosphamide rather than to drug-induced ISCs[23,121,146,147].

Cells lacking both AGT and MMR activity are more resistant to alkylating agents than cells lacking AGT alone[29,148,149]. It appears that MMR-proficient cells erroneously attempt to repair the O^6-methylguanine-thymine mismatches introduced during DNA replication. In the absence of AGT, such cells may be trapped in a futile repair cycle that leads to cytotoxicity. In MMR-deficient cells, there would be no attempt to repair these mismatches, and the cells can complete DNA replication (albeit with elevated mutation rates).

8. DNA DAMAGE TOLERANCE MECHANISMS IN DRUG RESISTANCE

In several instances, an increased ability of drug-resistant cells to "tolerate" DNA damage has been described which is not directly associated with a primary increase in the cells' ability to repair drug-induced DNA damage *per se*[150]. Several potential mechanisms for such tolerance effects were discussed in earlier sections. For example, the role of the loss of proteins that recognize DNA damage, such as the MMR proteins (section 6) and the HMG-domain family of proteins[151], in generating low-level cisplatin resistance by increasing the cell's ability to tolerate Pt-DNA lesions has been clearly recognized. The extension of this mechanism to other drugs is uncertain. Alterations in pathways that detect such damage and transmit signals to the apoptotic machinery may also contribute to tolerance[152,153].

Chapter 12 in this volume by Drs. M. Andreeff and M. Konopleva details changes in the apoptotic machinery itself that can lead to a drug-resistant phenotype. Replicative bypass, defined as the ability of the DNA replication machinery to synthesize past a DNA lesion, has also been demonstrated to occur for cisplatin[154–156]. Subsequent repair of the lesion could then be completed at the G_2 cell-cycle checkpoint prior to mitosis. The process of trans-lesion DNA synthesis was enhanced in two cisplatin-resistant human ovarian cancer cell lines[155].

The G_2 checkpoint itself provides a mechanism of tolerance to alkylating and platinating agents by providing time for lesions such as drug-induced ISCs to be repaired prior to mitosis[157]. In melphalan-treated human myeloma (RPMI 8226) cells, for example, resumption of cell progression following arrest at the G_2 checkpoint correlated with the removal of ISCs[158]. Similarly, melphalan resistant WSU-CLL B lymphoid cells underwent a progressive arrest in G_1 and G_2 phases following melphalan treatment, whereas WIL2 (melphalan sensitive) cells did not[62]. The ability to arrest in G_2 until DNA repair is completed was suggested to explain the resistance of a human lymphoma cell line to mechlorethamine[159]. Similarly, the sensitivity of some rodent cells to mafosfamide has been related to their failure to activate cell-cycle checkpoints[160].

Another aspect of resistance to chemotherapeutic drugs is the role of growth factors and signal transduction pathways[5,161]. These mechanisms have been reviewed in chapter 5 of this volume by Dr. S Grant and colleagues. Factors that promote proliferation will tend to block apoptosis[162] and might also influence drug sensitivity by altering the cells' DNA repair status[163]. Fan and Bertino[164], using an HCR assay involving cisplatin-treated pGL3luc plasmid, showed that the induction of p53 in SaOS-2 human osteosarcoma cells could enhance the repair of cisplatin-induced DNA damage. These authors suggested that the combined effect of p53-mediated apoptosis and DNA repair is a major determinant of drug resistance. In a study of drug-naïve sub-populations of the A2780 human ovarian cancer cell line, intrinsic resistance to cisplatin was associated with a defect in MMR (specifically, with silencing of the hMLH1 gene); however, the presence of an accompanying p53 mutation was the dominant determinant of cisplatin resistance in these cells[165].

9. DNA REPAIR INHIBITION

Because DNA repair can clearly contribute to tumor-cell resistance to chemotherapeutic platinating and alkylating agents, it is axiomatic that repair pathways are targets for pharmacological inhibition with the purpose of overcoming this resistance. The status of repair-inhibitor studies was recently reviewed[166], and will only be illustrated here by reference to a few selected examples. Commonly-used inhibitors include nucleoside analogs such as fludarabine or cytarabine[167,168], hydroxyurea (an inhibitor of ribonucleotide reductase), aphidicolin (an inhibitor of DNA polymerases α and γ), 3-aminobenzamide (an inhibitor of PARP), novobiocin and etoposide (topoisomerase II inhibitors)[169]. In some cases, repair inhibition and increased drug cytotoxicity is preferential for the resistant versus sensitive/parental cell line[53].

Novel inhibitors of specific targets are being developed. Molecules with AP endonuclease activity and which incorporate a DNA-intercalating moiety can inhibit BER and sensitize L1210 cells to nitrosoureas[170]. O^6-benzylguanine, a potent inhibitor of AGT, can increase the chemotherapeutic effectiveness of chloroethylating and methylating agents that alkylate O^6-guanine in both tumor cells and xenografts[171,172]. Clinical trials of the combination of O^6-benzylguanine and BCNU are ongoing[173]. Sensitization of brain tumor xenografts to other alkylating agents, such as cyclophosphamide, has been reported in animals treated with O^6-benzylguanine[121].

In cultured human ovarian cancer cells, the expression of *ERCC1* and *XPA* mRNA and ERCC1 protein (but not *XPB* mRNA or protein) is generally inducible by cisplatin[107,125]. Pharmacological agents have been evaluated for their ability to block induction of the *ERCC1* gene. Cyclosporin A and herbimycin A (which suppress c-*fos* and c-*jun* expression, respectively) blocked the cisplatin-induced increase in *ERCC1* mRNA and sensitized A2780/CP70 human ovarian carcinoma cells to cisplatin[174].

Other approaches to chemosensitization that are potentially mediated by repair-inhibitory mechanisms involve the manipulation of growth factor signaling pathways that appear to be coupled to DNA repair pathways[175,176].

10. DNA REPAIR GENES FOR BONE MARROW CYTOPROTECTION

The primary dose-limiting toxicity of most alkylating agents is bone marrow suppression. A number of investigators have considered the possibility of increasing the resistance of normal bone marrow stem cells to alkylating agents. Could DNA repair genes be used in this context? The answer appears to be both yes and no. Increased cellular resistance to a drug will only be achieved by over-expression if the repair protein either acts by itself or is rate limiting in the pathway in which it participates. Thus, AGT has been widely considered for this purpose[148,177–180]. A retroviral vector expressing the human *AGT* gene stably protected murine bone marrow, both *in vitro* and *in vivo*, from the toxic effects of BCNU[181,182]. Similar effects have been observed following retroviral transfer of the bacterial *ada* (*AGT*) gene into murine bone marrow cells[183]. A retroviral construct expressing a chimeric protein combining two repair proteins, AGT and the BER enzyme AP endonuclease, also protected HeLa cells against BCNU and MMS[184]. A number of clinical trials of AGT gene therapy in humans are in progress.

If a repair enzyme is a component of a rate-limiting multi-protein complex, then each protein in the complex may have to be up-regulated to cause cytoprotection. Such proteins would therefore probably be poor choices for gene therapy. The difficulties involved can be illustrated with respect to ERCC1. Transfecting mammalian cells with a cloned wild-type human *ERCC1* cDNA, such that expression of *ERCC1* is far above wild-type levels, generally fails to invoke resistance to UV or to drugs such as cisplatin, mitomycin C and cyclophosphamide[14,185–188]. In one study, highly over-expressing ERCC1 in a wild-type cell line actually *sensitized* the cells to melphalan and cisplatin, presumably because it imbalances the repair pathway[187].

The difficulty in conferring cellular resistance to DNA crosslinking agents is further illustrated in studies by Grombacher *et al.*[189], who transfected rodent cells with cDNAs whose absence is known to render cells more sensitive to such drugs. Over-expression of *FANCC*, *SPHAR*, *MPG*, *SNM1* or *HA3611* (a human homolog of the yeast crosslink repair gene *SNM1*) did not invoke resistance to mafosfamide, melphalan or mitomycin C. In one study, over-expressing the BER enzyme MPG increased cellular sensitivity to alkylating agents, suggesting that the initial glycosylase step in BER is not rate limiting and that the accumulation of AP sites can be cytotoxic[190]. Further discussion of the use of BER genes in cytoprotective gene therapy can be found elsewhere[179,191].

ACKNOWLEDGMENTS

We gratefully acknowledge the support of grant RO1 CA-67270 from the NIH/NCI (USA) and of Operating Grant RI-116 from the Alberta Cancer Board Research Initiative Program.

REFERENCES

1. Sladek NE. Aldehyde dehydrogenase-mediated cellular relative insensitivity to the oxazaphosphorines. Curr Pharm Design, 5:607-625, 1999.
2. Calsou P, Salles B. Role of DNA repair in the mechanisms of cell resistance to alkylating agents and cisplatin. Cancer Chemother Pharmacol, 32:85-89, 1993.
3. Zamble DB, Lippard SJ. Cisplatin and DNA repair in cancer chemotherapy. Trends Biochem Sci, 20:435-439, 1995.
4. Chaney SG, Sancar A. DNA repair: enzymatic mechanisms and relevance to drug response. J Natl Cancer Inst, 88:1346-1360, 1996.
5. Akiyama S, Chen ZS, Sumizawa T, Furukawa T. Resistance to cisplatin. Anticancer Drug Design, 14:143-151, 1999.
6. O'Connor PM, Kohn KW. Comparative pharmacokinetics of DNA lesion formation and removal following treatment of L1210 cells with nitrogen mustards. Cancer Commun, 2:387-394, 1990.
7. Plooy ACM, van Dijk M, Lohman PHM. Induction and repair of DNA cross-links in Chinese hamster ovary cells treated with various platinum coordination compounds in relation to platinum binding to DNA, cytotoxicity, mutagenicity and antitumor activity. Cancer Res, 44:2043-2051, 1984.

8. Pinto AL, Lippard SJ. Binding of the antitumor drug cis-diamminedichloroplatinum(II) (Cisplatin) to DNA. Biochim Biophys Acta, 708:167-180, 1985.
9. Roberts JJ, Knox RJ, Pera MF, *et al.* The role of platinum-DNA interactions in the cellular toxicity and anti-tumour effects of platinum co-ordination compounds. *In:* Platinum and other metal coordination compounds in cancer chemotherapy, M Nicolini (ed.), Nijhoff, Boston, MA, 16-31, 1987.
10. Friedberg EC, Walker GC, Siede W. DNA Repair and Mutagenesis, ASM Press, Washington, DC, 1995.
11. Petit C, Sancar A. Nucleotide excision repair: from E. coli to man. Biochimie, 81:15-25, 1999.
12. Hoy CA, Thompson LH, Mooney CL, Salazar EP. Defective DNA crosslink removal in Chinese hamster cell mutants hypersensitive to bifunctional alkylating agents. Cancer Res, 45:1737-1743, 1985.
13. Sorenson CM, Eastman A. Influence of *cis*-diamminedichloroplatinum(II) on DNA synthesis and cell cycle progression in excision repair proficient and deficient Chinese hamster ovary cells. Cancer Res, 48:6703-6707, 1988.
14. Andersson BS, Sadeghi T, Siciliano MJ, *et al.* Nucleotide excision repair genes as determinants of cellular sensitivity to cyclophosphamide analogs. Cancer Chemother Pharmacol, 38:406-416, 1996.
15. Damia G, Imperatori L, Stefanini M, D'Incalci M. Sensitivity of CHO mutant cell lines with specific defects in nucleotide excision repair to different anti-cancer agents. Int J Cancer, 66:779-783, 1996.
16. Bessho T, Mu D, Sancar A. Initiation of DNA interstrand cross-link repair in humans: the nucleotide excision repair system makes dual incisions 5' to the cross-linked base and removes a 22- to 28-nucleotide-long damage-free strand. Mol Cell Biol, 17:6822-6830, 1997.
17. Kuraoka I, Kobertz WR, Ariza RR, *et al.* Repair of an interstrand DNA cross-link initiated by ERCC1-XPF repair/recombination nuclease. J Biol Chem, 275:26632-26636, 2000.
18. De Silva IU, McHugh PJ, Clingen PH, Hartley JA. Defining the roles of nucleotide excision repair and recombination in the repair of DNA interstrand cross-links in mammalian cells. Mol Cell Biol, 20:7980-7990, 2000.
19. Mu D, Bessho T, Nechev LV, *et al.* DNA interstrand cross-links induce futile repair synthesis in mammalian cell extracts. Mol Cell Biol, 20:2446-2454, 2000.
20. Thompson LH. Evidence that mammalian cells possess homologous recombinational repair pathways. Mutat Res, 363:77-88, 1996.
21. Li L, Peterson CA, Zhang X, Legerski RJ. Requirement for PCNA and RPA in interstrand crosslink-induced DNA synthesis. Nucleic Acids Res, 28:1424-1427, 2000.
22. Liu N, Lamerdin JE, Tebbs RS, *et al.* XRCC2 and XRCC3, new human Rad51-family members, promote chromosome stability and protect against DNA cross-links and other damages. Mol Cell, 1:783-793, 1998.
23. Gamcsik MP, Dolan ME, Andersson BS, Murray D. Mechanisms of resistance to the toxicity of cyclophosphamide. Curr Pharm Design, 5:587-605, 1999.
24. Caldecott K, Jeggo P. Cross-sensitivity of gamma-ray-sensitive hamster mutants to cross-linking agents. Mutat Res, 255:111-121, 1991.
25. Pegg AE, Dolan ME, Moschel RC. Structure, function, and inhibition of O^6-alkylguanine-DNA alkyltransferase. Progr Nucleic Acid Res Mol Biol, 51:167-223, 1995.
26. Pegg AE. Repair of O^6-alkylguanine by alkyltransferases. Mutat Res, 462:83-100, 2000.

27. Pegg AE. Mammalian O^6-alkylguanine-DNA alkyltransferase: regulation and importance in response to alkylating carcinogenic and therapeutic agents. Cancer Res, 50:6119-6129, 1990.
28. Karran P, Bignami M. Drug-related killings: a case of mistaken identity. Chem Biol, 3:875-879, 1996.
29. Fink D, Aebi S, Howell SB. The role of DNA mismatch repair in drug resistance. Clin Cancer Res, 4:1-6, 1998.
30. Lage H, Dietel M. Involvement of the DNA mismatch repair system in antineoplastic drug resistance. J Cancer Res Clin Oncol, 125:156-165, 1999.
31. Seeberg E, Eide L, Bjøras M. The base excision repair pathway. Trends Biochem Sci, 20:391-397, 1995.
32. Lindahl T, Karran P, Wood RD. DNA excision repair pathways. Curr Opin Genet Dev, 7:158-169, 1997.
33. Memisoglu A, Samson L. Base excision repair in yeast and mammals. Mutat Res, 451:39-51, 2000.
34. Krokan HE, Nilsen H, Skorpen F, *et al.* Base excision repair of DNA in mammalian cells. FEBS Lett, 476:73-77, 2000.
35. Wyatt MD, Allan JM, Lau AY, *et al.* 3-methyladenine DNA glycosylases: structure, function, and biological importance. Bioessays, 21:668-676, 1999.
36. Ross WE, Ewig RA, Kohn KW. Differences between melphalan and nitrogen mustard in the formation and removal of DNA cross-links. Cancer Res, 38:1502-1506, 1978.
37. De Jong S, Zijlstra JG, Timmer-Bosscha H, *et al.* Detection of DNA crosslinks in tumor cells with the ethidium bromide fluorescence assay. Int J Cancer, 37:557-561, 1986.
38. Batist G, Torres-Garcia S, Demuys J-M, *et al.* Enhanced DNA cross-link removal: The apparent mechanism of resistance in a clinically relevant melphalan-resistant human breast cancer cell line. Mol Pharmacol, 36:224-230, 1989.
39. Hartley JM, Spanswick VJ, Gander M, *et al.* Measurement of DNA cross-linking in patients on ifosfamide therapy using the single cell gel electrophoresis (comet) assay. Clin Cancer Res, 5:507-512, 1999.
40. Ball LM, Lannon CL, Langley GR, *et al.* Differential kinetics of drug resistance in human leukaemic cells measured by SCGE/CLSM. Adv Exp Med Biol, 457:501-508, 1999.
41. Dong Q, Bullock N, Ali-Osman F, *et al.* Repair analysis of 4-hydroperoxycyclophosphamide-induced DNA interstrand crosslinking of the c-*myc* gene in 4-hydroperoxycyclophosphamide-sensitive and -resistant medulloblastoma cell lines. Cancer Chemother Pharmacol, 37:242-246, 1996.
42. Grimaldi KA, Bingham JP, Hartley JA. PCR-based assays for strand-specific measurement of DNA damage and repair. I. Strand-specific quantitative PCR. Methods Mol Biol, 113:227-240, 1999.
43. Grimaldi KA, McAdam SR, Hartley JA. PCR-based assays for strand-specific measurement of DNA damage and repair. II. Single-strand ligation-PCR. Methods Mol Biol, 113:241-255, 1999.
44. Fichtinger-Schepman AM, Dijt FJ, Bedford P, *et al.* Induction and removal of cisplatin-DNA adducts in human cells in vivo and in vitro as measured by immunochemical techniques. IARC Sci Publ, 89:321-328, 1988.
45. Tilby MJ, McCartney H, Gould KA, *et al.* A monofunctional derivative of melphalan: preparation, DNA alkylation products, and determination of the specificity of monoclonal antibodies that recognize melphalan-DNA adducts. Chem Res Toxicol, 11:1162-1168, 1998.

46. Kelland LR. Preclinical perspectives on platinum resistance. Drugs, 59 Suppl 4:1-8, 2000.
47. Bedford P, Fichtinger-Schepman AM, Shellard SA, *et al.* Differential repair of platinum-DNA adducts in human bladder and testicular tumor continuous cell lines. Cancer Res, 48:3019-3024, 1988.
48. Hill BT, Scanlon KJ, Hansson J, *et al.* Deficient repair of cisplatin-DNA adducts identified in human testicular teratoma cell lines established from tumours from untreated patients. Eur J Cancer, 30A:832-837, 1994.
49. Hill BT, Shellard SA, Hosking LK, *et al.* Enhanced DNA repair and tolerance of DNA damage associated with resistance to cis-diammine-dichloroplatinum (II) after in vitro exposure of a human teratoma cell line to fractionated X-irradiation. Int J Radiat Oncol Biol Phys, 19:75-83, 1990.
50. Hill BT, Shellard SA, Fichtinger-Schepman AM, *et al.* Differential formation and enhanced removal of specific cisplatin-DNA adducts in two cisplatin-selected resistant human testicular teratoma sublines. Anticancer Drugs, 5:321-328, 1994.
51. Koberle B, Masters JR, Hartley JA, Wood RD. Defective repair of cisplatin-induced DNA damage caused by reduced XPA protein in testicular germ cell tumours. Curr Biol, 9:273-276, 1994.
52. Shellard SA, Fichtinger-Schepman AM, Lazo JS, Hill BT. Evidence of differential cisplatin-DNA adduct formation, removal and tolerance of DNA damage in three human lung carcinoma cell lines. Anticancer Drugs, 4:491-500, 1993.
53. Masuda H, Ozols RF, Lai GM, *et al.* Increased DNA repair as a mechanism of acquired resistance to cis-diamminedichloroplatinum (II) in human ovarian cancer cell lines. Cancer Res, 48:5713-5716, 1988.
54. Lai GM, Ozols RF, Smyth JF, *et al.* Enhanced DNA repair and resistance to cisplatin in human ovarian cancer. Biochem Pharmacol, 37:4597-4600, 1988.
55. Johnson SW, Swiggard PA, Handel LM, *et al.* Relationship between platinum-DNA adduct formation and removal and cisplatin cytotoxicity in cisplatin-sensitive and –resistant human ovarian cancer cells. Cancer Res, 54:5911-5916, 1994.
56. Johnson SW, Perez RP, Godwin AK, *et al.* Role of platinum-DNA adduct formation and removal in cisplatin resistance in human ovarian cancer cell lines. Biochem Pharmacol, 47:689-697, 1994.
57. Zhen W, Link CJ Jr, O'Connor PM, *et al.* Increased gene-specific repair of cisplatin interstrand cross-links in cisplatin-resistant human ovarian cancer cell lines. Mol Cell Biol, 12:3689-3698, 1992.
58. Johnson SW, Laub PB, Beesley JS, *et al.* Increased platinum-DNA damage tolerance is associated with cisplatin resistance and cross-resistance to various chemotherapeutic agents in unrelated human ovarian cancer cell lines. Cancer Res, 57:850-856, 1997.
59. Johnson SW, Ferry KV, Hamilton TC. Recent insights into platinum drug resistance in cancer. Drug Resist Updates, 1:243-254, 1998.
60. Gornati D, Zaffaroni N, Villa R, *et al.* Modulation of melphalan and cisplatin cytotoxicity in human ovarian cancer cells resistant to alkylating drugs. Anticancer Drugs, 8:509-516, 1997.
61. Torres-Garcia SJ, Cousineau L, Caplan S, Panasci L. Correlation of resistance to nitrogen mustards in chronic lymphocytic leukemia with enhanced removal of melphalan-induced DNA cross-links. Biochem Pharmacol, 38:3122-3123, 1989.
62. Pu Q, Bianchi P, Bezwoda WR. Alkylator resistance in human B lymphoid cell lines: (1). Melphalan accumulation, cytotoxicity, interstrand-DNA-crosslinks, cell cycle analysis, and glutathione content in the melphalan-sensitive B-lymphocytic cell line (WIL2) and in the melphalan-resistant B-CLL cell line (WSU-CLL). Anticancer Res, 20:2561-2568, 2000.

63. Friedman HS, Colvin OM, Kaufmann SH, *et al.* Cyclophosphamide resistance in medulloblastoma. Cancer Res, 52:5373-5378, 1992.
64. Andersson BS, Mroue M, Britten R, Murray D. The role of DNA damage in the resistance of human chronic myeloid leukemia cells to cyclophosphamide analogs. Cancer Res, 54:5394-5400, 1994.
65. Andersson BS, Mroue M, Britten RA, *et al.* Mechanisms of cyclophosphamide resistance in a human myeloid leukemia cell line. Acta Oncol, 34:247-251, 1995.
66. Petersen LN, Mamenta EL, Stevnsner T, *et al.* Increased gene specific repair of cisplatin induced interstrand crosslinks in cisplatin resistant cell lines, and studies on carrier ligand specificity. Carcinogenesis, 17:2597-2602, 1996.
67. O'Neill CF, Koberle B, Masters JR, Kelland LR. Gene-specific repair of Pt/DNA lesions and induction of apoptosis by the oral platinum drug JM216 in three human ovarian carcinoma cell lines sensitive and resistant to cisplatin. Br J Cancer, 81:1294-1303, 1999.
68. Koberle B, Payne J, Grimaldi KA, *et al.* DNA repair in cisplatin-sensitive and resistant human cell lines measured in specific genes by quantitative polymerase chain reaction. Biochem Pharmacol, 52:1729-1734,1996.
69. Koberle B, Grimaldi KA, Sunters A, *et al.* DNA repair capacity and cisplatin sensitivity of human testis tumour cells. Int J Cancer, 70:551-555, 1997.
70. Yarosh DB, Foote RS, Mitra S, Day RS III. Repair of O^6-methylguanine in DNA by demethylation is lacking in Mer^- human tumor cell strains. Carcinogenesis, 4:199-205, 1983.
71. Moorehead RA, Armstrong SG, Rainbow AJ, Singh G. Nucleotide excision repair in the human ovarian carcinoma cell line (2008) and its cisplatin-resistant variant (C13*). Cancer Chemother Pharmacol, 38:245-253, 1996.
72. Day RS III. Adenovirus: A probe for human cells deficient in DNA repair. Biosci, 31:807-813, 1981.
73. Day RS III. Use of human adenoviruses 2 and 5: Purification, plaque assay, and inactivation. *In*: DNA Repair. A Laboratory Manual of Research Procedures, Vol 1, EC Friedberg, PC Hanawalt (eds.), Marcel Dekker, New York, NY, 587-604, 1981.
74. Day RS III, Rasouli-Nia A, Meservy J, *et al.* Decreased host-cell reactivation of UV-irradiated adenovirus in human colon tumor cell lines that have normal post-UV survival. Photochem Photobiol, 70:217-227, 1999.
75. Day RS III, Ziolkowski C, DiMattina M. Decreased host cell reactivation of UV-irradiated adenovirus 5 by fibroblasts from Cockayne's syndrome patients. Photochem Photobiol, 34:603-607, 1981.
76. Valerie K, Singhal A. Host-cell reactivation of reporter genes introduced into cells by adenovirus as a convenient way to measure cellular DNA repair. Mutat Res, 336:91-100, 1995.
77. Arnold WR, Rainbow AJ. Host cell reactivation of irradiated adenovirus in UV-sensitive Chinese hamster ovary cell mutants. Mutagenesis, 11:89-94, 1996.
78. Protic-Sabljic M, Kraemer KH. Host cell reactivation by human cells of DNA expression vectors damaged by ultraviolet radiation or by acid-heat treatment. Carcinogenesis, 7:1765-1770, 1986.
79. Sheibani N, Jennerwein M, Eastman A. DNA repair in cells sensitive and resistant to *cis*-diamminedichloroplatinum (II): Host cell reactivation of damaged plasmid DNA. Biochem, 28:3120-3124, 1989.
80. Knox RJ, Lydall DA, Friedlos F, *et al.* The effect of monofunctional or difunctional platinum adducts and of various other associated DNA damage on the expression of

transfected DNA in mammalian cell lines sensitive or resistant to difunctional agents. Biochim Biophys Acta, 908:214-223, 1987.

81. Chao CC, Lee YL, Lin-Chao S. Phenotypic reversion of cisplatin resistance in human cells accompanies reduced host cell reactivation of damaged plasmid. Biochem Biophys Res Commun, 170:851-859, 1990.
82. Chao CC, Lee YL, Cheng PW, Lin-Chao S. Enhanced host cell reactivation of damaged plasmid DNA in HeLa cells resistant to cis-diamminedichloroplatinum(II). Cancer Res, 51:601-605, 1991.
83. Chao CC. Decreased accumulation as a mechanism of resistance to cis-diamminedichloroplatinum(II) in cervix carcinoma HeLa cells: Relation to DNA repair. Mol Pharmacol, 45:1137-1144, 1994.
84. Chao CC. Enhanced excision repair of DNA damage due to cis-diamminedichloroplatinum(II) in resistant cervix carcinoma HeLa cells. Eur J Pharmacol, 268:347-355, 1994.
85. Parker RJ, Eastman A, Bostick-Bruton F, Reed E. Acquired cisplatin resistance in human ovarian cancer cells is associated with enhanced repair of cisplatin-DNA lesions and reduced drug accumulation. J Clin Invest, 87:772-777, 1991.
86. Zeng-Rong N, Paterson J, Alpert L, *et al.* Elevated DNA repair capacity is associated with intrinsic resistance of lung cancer to chemotherapy. Cancer Res, 55:4760-4764, 1995.
87. Damia G, Guidi G, D'Incalci M. Expression of genes involved in nucleotide excision repair and sensitivity to cisplatin and melphalan in human cancer cell lines. Eur J Cancer, 11:1783-1788, 1998.
88. Runger TM, Emmert S, Schadendorf D, *et al.* Alterations of DNA repair in melanoma cell lines resistant to cisplatin, fotemustine, or etoposide. J Invest Dermatol, 114:34-39, 2000.
89. Wood RD, Robins P, Lindahl T. Complementation of the xeroderma pigmentosum DNA repair defect in cell-free extracts. Cell, 53:97-106, 1988.
90. Hansson J, Wood RD. Repair synthesis by human cell extracts in DNA damaged by cis- and trans-diamminedichloroplatinum(II). Nucleic Acids Res, 17:8073-8091, 1989.
91. Jones SL, Hickson ID, Harris AL, Harnett PR. Repair of cisplatin-DNA adducts by protein extracts from human ovarian carcinoma. Int J Cancer, 59:388-393, 1994.
92. Barret J-M, Calsou P, Laurent G, Salles B. DNA repair activity in protein extracts of fresh human malignant lymphoid cells. Mol Pharmacol, 49:766-771, 1996.
93. Ferry KV, Hamilton TC, Johnson SW. Increased nucleotide excision repair in cisplatin-resistant ovarian cancer cells. Role of ERCC1-XPF. Biochem Pharmacol, 60:1305-1313, 2000.
94. Parsons PG, Lean J, Kable EPW, *et al.* Relationships between resistance to cross-linking agents and glutathione metabolism, aldehyde dehydrogenase isozymes and adenovirus replication in human tumour cell lines. Biochem Pharmacol, 40:2641-2649, 1990.
95. Maynard KR, Hosking LK, Hill BT. Use of host cell reactivation of cisplatin-treated adenovirus 5 in human cell lines to detect repair of drug-treated DNA. Chem-Biol Interact, 71:353-365, 1989.
96. Dean SW, Sykes HR, Lehmann AR. Inactivation by nitrogen mustard of plasmids introduced into normal and Fanconi's anaemia cells. Mutat Res, 194:57-63, 1988.
97. Day RS III, Giuffrida AS, Dingman CW. Repair by human cells of adenovirus-2 damaged by psoralen plus near ultraviolet light treatment. Mutat Res, 33:311-320, 1975.

98. Poll EH, Abrahams PJ, Arwert F, Eriksson AW. Host-cell reactivation of cis-diamminedichloroplatinum(II)-treated SV40 DNA in normal human, Fanconi anaemia and xeroderma pigmentosum fibroblasts. Mutat Res, 132:181-187, 1984.
99. Hall JD, Scherer K. Repair of psoralen-treated DNA by genetic recombination in human cells infected with herpes simplex virus. Cancer Res, 41:5033-5038, 1981.
100. Hall JD. Repair of psoralen-induced crosslinks in cells multiply infected with SV40. Mol Gen Genet, 188:135-138, 1982.
101. Das SK. Multiplicity reactivation of alkylating agent damaged herpes simplex virus (type I) in human cells. Mutat Res, 105:15-18, 1982.
102. Yen L, Woo A, Christopoulopoulos G, *et al.* Enhanced host cell reactivation capacity and expression of DNA repair genes in human breast cancer cells resistant to bi-functional alkylating agents. Mutat Res, 337:179-189, 1995.
103. Grant DF, Bessho T, Reardon JT. Nucleotide excision repair of melphalan monoadducts. Cancer Res, 58:5196-5200, 1998.
104. van Duin M, de Wit J, Odijk H, *et al.* Molecular characterization of the human excision repair gene ERCC-1: cDNA cloning and amino acid homology with the yeast DNA repair gene RAD10. Cell, 44:913-923, 1986.
105. Dabholkar M, Bostick-Bruton F, Weber C, *et al.* ERCC1 and ERCC2 expression in malignant tissues from ovarian cancer patients. J Natl Cancer Inst, 84:1512-1517, 1992.
106. Dabholkar M, Vionnet J, Bostick-Bruton F, *et al.* Messenger RNA levels of XPAC and ERCC1 in ovarian cancer tissue correlate with response to platinum-based chemotherapy. J Clin Invest, 84:703-708, 1994.
107. Reed E. Ovarian cancer: Molecular abnormalities. *In*: Encyclopedia of Cancer, Vol. II, JR Bertino (ed.), Academic Press, San Diego, CA, 1192-1200, 1997.
108. Yu JJ, Mu C, Dabholkar M, *et al.* Alternative splicing of ERCC1 and cisplatin-DNA adduct repair in human tumor cell lines. Int J Mol Med, 1:617-620, 1988.
109. Yu JJ, Bicher A, Ma YK, *et al.* Absence of evidence for allelic loss or allelic gain for ERCC1 or for XPD in human ovarian cancer cells and tissues. Cancer Lett, 151:127-132, 2000.
110. Codegoni AM, Broggini M, Pitelli MR, *et al.* Expression of genes of potential importance in the response to chemotherapy and DNA repair in patients with ovarian cancer. Gynecol Oncol, 65:130-137, 1997.
111. Matijasevic Z, Boosalis M, Mackay W, *et al.* Protection against chloroethylnitrosourea cytotoxicity by eukaryotic 3-methyladenine DNA glycosylase. Proc Natl Acad Sci USA, 90:11855-11859, 1993.
112. Klungland A, Fairbairn L, Watson AJ, *et al.* Expression of the E. coli 3-methyladenine DNA glycosylase I gene in mammalian cells reduces the toxic and mutagenic effects of methylating agents. EMBO J, 11:4439-4444, 1992.
113. Damia G, Imperatori L, Citti L, *et al.* 3-methyladenine-DNA-glycosylase and O^6-alkyl guanine-DNA-alkyltransferase activities and sensitivity to alkylating agents in human cancer cell lines. Br J Cancer, 73:861-865, 1996.
114. Metzger R, Leichman CG, Danenberg KD, *et al.* *ERCC1* mRNA levels complement thymidylate synthase mRNA levels in predicting response and survival for gastric cancer patients receiving combination cisplatin and fluorouracil chemotherapy. J Clin Oncol, 16:309-316, 1998.
115. Taverna P, Hansson J, Scanlon KJ, Hill BT. Gene expression in X-irradiated human tumour cell lines expressing cisplatin resistance and altered DNA repair capacity. Carcinogenesis, 15:2053-2056, 1994.

116. Britten RA, Liu D, Tessier A, *et al.* ERCC1 expression as a molecular marker of cisplatin resistance in human cervical tumor cells. Int J Cancer (Predict Oncol), 89:453-457, 2000.
117. Geleziunas R, McQuillan A, Malapetsa A, *et al.* Increased DNA synthesis and repair-enzyme expression in lymphocytes from patients with chronic lymphocytic leukemia resistant to nitrogen mustards. J Natl Cancer Inst, 83:557-564, 1991.
118. Bramson J, McQuillan A, Panasci LC. DNA repair enzyme expression in chronic lymphocytic leukemia vis-a-vis nitrogen mustard drug resistance. Cancer Lett, 90:139-148, 1995.
119. Panasci L, Paiement JP, Christopoulopoulos G, *et al.* Chlorambucil drug resistance in chronic lymphocytic leukemia: the emerging role of DNA repair. Clin Cancer Res, 7:454-461, 2001.
120. Dong Q, Johnson SP, Colvin OM, *et al.* Multiple DNA repair mechanisms and alkylator resistance in the human medulloblastoma cell line D-283 Med (4-HCR). Cancer Chemother Pharmacol, 43:73-79, 1999.
121. Friedman HS, Pegg AE, Johnson SP, *et al.* Modulation of cyclophosphamide activity by O^6-alkylguanine-DNA alkyltransferase. Cancer Chemother Pharmacol, 43:80-85,1999.
122. Liang BC, Ross DA, Reed E. Genomic copy number changes of DNA repair genes ERCC1 and ERCC2 in human gliomas. J Neurooncol, 26:17-23, 1995.
123. Dabholkar MD, Berger MS, Vionnet JA, *et al.* Malignant and nonmalignant brain tissues differ in their messenger RNA expression patterns for ERCC1 and ERCC2. Cancer Res, 55:1261-1266, 1995.
124. Dabholkar MD, Berger MS, Vionnet JA, *et al.* Comparative analyses of relative ERCC3 and ERCC6 mRNA levels in gliomas and adjacent non-neoplastic brain. Mol Carcinogenesis, 17:1-7, 1996.
125. Ferry KV, Ozols RF, Hamilton TC, Johnson SW. Expression of nucleotide excision repair genes in CDDP-sensitive and resistant human ovarian cancer cell lines. Proc Amer Assoc Cancer Res, Abstract 2492, 1996.
126. Li Q, Yu JJ, Mu C, *et al.* Association between the level of ERCC-1 expression and the repair of cisplatin-induced DNA damage in human ovarian cancer cells. Anticancer Res, 20:645-652, 2000.
127. Yu JJ, Lee KB, Mu C, *et al.* Comparison of two human ovarian carcinoma cell lines (A2780/CP70 and MCAS) that are equally resistant to platinum, but differ at codon 118 of the ERCC1 gene. Int J Oncol, 16:555-560, 2000.
128. Cenni B, Kim HK, Bubley GJ, *et al.* Loss of DNA mismatch repair facilitates reactivation of a reporter plasmid damaged by cisplatin. Br J Cancer, 80:699-704, 1999.
129. Friedman HS, Johnson SP, Dong Q, *et al.* Methylator resistance mediated by mismatch repair deficiency in a glioblastoma multiforme xenograft. Cancer Res, 57:2933-2936, 1997.
130. Aebi S, Fink D, Gordon R, *et al.* Resistance to cytotoxic drugs in DNA mismatch repair-deficient cells. Clin Cancer Res, 10:1763-1767, 1997.
131. Day RS III, Ziolkowski CHJ. Human brain tumor cell strains with deficient host-cell reactivation of N-methyl-N'-nitro-N-nitrosoguanidine-damaged adenovirus 5. Nature, 279:797-799, 1979.
132. Day RS III, Ziolkowski CHJ, Scudiero DA, *et al.* Defective repair of alkylated DNA by human tumor and SV40-transformed human cell strains. Nature, 288:724-727, 1980.
133. Walker MC, Masters JR, Margison GP. O^6-alkylguanine-DNA-alkyltransferase activity and nitrosourea sensitivity in human cancer cell lines. Br J Cancer, 66:840-843, 1992.
134. Feun LG, Savaraj N, Landy HJ. Drug resistance in brain tumors. J Neurooncol, 20:165-176, 1994.

135. Lee SM, Reid H, Elder RH, *et al.* Inter- and intracellular heterogeneity of O^6-alkylguanine-DNA alkyltransferase expression in human brain tumors: possible significance in nitrosourea therapy. Carcinogenesis, 17:637-641, 1996.
136. Beith J, Hartley J, Darling J, Souhami R. DNA interstrand cross-linking and cytotoxicity induced by chloroethylnitrosoureas and cisplatin in human glioma cell lines which vary in cellular concentration of O^6-alkylguanine-DNA alkyltransferase. Br J Cancer, 75:500-505, 1997.
137. Vassal G, Boland I, Terrier-Lacombe MJ, *et al.* Activity of fotemustine in medulloblastoma and malignant glioma xenografts in relation to O^6-alkylguanine-DNA alkyltransferase and alkylpurine-DNA N-glycosylase activity. Clin Cancer Res, 4:463-468, 1998.
138. Preuss I, Thust R, Kaina B. Protective effect of O^6-methylguanine-DNA methyltransferase (MGMT) on the cytotoxic and recombinogenic activity of different antineoplastic drugs. Int J Cancer, 65:506-512, 1996.
139. Yu Z, Chen J, Ford BN, *et al.* Human DNA repair systems: An overview. Environ Mol Mutagen, 33:3-20, 1999.
140. Belanich M, Pastor M, Randall T, *et al.* Retrospective study of the correlation between the DNA repair protein alkyltransferase and survival of brain tumor patients treated with carmustine. Cancer Res, 56:783-788, 1996.
141. Jaeckle KA, Eyre HJ, Townsend JJ, *et al.* Correlation of tumor O^6 methylguanine-DNA methyltransferase levels with survival of malignant astrocytoma patients treated with bis-chloroethylnitrosourea: a Southwest Oncology Group study. J Clin Oncol, 16:3310-3315, 1998.
142. Lee SM, Harris M, Rennison J, *et al.* Expression of O^6-alkylguanine-DNA-alkyltransferase in situ in ovarian and Hodgkin's tumours. Eur J Cancer, 29A:1306-1312, 1993.
143. Chen SS, Citron M, Spiegel G, Yarosh D. O^6-methylguanine-DNA methyltransferase in ovarian malignancy and its correlation with postoperative response to chemotherapy. Gynecol Oncol, 52:172-174, 1994.
144. Mattern J, Eichhorn U, Kaina B, Volm M. O^6-methylguanine-DNA methyltransferase activity and sensitivity to cyclophosphamide and cisplatin in human lung tumor xenografts. Int J Cancer, 77:919-922, 1998.
145. D'Incalci M, Bonfanti M, Pifferi A, *et al.* The antitumour activity of alkylating agents is not correlated with the levels of glutathione, glutathione transferase and O^6-alkylguanine-DNA-alkyltransferase of human tumour xenografts. EORTC SPG and PAMM groups. Eur J Cancer, 34:1749-1755, 1998.
146. Cai Y, Wu MH, Ludeman SM, *et al.* Role of O^6-alkylguanine-DNA alkyltransferase in protecting against cyclophosphamide-induced toxicity and mutagenicity. Cancer Res, 59:3059-3063, 1999.
147. Friedman HS, Pegg AE, Johnson SP, *et al.* Modulation of cyclophosphamide activity by O^6-alkylguanine-DNA alkyltransferase. Cancer Chemother Pharmacol, 43:80-85, 1999.
148. Hansen WK, Kelley MR. Review of mammalian DNA repair and translational implications. J Pharmacol Exp Ther, 295:1-9, 2000.
149. Kawate H, Sakumi K, Tsuzuki T, *et al.* Separation of killing and tumorigenic effects of an alkylating agent in mice defective in two of the DNA repair genes. Proc Natl Acad Sci USA, 95:5116-5120, 1998.
150. Karran P, Bignami M. Self-destruction and tolerance in resistance of mammalian cells to alkylation damage. Nucleic Acids Res, 20:2933-2940, 1992.

151. Huang JC, Zamble DB, Reardon JT, *et al.* HMG-domain proteins specifically inhibit the repair of the major DNA adduct of the anticancer drug cisplatin by human excision nuclease. Proc Natl Acad Sci USA, 91:10394-10398, 1994.
152. Perez RP. Cellular and molecular determinants of cisplatin resistance. Eur J Cancer, 34:1535-1542, 1998.
153. Segal-Bendirdjian E, Mannone L, Jacquemin-Sablon A. Alteration in p53 pathway and defect in apoptosis contribute independently to cisplatin-resistance. Cell Death Differ, 5:390-400, 1998.
154. Hoffmann JS, Pillaire MJ, Maga G, *et al.* DNA polymerase beta bypasses in vitro a single d(GpG)-cisplatin adduct placed on codon 13 of the HRAS gene. Proc Natl Acad Sci USA, 92:5356-5360, 1995.
155. Mamenta EL, Poma EE, Kaufmann WK, *et al.* Enhanced replicative bypass of platinum-DNA adducts in cisplatin-resistant human ovarian carcinoma cell lines. Cancer Res, 54:3500-3505, 1994.
156. Haq R, Zanke B. Inhibition of apoptotic signaling pathways in cancer cells as a mechanism of chemotherapy resistance. Cancer Metastasis Rev, 17:233-239, 1998.
157. Meyn RE, Murray D. Cell cycle effects of alkylating agents. Pharmacol Ther, 24:147-163, 1984.
158. Fernberg JO, Lewensohn R, Skog S. Cell cycle arrest and DNA damage after melphalan treatment of the human myeloma cell line RPMI 8226. Eur J Haematol, 47:161-167, 1991.
159. O'Connor PM, Ferris DK, White GA, *et al.* Relationships between cdc2 kinase, DNA cross-linking, and cell cycle perturbations induced by nitrogen mustard. Cell Growth Differ, 3:43-52, 1992.
160. Fritz G, Hengstler JG, Kaina B. High-dose selection with mafosfamide results in sensitivity to DNA cross-linking agents: characterization of hypersensitive cell lines. Cancer Res, 57:454-460, 1997.
161. Dent P, Jarvis WD, Birrer MJ, *et al.* The roles of signaling by the p42/p44 mitogen-activated protein (MAP) kinase pathway; a potential route to radio- and chemo-sensitization of tumor cells resulting in the induction of apoptosis and loss of clonogenicity. Leukemia, 12:1843-1850, 1998.
162. Frankel A, Mills GB. Peptide and lipid growth factors decrease cis-diamminedichloroplatinum-induced cell death in human ovarian cancer cells. Clin Cancer Res, 2:1307-1313, 1996.
163. Christen RD, Isonishi S, Jones JA, *et al.* Signaling and drug sensitivity. Cancer Metastasis Rev, 13:175-189, 1994.
164. Fan J, Bertino JR. Modulation of cisplatinum cytotoxicity by p53: effect of p53-mediated apoptosis and DNA repair. Mol Pharmacol, 56:966-972, 1999.
165. Branch P, Masson M, Aquilina G, *et al.* Spontaneous development of drug resistance: mismatch repair and p53 defects in resistance to cisplatin in human tumor cells. Oncogene, 19:3138-3145, 2000.
166. Barret JM, Hill BT. DNA repair mechanisms associated with cellular resistance to antitumor drugs: potential novel targets. Anticancer Drugs, 9:105-123, 1998.
167. Li L, Keating MJ, Plunkett W, Yang LY. Fludarabine-mediated repair inhibition of cisplatin-induced DNA lesions in human chronic myelogenous leukemia-blast crisis K562 cells: induction of synergistic cytotoxicity independent of reversal of apoptosis resistance. Mol Pharmacol, 52:798-806, 1997.
168. Giles FJ, O'Brien SM, Santini V, *et al.* Sequential cis-platinum and fludarabine with or without arabinosyl cytosine in patients failing prior fludarabine therapy for chronic lymphocytic leukemia: a phase II study. Leukemia Lymphoma, 36:57-65, 1999.

169. Alaoui-Jamali M, Loubaba BB, Robyn S, *et al.* Effect of DNA-repair-enzyme modulators on cytotoxicity of L-phenylalanine mustard and cis-diamminedichloroplatinum (II) in mammary carcinoma cells resistant to alkylating drugs. Cancer Chemother Pharmacol, 34:153-158, 1994.
170. Barret JM, Etievant C, Fahy J, *et al.* Novel artificial endonucleases inhibit base excision repair and potentiate the cytotoxicity of DNA-damaging agents on L1210 cells. Anticancer Drugs, 10:55-65, 1999.
171. Dolan ME, Pegg AE. O^6-benzylguanine and its role in chemotherapy. Clin Cancer Res, 3:837-847, 1997.
172. Spiro T, Liu L, Gerson S. New cytotoxic agents for the treatment of metastatic malignant melanoma: temozolomide and related alkylating agents in combination with guanine analogues to abrogate drug resistance. Forum (Genova), 10:274-285, 2000.
173. Friedman HS, Kokkinakis DM, Pluda J, *et al.* Phase I trial of O^6-benzylguanine for patients undergoing surgery for malignant glioma. J Clin Oncol, 16:3570-3575, 1998.
174. Li Q, Tsang B, Bostick-Bruton F, Reed E. Modulation of excision repair cross complementation group 1 (ERCC-1) mRNA expression by pharmacological agents in human ovarian carcinoma cells. Biochem Pharmacol, 57:347-353, 1999.
175. Pietras RJ, Fendly BM, Chazin VR, *et al.* Antibody to HER-2/neu receptor blocks DNA repair after cisplatin in human breast and ovarian cancer cells. Oncogene, 9:1829-1838, 1994.
176. Benchekroun MN, Parker R, Dabholkar M, *et al.* Effects of interleukin-1 alpha on DNA repair in human ovarian carcinoma (NIH:OVCAR-3) cells: implications in the mechanism of sensitization of cis-diamminedichloroplatinum(II). Mol Pharmacol, 47:1255-1260, 1995.
177. Kleibl K, Margison GP. Increasing DNA repair capacity in bone marrow by gene transfer as a prospective tool in cancer therapy. Neoplasma, 45:181-186, 1998.
178. Moritz T, Mackay W, Glassner BJ, *et al.* Retrovirus-mediated expression of a DNA repair protein in bone marrow protects hematopoietic cells from nitrosourea-induced toxicity in vitro and in vivo. Cancer Res, 55:2608-2614, 1995.
179. Frosina G. Overexpression of enzymes that repair endogenous damage to DNA. Eur J Biochem, 267:2135-2149, 2000.
180. Fairbairn LJ, Rafferty JA, Lashford LS. Engineering drug resistance in human cells. Bone Marrow Transplant, 25 Suppl 2:S110-113, 2000.
181. Maze R, Carney JP, Kelley MR, *et al.* Increasing DNA repair methyltransferase levels via bone marrow stem cell transduction rescues mice from the toxic effects of 1,3-bis(2-chloroethyl)-1-nitrosourea, a chemotherapeutic alkylating agent. Proc Natl Acad Sci USA, 93:206-210, 1996.
182. Maze R, Hanenberg H, Williams DA. Establishing chemoresistance in hematopoietic progenitor cells. Mol Med Today, 3:350-358, 1997.
183. Harris LC, Marathi UK, Edwards CC, *et al.* Retroviral transfer of a bacterial alkyltransferase gene into murine bone marrow protects against chloroethylnitrosourea cytotoxicity. Clin Cancer Res, 1:1359-1368, 1995.
184. Hansen WK, Deutsch WA, Yacoub A, *et al.* Creation of a fully functional human chimeric DNA repair protein. Combining O^6-methylguanine DNA methyltransferase (MGMT) and AP endonuclease (APE/redox effector factor 1 (Ref 1)) DNA repair proteins. J Biol Chem, 273:756-762, 1998.
185. Zdzienicka MZ, Roza L, Westerveld A, *et al.* Biological and biochemical consequences of the human ERCC-1 repair gene after transfection into a repair-deficient CHO cell line. Mutat Res, 183:69-74, 1987.

186. van Duin M, Janssen JH, de Wit J, *et al.* Transfection of the cloned human excision repair gene *ERCC-1* to UV-sensitive CHO mutants only corrects the repair defect in complementation group-2 mutants. Mutat Res, 193:123-130, 1988.
187. Bramson J, Panasci LC. Effect of ERCC-1 overexpression on sensitivity of Chinese hamster ovary cells to DNA damaging agents. Cancer Res, 53:3237-3240, 1993.
188. Belt PBGM, van Oosterwijk MF, Odjik H, *et al.* Induction of a mutant phenotype in human repair proficient cells after overexpression of a mutated human DNA repair gene. Nucleic Acids Res, 19:5633-5637, 1991.
189. Grombacher T, Tomicic M, Digweed M, *et al.* Overexpression of cDNA encoding FANCC, SPHAR, MPG, SNM1 or HA 3611 does not render CHO cells more resistant to DNA crosslinking agents. Anticancer Res, 19:1729-1735, 1999.
190. Coquerelle T, Dosch J, Kaina B. Overexpression of N-methylpurine-DNA glycosylase in Chinese hamster ovary cells renders them more sensitive to the production of chromosomal aberrations by methylating agents–a case of imbalanced DNA repair. Mutat Res, 336:9-17, 1995.
191. Limp-Foster M, Kelley MR. DNA repair and gene therapy: Implications for translational uses. Environ Mol Mutagen, 35:71-81, 2000.
192. Allalunis-Turner MJ, Barron GM, Day RS III, *et al.* Radiosensitivity testing of human primary brain tumor specimens. Int J Radiat Oncol Biol Phys, 23:339-343, 1992.

Chapter 8

LEUKEMIC CELL INSENSITIVITY TO CYCLOPHOSPHAMIDE AND OTHER OXAZAPHOSPHORINES MEDIATED BY ALDEHYDE DEHYDROGENASE(S)

Norman E. Sládek
Department of Pharmacology, University of Minnesota Medical School Minneapolis, Minnesota, USA

1. INTRODUCTION

"Acquired" insensitivity to cyclophosphamide and other oxazaphosphorines, e.g., 4-hydroperoxycyclophosphamide (4HC), mafosfamide, ifosfamide and 4-hydroperoxyifosfamide, on the part of the leukemias for which these agents are used is encountered all too often clinically. Increased detoxification of the oxazaphosphorines catalyzed by relatively elevated levels of any of several aldehyde dehydrogenases (ALDHs) present in target (malignant) cells could, at least in some cases, account for the relative insensitivity to these agents. Presently, however, there is no direct evidence (as would be provided by a prospective study, or even retrospective analysis, comparing [1] therapeutic responses to therapeutic strategies of which an oxazaphosphorine is a part with [2] cellular levels of relevant ALDH activity) to support that notion. By the same token, there is little direct evidence disputing it. Herein summarized is the indirect evidence consistent, as well as inconsistent, with the aforementioned possibility.

Leukemias are widely disseminated malignancies and are thus not amenable (as are localized solid tumors) to complete surgical removal or total eradication with local irradiation. Thus, systemic strategies must be devised to treat these malignancies. Currently, induction of remission, post-remission consolidation/intensification, and maintenance of remission are attempted largely with cytotoxic drugs, usually in combinations of two or more (combination chemotherapy), thereby minimizing the cultivation of relatively drug-insensitive malignant cell subpopulations.

Fortunately, leukemias are amongst the most chemotherapy-responsive malignancies. At a minimum, essentially all patients go into partial remission (reduction of malignant cell number, but not to less than detectable amounts) when a chemotherapeutic strategy is initiated. Many go on to complete remission (no detectable malignant cells), e.g., >95% of children with acute lymphocytic leukemia (ALL), 60-90% of adults with ALL, 75-85% of children with acute myeloid leukemia (AML, also known as acute myelogenous leukemia and as acute nonlymphocytic leukemia or ANLL), and 60-70% of adults with AML. Nonetheless, "cures" (eradication of all malignant cells), as judged by 5-year survival rates (valid except in the cases of chronic lymphocytic leukemia (CLL) and chronic myelogenous leukemia (CML), where 5-year survival often does not translate into cures as defined herein), are achieved far less often, e.g., in ~80% of children with ALL, ~41% of adults with ALL, ~40% of children with AML, and ~13% of adults with AML[6,7]. Overall, the 5-year survival rate for all leukemia patients is only ~44%[7]. It follows that since [1] chemotherapy is the initial treatment strategy of choice in the case of virtually all leukemias, and [2] cures are achieved in <44% of cases, leukemias are not fully chemotherapy-responsive in >56% of cases.

Failure to achieve cures after obtaining partial or even complete responses is due to the expansion of a subpopulation of malignant cells that escapes the cytotoxic action of the therapeutic regimen, i.e., these cells are insensitive to all of the drugs, at the concentrations achieved, to which they are exposed. Residence in a "sanctuary" and inadequate systemic drug availability aside, such malignant cell populations arise from a minority population of drug-insensitive malignant cells, or even one such cell, already present in a majority population of drug-sensitive cells, or from a drug-induced drug-insensitive malignant cell. In the case of the former, the drug(s) acts only as a selecting agent, i.e., to create an environment relatively favorable to expansion of the drug-insensitive subpopulation. In the case of the latter, the drug(s) acts first as a mutagen, i.e., to create the drug-insensitive progenitor, and then as a selecting agent. Regardless, the end result is the same: a malignancy that stops responding to a chemotherapeutic regimen after initially doing so, i.e., chronologically, drug-insensitivity presents as being "acquired" in both scenarios.

Perusal of the treatment options listed by the National Cancer Institute (http://cancernet.nci.nih.gov/Cancer_Types/Leukemia.shtml#toc2) at the start of this millennium reveals that the oxazaphosphorines such as cyclophosphamide are viewed as agents of first choice in the cases of only a few leukemias when the strategy is a conventional attempt to induce remissions, i.e., conventional treatment. Thus, they are generally not used in the conventional treatment of CML or childhood or adult AML. Further, limited use of the oxazaphosphorines in the conventional treatment of childhood ALL, indeed, all childhood malignancies, is advised because of their genotoxic action and association with an increased risk of late adverse effects. Initial systemic treatment of adult ALL sometimes does include an oxazaphosphorine as part of a 4- or 5-drug regimen; oxazaphosphorine-containing regimens are particularly of relative advantage in the treatment of two adult ALL subsets, viz., B- and T-cell ALL. Currently preferred treatment options for CLL do include an oral alkylating agent, e.g., chlorambucil or cyclophosphamide, with or without corticosteroids.

On the other hand, the oxazaphosphorines are viewed as useful drugs in the treatment of all of the leukemias in the setting of high-dose myeloablative therapy/allogeneic and autologous bone marrow transplantation (BMT) (hematopoietic stem cell rescue) strategies that are used following chemotherapy-induced first and subsequent remissions and in otherwise drug-insensitive recurrent disease; included is their *ex vivo* use to purge autologous marrow of residual leukemic cells prior to its reintroduction into the patient. Indeed, high-dose cyclophosphamide and total body irradiation, or high-dose busulfan and cyclophosphamide, followed by allogeneic BMT, is currently the only consistently successful curative treatment for CML.

Given their initial value in the conventional treatment of some leukemias and in the setting of high-dose therapy/BMT strategies for all leukemias, an understanding of the basis for "acquired" relative drug-insensitivity to cyclophosphamide and other oxazaphosphorines would seem to be important, especially since such an understanding could provide the basis for strategies designed to reverse or circumvent it, or, at a minimum, point the way to prognostic tests that could be used to identify patients in whom the use of the oxazaphosphorines would be invariably fruitless, thereby sparing them needless oxazaphosphorine-induced morbidity.

Cellular sensitivity to any given cytotoxic agent is governed by molecular determinants thereof. Potentially, a decrease or an increase in the cellular level of those determinants that increase or decrease, respectively, cellular sensitivity to a given agent, could account for relative insensitivity to that agent.

Molecular determinants of cellular sensitivity to any given cytotoxic agent are found at the molecular site of cytotoxic action, i.e., at the site of drug-target interaction, as well as upstream and downstream thereof. Since a number of these determinants are likely to be operative in the case of any given cytotoxic agent, intrinsic and acquired insensitivity to any given antitumor agent is likely to be multifactorial; on occasion, even in a single malignant cell population.

Like other bifunctional alkylating agents of the nitrogen mustard type, oxazaphosphorines are thought to effect their cytotoxic action primarily by cross-linking the two strands of DNA, although ring cleavage and depurination may also be important[8]. As judged by preclinical models, there are at least two upstream, and one downstream, molecular determinants of cellular sensitivity to the oxazaphosphorines, the cellular levels of which can vary. Demonstrated upstream determinants are glutathione[9] and certain

ALDHs[10]; cellular sensitivity to the oxazaphosphorines decreases as cellular levels of glutathione or operative ALDHs increase. A demonstrated downstream determinant is DNA repair capacity; cellular sensitivity to the oxazaphosphorines decreases as cellular DNA repair capacity increases[9].

Table 1. Cultured cell lines exhibiting acquired, ALDH-mediated, relative insensitivity to the oxazaphosphorines.

Preclinical Model				
Species	**Cell Line**	**Stability**	**Aldehyde Dehydrogenase**[a]	**References**
Mouse	L1210/OAP lymphocytic leukemia[b]	Stable	ALDH1A1	8, 12-23
	P388/CLA lymphocytic leukemia[b]	Stable	ALDH1A1	8, 12, 15, 18, 20, 21
Rat	BNML/CPR acute myeloid leukemia[c]	Unstable	ALDH[d]	24, 25
	LBN/R acute myeloid leukemia[c]	Apparently Stable	ALDH[d,e]	26
Human	KBM-7/B5-180[3] myeloid leukemia[f]	Stable	ALDH1A1	27-29
	K562/R erythroleukemia[g]	Stable	ALDH1A1	30

[a]ALDH1A1 (formerly ALDH-1) and ALDH3A1 (formerly ALDH-3), human cytosolic aldehyde dehydrogenases; Mouse and rat aldehyde dehydrogenase homologues of human ALDH1A1 and ALDH301 are also termed ALDH1A and ALDH3A1, respectively. Amino acid sequences deduced from mouse and rat ALDH1A1 cDNAs are each 87% identical with the amino acid sequence of human ALDH1A1[1-5]. Mouse ALDH1A1 is also known as AHD2.

[b]Relative insensitivity to the oxazaphosphorines was induced *in vivo* when L1210/0[31] or P388/0[32] lymphocytic leukemia cells were serially passaged in mice, and mice thus inoculated were serially injected with cyclophosphamide. The L1210/OAP and P388/CLA sublines have also been referred to as L1210/CPA and P388/CPA sublines, respectively. Relative insensitivity of P388/CLA leukemia cells to the oxazaphosphorines appeared to be multifactorial, but ALDH1A2 was clearly the most important mediator thereof[15,35].

[c]Relative insensitivity to the oxazaphosphorines was induced *in vivo* when BNML AML cells were serially passaged in rats, and rats thus inoculated were serially injected with cyclophosphamide[24,26]. Relative insensitivity of BNML/CPR

leukemia cells to the oxazaphosphorines may have been multifactorial, but ALDH was the most important, if not the sole, mediator thereof[25].

[d]The specific identity of the relevant ALDH was not determined, but was probably the rat homologue of human ALDH1A1, i.e., rat ALDH1A1, given that propionaldehyde and NAD were used to quantify enzyme activity, and that propionaldehyde is a good substrate, and NAD is a good cofactor, for ALDH1A1[34-36].

[e]To a lesser extent, ALDH activity was also found to be elevated when NADP was used as the cofactor, and benzaldehyde was used as the substrate, to quantify enzyme activity, suggesting that cellular levels of the rat homologue of human ALDH3A1, i.e., rat ALDH3A1, may also have been operative since [1] benzaldehyde is a good substrate for ALDH3A1 and [2] ALDH3A1 can utilize NADP, as well as NAD, as a proton acceptor; in contrast, propionaldehyde is a poor substrate for ALDH3A1, benzaldehyde is a poor substrate for ALDH1A1, and ALDH1A1 does not utilize NADP as a proton acceptor[34-36].

[f]Relative insensitivity to the oxazaphosphorines was induced when a subclone of cultured human KBM-7 myeloid leukemia cells, viz., KBM-7/B5, was grown in the intermittent presence of gradually increasing concentrations of 4HC for several months[27]; relative insensitivity to the oxazaphosphorines was multifactorial, but ALDH was the most important mediator thereof[27,28]. Relative insensitivity to the oxazaphosphorines was also induced when cultured human KBM-7/B5 cells were exposed once to a relatively high concentration of 4HC (60 μg/ml) for 1 h and then cultured in drug-free medium for 4-6 weeks. Surviving clonogenic cells (~5 x 10^{-6}) were then each further expanded in drug-free culture medium; 64% were found to be stably relatively insensitive to the oxazaphosphorines[29].

[g]Relative insensitivity to the oxazaphosphorines was induced when cultured human K562/0 erythroleukemia cells were grown in the presence of gradually increasing concentrations of 4HC for several months[30].

All of the clinically useful oxazaphosphorines are prodrugs. Each gives rise to a pivotal metabolite that is also without cytotoxic activity, viz., an aldehyde (aldophosphamide/aldoifosfamide) that undergoes one of two systemic fates: base-catalyzed hydrolysis to a cytotoxic metabolite (phosphoramide mustard/iphosphoramide mustard), or, alternatively, enzyme-catalyzed oxidation to an acid (carboxyphosphamide/carboxyifosfamide) that is without cytotoxic activity and that does not, under physiological conditions, give rise to a cytotoxic metabolite; the latter reaction is, therefore, properly viewed as enzyme-catalyzed bio-inactivation (detoxification) of the oxazaphosphorines[8].

Oxidation of the aldehyde to the acid is catalyzed by NAD(P)-dependent aldehyde dehydrogenases, but not all ALDHs catalyze this reaction. At least 17 members of the ALDH superfamily are found in human tissues[11]. One, ALDH1A1, is known to catalyze the oxidation of aldophosphamide to carboxyphosphamide with a favorable apparent K_m[8,10]. Three others,

ALDH2, ALDH3A1 and ALDH5A1, have also been shown to catalyze this reaction, but not very efficaciously as judged by apparent K_m values. Two, ALDH1B1 and ALDH4A1, do not catalyze the reaction. Not known is whether any of the other eight identified ALDHs do so.

Several experimental approaches have established that cellular sensitivity to the oxazaphosphorines decreases as cellular levels of ALDH1A1 increase, and that the latter is causal of the former. Especially germane are experiments in which stable ALDH1A1-mediated relative insensitivity to the oxazaphosphorines was induced in mouse, rat and human leukemia cells as a consequence of long-term (months) exposure to an oxazaphosphorine (Table 1). Perhaps of particular clinical relevance in view of their 2- and 4-day use at high doses prior to BMT, stable ALDH1A1-mediated relative insensitivity to the oxazaphosphorines was also induced in human leukemia cells as a consequence of very brief (1 h) exposure to a high concentration of an oxazaphosphorine[29] (see also chapter 11 in this volume by Drs. B. Andersson and D. Murray).

Further evidence supporting the contention that cellular sensitivity to the oxazaphosphorines decreases as cellular levels of ALDH1A1 increase has been reported. Thus: [1] expression of ALDH1A1 antisense RNA in human K562 erythroleukemia cells effected a decrease in ALDH1A1 mRNA expression and catalytic activity, and an increase in sensitivity to 4HC[37]; [2] sensitivity to 4HC, as indicated by clonogenic survival, on the part of four human nonlymphocytic leukemia cell lines (K562, HEL, HL-60, ML-1) was inversely related to their content of an ALDH of undetermined identity, but most probably ALDH1A1[17,18]; and [3] human K562/0 erythroleukemia[38] and V79/SD1 Chinese hamster lung fibroblast[39] cells transfected with human ALDH1A1 cDNA, and [4] mouse L1210/0 leukemia, human U937/0 monoblastic leukemia and human $CD34^+$ primary hematopoietic cells transduced with human ALDH1A1 cDNA[40], were each rendered relatively insensitive to the oxazaphosphorines.

Still further evidence supporting the contention that cellular sensitivity to the oxazaphosphorines decreases as cellular levels of ALDH1A1 increase has been generated. Thus: [1] Friedman and coworkers[41] found that relative insensitivity to 4HC on the part of cultured human medulloblastoma Daoy (4-HCR) cells (relative insensitivity to the oxazaphosphorines was induced by intermittently exposing the cultured parent line to progressively increasing concentrations of 4HC) was mediated, in large part, by elevated levels of an ALDH of undetermined identity, but most probably ALDH1A1 given the substrate (propionaldehyde) and cofactor (NAD) that were used to quantify enzyme activity (see footnote to Table 1) in this investigation; and [2] Yoshida and coworkers[42] reported that relative insensitivity to 4HC and cyclophosphamide on the part of cultured human A2780/R ovarian carcinoma cells (relative insensitivity to the oxazaphosphorines was induced by growing the parent human A2780 ovarian carcinoma cells in gradually increasing concentrations of cyclophosphamide for 12 weeks) was mediated by elevated levels of ALDH1A1.

Similarly, several experimental approaches have established that cellular sensitivity to the oxazaphosphorines decreases as cellular levels of ALDH3A1 increase, and that the latter is causal of the former. Thus, stable ALDH3A1-mediated relative insensitivity to the oxazaphosphorines was induced in cultured human MCF-7 breast adenocarcinoma cells as a consequence of long-term (months) exposure to gradually increasing concentrations of 4HC[43–46] or benz(a)pyrene[47], or, again, perhaps of particular clinical relevance, even brief (30 min) exposure to a high concentration of mafosfamide[47]. Potentially of substantial clinical significance, too, was that transient ALDH3A1-mediated relative insensitivity to the oxazaphosphorines could be induced in cultured human MCF-7 breast adenocarcinoma cells by agents commonly found in the diet/environment, e.g., 3-methylcholanthrene, benz(a)pyrene, 7,12-dimethylbenzanthracene, indole-3-carbinol, catechol, *t*-butyl-hydroquinone, 2,6-di-*t*-butyl-4-hydroxytoluene (BHT) and 3(5)-di-*t*-butyl-4-hydroxyanisole (BHA)[45,46,48–51]; [G. K. Rekha and N. E. Sladek, unpublished observations]. Relevant to the issue at hand, transient ALDH3A1-mediated relative insensitivity to the oxazaphosphorines could not be induced by these agents in cultured human K562 pre-erythroid blast leukemia, or in cultured mouse L1210 lymphocytic leukemia, cells [L. Sreerama and N. E. Sladek, unpublished observations].

Further evidence supporting the contention that cellular sensitivity to the oxazaphosphorines decreases as cellular levels of ALDH3A1 increase has been generated. Thus, [1] human MCF-7 breast adenocarcinoma cells electroporated with human ALDH3A1[52], [2] human MCF-7 breast adenocarcinoma[53] and V79/SD1 Chinese hamster lung fibroblast[54] cells transfected with rat ALDH3A1 cDNA, and [3] V79/SD1 Chinese hamster lung fibroblast cells transfected with human ALDH3A1 cDNA[54], were each rendered relatively insensitive to the oxazaphosphorines.

Although intrinsic or "acquired" relative cellular insensitivity to the oxazaphosphorines mediated by other ALDHs known to catalyze the oxidation of aldophosphamide/aldoifosfamide to carboxyphosphamide/carboxyifosfamide, e.g., ALDH5A1, or by ALDHs that have yet to be evaluated with respect to their ability to catalyze this reaction, e.g., ALDH1A6, has never been demonstrated in pre-clinical rodent, human, transgenic or other models, the possibilities that [1] one or more of these enzymes can catalyze the oxidation of aldophosphamide/aldoifosfamide to carboxyphosphamide/carboxyifosfamide *in situ* at a pharmacologically significant rate, and that [2] elevated levels of one or more enzymes that have such capability can be induced in tumor cells, thereby decreasing their sensitivity to the oxazaphosphorines, cannot be dismissed.

All else being equal, for a given molecular determinant of cellular sensitivity to a given agent to account for the variation in the therapeutic response to that agent, tumor cell levels of the putative determinant must vary significantly at magnitudes sufficient to have a pharmacological impact. Further, given that ALDH1A1 and/or ALDH3A1 are operational molecular determinants of cellular sensitivity to the oxazaphosphorines clinically, the expectation is that low tumor cell levels of these enzymes would predict for a more favorable therapeutic response to this agent as compared to that obtained when tumor cell levels of these enzymes are high.

Thus, ALDH1A1 levels vary substantially, ~276 fold, as do those of ALDH3A1, ~356 fold, in human breast tumor (largely, infiltrating ductal carcinomas) tissue[10], and retrospective analyses by our laboratory revealed a statistically significant inverse relationship between favorable therapeutic outcomes of cyclophosphamide-based chemotherapy of breast cancers and ALDH1A1, although not ALDH3A1, levels[55]. Further, relatively high ALDH1A1 and/or ALDH3A1 levels may be one reason why the oxazaphosphorines are of limited or no clinical value in the treatment of the vast majority of lung, gastrointestinal, salivary gland and renal cancers, i.e., many of these cancers may be intrinsically insensitive to the oxazaphosphorines, at least in part, because they express large amounts of ALDH1A1 and/or ALDH3A[10].

As judged by the results of experiments with known, but less than specific, inhibitors of ALDH1A1, viz., cyanamide and disulfiram, various human normal multipotent and committed hematopoietic progenitor cells, viz., CFU-Mix, CFU-Mk, CFU-GM and BFU-E, possess an inhibitor-sensitive ALDH, most probably ALDH1A1[16]. Direct demonstration of ALDH1A1 in human normal erythroid progenitor[56], bone marrow mononuclear[57], and $CD34^+$ hematopoietic progenitor[56] cells has been reported.

Low levels of ALDH1A1 are known to be present in human normal mature erythrocytes[58,59]. Approximately equal amounts of a cytosolic ALDH, most probably ALDH1A1, were reportedly present in human nonmalignant leukocytes, but, according to an anecdotal comment by the investigator, ALDH activity varied substantially between different leukocyte subpopulations, viz., as compared to those in lymphocytes, levels were much higher in granulocytes and monocytes[58]. Another laboratory[56] found ALDH1A1 to be present in human normal monocytes (highest level), B-lymphoid cells and T-lymphoid (lowest level) cells. Perhaps not coincidentally, ALDH1A1 levels in stable human leukemic cell lines were of largest magnitude in K562 (pre-erythroid blast leukemia)[17,18,36], HEL (human erythroleukemia)[17,18], KBM-7 (CML)[29] and TF-1 (CML), cells[57], *vide infra*. ALDH3A1 is not found in mature erythrocytes[34].

Detectable, but relatively low, levels of both ALDH1A1 and ALDH3A1 were found in each of the 6 human leukemia cell lines used by the National Cancer Institute in the middle of the past decade to screen for potentially useful antitumor agents; by far, the highest level was that of ALDH1A1 in K562 erythroleukemia cells[36]. Others[16–18,57,60] report undetectable or relatively low to moderate levels of ALDH1A1 and/or ALDH3A1, or an ALDH of undetermined identity, but most probably ALDH1A1, in a variety of human lymphocytic and myelocytic leukemia cell lines. A relatively high level of ALDH1A1, viz., 1.6 mIU/million cells, was reported for a stable, growth factor-dependent cell line, TF-1, originating from cells taken from a CML patient[57].

Neither the greater *ex vivo* sensitivity to mafosfamide of primary clonogenic blasts present in samples obtained from oxazaphosphorine-naïve B-lineage ALL patients relative to that of primary clonogenic blasts present in samples obtained from oxazaphosphorine-naïve T-lineage ALL patients, nor the marked interpatient variation in *ex vivo* sensitivity to mafosfamide in each subset, could be attributed to variation in the rates of ALDH-catalyzed oxidation of aldophosphamide to carboxyphosphamide[61]. Indeed, the presence of ALDH catalytic activity was not detected in the majority of samples, and was only borderline, and questionably, detectable in the remaining samples. Further, ALDH-catalyzed oxidation of aldophosphamide to carboxyphosphamide was not detected in malignant cell samples obtained from each of 6 relapsed B-lineage ALL patients who had been previously treated with cyclophosphamide, even though, in the two cases where the determination was made, primary clonogenic blasts emerging therefrom were relatively insensitive to mafosfamide[61]. Similarly, ALDH-catalyzed oxidation of aldophosphamide to carboxyphosphamide was, at best, marginally detectable in only two of the malignant cell samples obtained from each of 15 CLL patients[e]. Others[56] reported the presence of a measurable level of ALDH1A1 in a B-lineage ($CD10^+$) primary lymphocytic leukemia; ALDH1A1 levels at the time of initial diagnosis and at relapse were essentially identical and were similar to that in normal B-lineage cells.

ALDH-catalyzed aldophosphamide oxidation was, at best, marginally detectable in about half of the leukemic cell samples obtained from each of 10 AML and 16 CML (all but one AML, oxazaphosphorine-naïve) patients [N. E. Sladek, L. Sreerama and P. A. Dockham, unpublished observations].

Most directly germane to the topic at hand, Miller and coworkers[62] demonstrated a direct correlation between [1] the *ex vivo* sensitivity to 4HC of occult leukemic cells present in pre-transplant remission bone marrow obtained from AML and ALL patients and [2] the subsequent therapeutic response to a conditioning regimen of high-dose cyclophosphamide and busulfan or total body irradiation followed by autologous transplantation of the 4HC-purged marrow. Occult leukemic cells present in pre-transplant remission bone marrow obtained from AML patients were more sensitive to 4HC than were those obtained from ALL patients. Sensitivity to 4HC was independent of previous exposure to cyclophosphamide. Decreased *ex vivo* sensitivity of the leukemic cells to 4HC was associated with elevated levels of ALDH activity in about one-third of the non-responders [Colvin, O. M., personal communication to B. S. Andersson and D. Murray quoted in ref. 9].

Given that [1] ALDH1A1 is constitutively present, albeit at seemingly low levels, in human normal multipotent and committed hematopoietic progenitor cells as well as in mature erythrocytes and leukocytes, and that [2] ALDH1A1-mediated insensitivity to the oxazaphosphorines is evidently easy to induce, as reflected by the fact that, in pre-clinical models, ALDH1A1-mediated insensitivity to the oxazaphosphorines has been experimentally induced *ex vivo* and/or *in vivo* in leukemias of three different species, viz., mouse, rat and human (Table 1), it is likely that, in some cases, the "acquired" relative insensitivity to the oxazaphosphorines exhibited by various leukemias in the clinic is ALDH1A1-mediated, perhaps more so in those of erythroid-, or even myeloid-, as opposed to lymphoid-, lineage. Arguing against this notion is that, in the few cases where the determination has been attempted, the ALDH1A1 content of primary leukemic cells was quite low, often below, or, at best, just at, detectable levels, and in any case, did not, with one notable (but unpublished) exception, *vide supra*, inversely correlate with sensitivity to the oxazaphosphorines.

On the other hand, there is essentially no evidence indicating that the "acquired" relative insensitivity exhibited by various leukemias in the clinic is ever mediated by ALDH3A1 or any ALDH other than ALDH1A1. Further, there is no evidence indicating that the intrinsic relative insensitivity occasionally exhibited by various leukemias in the clinic is ever mediated by ALDH1A1, ALDH3A1 or any other ALDH.

At least one potentially useful clinical strategy can be envisioned and might be pursued if it turns out that, in some cases, relatively elevated levels of ALDH1A1 do, indeed, account for leukemic cell insensitivity to the oxazaphosphorines, viz., individualization of cancer chemotherapeutic regimens on the basis of, at least in part, the level of this enzyme in the leukemia of interest. Thus, cyclophosphamide and other oxazaphosphorines may well be the drugs of choice when ALDH1A1 levels are low, but they likely would not be when the levels of this enzyme are high since their use in that case would likely be in vain and only contribute to morbidity. Sensitization of malignant cells that express relatively large amounts of ALDH1A1 to the oxazaphosphorines by preventing the synthesis of this enzyme, e.g., with ALDH1A1 antisense oligonucleotides, or by introducing an agent, e.g., disulfiram, that directly inhibits the catalytic action of ALDH1A1, is not likely to be a rewarding strategy because certain critical normal cells, e.g., multipotent and committed hematopoietic progenitor cells, appear to be relatively insensitive to the oxazaphosphorines precisely because they express relatively elevated levels of ALDH1A1 or a very closely related enzyme[8,10,57,63].

The therapeutic potential of a given anticancer agent is governed not only by factors that impact on its uptake, distribution and clearance by/in the targeted malignant cell (cellular pharmacokinetics), but also by factors that impact on its absorption, distribution and clearance by/in the host organism (systemic pharmacokinetics). Variability in cellular pharmacokinetics provides an easily defensible rationale for individualized chemotherapeutic regimens with regard to drug choice. Variability in systemic pharmacokinetics provides an equally easily defensible rationale for individualized chemotherapeutic regimens with regard to drug amount/schedule. Relevant to the latter is the observation of Evans and associates[64] that "recommended/conventional doses of [cancer] chemotherapeutic drugs are typically within the limits that essentially all patients can tolerate, regardless of the rate at which the drug is [activated and/or cleared from the body]. For this reason, it is not surprising that such doses may be sub-optimal in some patients."

ALDH1A1 is abundantly present in liver and other organs[34,35]. It is also found in erythrocytes, albeit at low levels, but they are many in number (about 3.3 x 10^{13} in an average 70-kg human male)[59]. The tissue distribution of ALDH3A1 is more limited, but large amounts of it are also found in non-malignant tissues, e.g., stomach mucosa[45]. Thus, in theory at least, variability in the therapeutic effectiveness of the oxazaphosphorines, as well as in the incidence and extent of unacceptable oxazaphosphorine-induced host toxicity, could be due to variability in non-malignant tissue levels of these enzymes or in their functional capacity. For example, erythrocyte ALDH1A1 levels are known to distribute over at least a 3 fold range[59]. Further, phenotypic variants of ALDH1A1 have been identified in human tissues[34], although the incidence is apparently rare and it is unknown as to whether the variant forms of ALDH1A1 catalyze the oxidation of aldophosphamide/aldoifosfamide as does the wild type, and whether they are the consequence of genetic polymorphisms. Interestingly, AUC (area under the whole blood/plasma/serum concentration versus time curve) values for aldophosphamide and the tautomer with which it is in equilibrium, viz., 4-hydroxycyclophosphamide, varied several fold even when normalized for dose of cyclophosphamide[8]. Assuming first-order kinetics, and that essentially all of the administered cyclophosphamide is ultimately oxidized to 4-hydroxycyclophosphamide/aldophosphamide, the argument can be made that the observed variability in AUC values must have been due to differences in the rate at which 4-hydroxycyclophosphamide/aldophosphamide was removed, e.g., as a consequence of ALDH-catalyzed oxidation to carboxyphosphamide, from the systemic circulation. Regardless, pretreatment assessment of functional (catalysis of aldophosphamide/ aldophosphamide) ALDH1A1 levels in erythrocytes, especially if such levels reflect functional ALDH1A1 levels in other tissues, may be of value in terms of individualizing, and therefore optimizing, oxazaphosphorine doses and schedules.

ACKNOWLEDGEMENTS

Investigations conducted by the author and reviewed herein were funded by USPHS Grants CA 67270, CA 21737, CA 26357, CA 70383, and GM 15477; USPHS DOA DAMD Grant 17-94-J-4057; ACS Grant CH-106; Bristol-Myers Squibb Grant 100-R220; and the University of Minnesota Bone Marrow Transplant Research Fund.

REFERENCES

1. Hempel J, von Bahr-Lindstrom H, Jömvall H. Aldehyde dehydrogenase from human liver: primary structure of the cytoplasmic isoenzyme. Eur J Biochem, 141:21-35, 1984.
2. Hsu LC, Tani K, Fujiyoshi T, *et al.* Cloning of cDNAs for human aldehyde dehydrogenases 1 and 2. Proc Natl Acad Sci USA, 82:3771-3775, 1985.
3. Rongnoparut P, Weaver S. Isolation and characterization of a cytosolic aldehyde dehydrogenase-encoding cDNA from mouse liver. Gene, 101:261-265, 1991.
4. Bhat PV, Labrecque J, Boutin JM, *et al.* Cloning of a cDNA encoding rat aldehyde dehydrogenase with high activity for retinal oxidation. Gene, 166:303-306, 1995.
5. Kathmann EC, Lipsky JJ. Cloning of a cDNA encoding a constitutively expressed rat liver cytosolic aldehyde dehydrogenase. Biochem Biophys Res Commun, 236:527-531, 1997.
6. Smith MA, Ries LAG, Gurney JG, Ross JA. Leukemia. *In*: Cancer incidence and Survival Among Children and Adolescents: United States SEER (Surveillance, Epidemiology, and End Results) Program, 1975-1995. LAG Ries, LA Smith, JG Gurney, *et al.* (eds.), Bethesda, MD:National Cancer Institute, NIH Pub, No. 99-4649:17-34, 1999.
7. Ries LAG, Eisner MP, Kosary CL, *et al.* (eds.) SEER (Surveillance, Epidemiology, and End Results) Cancer Statistics Review, 1973-1997. Bethesda, MD:National Cancer Institute 2000.
8. Sladek NE. Metabolism and pharmacokinetic behavior of cyclophosphamide and related oxazaphosphorines. *In*: Anticancer Drugs: Reactive Metabolism and Drug Interactions, G Powis (ed.), Pergamon Press, United Kingdom, 79-156, 1994.
9. Gamcsik MP, Dolan ME, Andersson BS, Murray D. Mechanisms of resistance to the toxicity of cyclophosphamide. Curr Pharm Design, 5:587-605, 1999.
10. Sladek NE. Aldehyde dehydrogenase-mediated cellular relative insensitivity to the oxazaphosphorines. Curr Pharm Design, 5:607-625, 1995.
11. Sophos NA, Pappa A, Ziegler IL, Vasiliou V. Aldehyde dehydrogenase gene superfamily: the 2000 update. Chem-Biol Interact, 130-132:323-337, 2001.
12. Sladek NE. Oxazaphosphorine-specific acquired cellular resistance. *In*: Drug Resistance in Oncology. BA Teicher (ed.), Marcel Dekker, New York, NY, 375-411, 1993.
13. Hilton J. Deoxyribonucleic acid crosslinking by 4-hydroperoxycyclophosphamide in cyclophosphamide-sensitive and -resistant L1210 cells. Biochem Pharmacol, 33:1867-1872, 1984.
14. Hilton J. Role of aldehyde dehydrogenase in cyclophosphamide-resistant L1210 leukemia. Cancer Res, 44:5156-5160, 1984.
15. Sladek NE, Landkamer GJ. Restoration of sensitivity to oxazaphosphorines by inhibitors of aldehyde dehydrogenase activity in cultured oxazaphosphorine-resistant L1210 and cross-linking agent-resistant P388 cell lines. Cancer Res, 45:1549-1555, 1985.
16. Kohn FR, Landkamer GJ, Manthey, *et al.* Effect of aldehyde dehydrogenase inhibitors on the ex vivo sensitivity of human multipotent and committed hematopoietic progenitor cells and malignant blood cells to oxazaphosphorines. Cancer Res, 47:3180-3185, 1987.
17. Colvin M, Hilton J. Cellular resistance to cyclophosphamide. *In*: Mechanisms of Drug Resistance in Neoplastic Cells, PV Woolley III, KD Tew (eds.), Academic Press, New York, NY, 161-171, 1988.
18. Colvin M, Russo JE, Hilton J. *et al.* Enzymatic mechanisms of resistance to alkylating agents in tumor cells and normal tissues. Adv Enz Regulat, 27:211-221, 1988.

19. Russo JE, Hauquitz D, Hilton J. Inhibition of mouse cytosolic aldehyde dehydrogenase by 4-(diethylamino)benzaldehyde. Biochem Pharmacol, 37:1639-1642, 1988.
20. Russo JE, Hilton J. Characterization of cytosolic aldehyde dehydrogenase from cyclophosphamide resistant L1210 cells. Cancer Res, 48:2963-2968, 1988.
21. Russo SE, Hilton J, Colvin OM. The role of aldehyde dehydrogenase isozymes in cellular resistance to the alkylating agent cyclophosphamide. Progr Clin Biol Res, 290:65-79, 1989.
22. Radin AT, Zhao X-L, Woo TH, *et al.* Structure and expression of the cytosolic aldehyde dehydrogenase gene in cyclophosphamide-resistant murine leukemia L1210 cells. Biochem Pharmacol, 42:1933-1939, 1991.
23. Habib AD, Boal JH, Hilton J, *et al.* Effect of stereochemistry on the oxidative metabolism of the cyclophosphamide metabolite aldophosphamide. Biochem Pharmacol, 50:429-433, 1995.
24. Martens ACM, de Groot CI, Hagenbeek A. Development and characterization of a cyclophosphamide resistant variant of the BNML rat model for acute myelocytic leukaemia. Eur J Cancer, 27:161-166, 1991.
25. de Groot CI, Martens ACM, Hagenbeek A. Aldehyde dehydrogenase involvement in a variant of the Brown Norway rat acute myelocytic leukaemia (BNML) that acquired cyclophosphamide resistance in vivo. Eur J Cancer, 30A:2137-2143, 1994.
26. Koelling TM, Yeager AM, Hilton J, *et al.* Development and characterization of a cyclophosphamide-resistant subline of acute myeloid leukemia in the Lewis x Brown Norway hybrid rat. Blood, 76:1209-1213, 1990.
27. Andersson BS, Mroue M, Britten RA, Murray D. The role of DNA damage in the resistance of human chronic myeloid leukemia cells to cyclophosphamide analogues. Cancer Res, 54:5394-5400, 1994.
28. Andersson BS, Mroue M, Britten RA, *et al.* Mechanisms of cyclophosphamide resistance in a human myeloid leukemia cell line. Acta Oncol, 34:247-251, 1995.
29. Andersson BS, Khajavi K, Sadeghi T, *et al.* Clinically relevant cyclophosphamide analog resistance can be induced by single drug exposure in human leukemic cells. Proc Amer Assoc Cancer Res, 37:317, 1996.
30. Tsukamoto N, Chen I, Yoshida A. Enhanced expressions of glucose-6-phosphate dehydrogenase and cytosolic aldehyde dehydrogenase, and elevation of reduced glutathione level in cyclophosphamide-resistant human leukemia cells. Blood Cells Molecules Diseases, 24:231-238, 1998.
31. De Wys WD. A dose-response study of resistance of leukemia L1210 to cyclophosphamide. J Natl Cancer Inst, 50:783-789, 1973.
32. Lane M, Yancey ST. Development of a leukaemia resistant to cyclophosphamide ("Cytoxan"). Nature (London), 188:756-757, 1960.
33. Sladek NE, Low JE, Landkamer GJ. Collateral sensitivity to cross-linking agents exhibited by cultured L1210 cells resistant to oxazaphosphorines. Cancer Res, 45:625-629, 1985.
34. Goedde HW, Agarwal DP. Pharmacogenetics of aldehyde dehydrogenase [ALDH]. Pharmacol Ther, 45:345-371, 1990.
35. Lindahl R. Aldehyde dehydrogenases and their role in carcinogenesis. Crit Rev Biochem Mol Biol, 27:283-335, 1992.
36. Sreerama L, Sladek NE. Class 1 and class 3 aldehyde dehydrogenase levels in the human

tumor cell lines currently used by the National Cancer Institute to screen for potentially useful antitumor agents. Adv Exp Med Biol, 414:81-94, 1997.

37. Moreb JS, Maccow C, Schweder M. Successful expression of antisense RNA to aldehyde dehydrogenase class-1 results in significant increase in the sensitivity to cyclophosphamide derivative. Proc Amer Assoc Cancer Res, 40:437, 1999.
38. Moreb J, Schweder M, Suresh A, Zucali JR. Overexpression of the human aldehyde dehydrogenase class I results in increased resistance to 4-hydroperoxycyclophosphamide. Cancer Gene Ther, 3:24-30, 1996.
39. Bunting KD, Townsend AJ. De novo expression of transfected human class 1 aldehyde dehydrogenase (ALDH) causes resistance to oxazaphosphorine anti-cancer alkylating agents in hamster V79 cell lines. Elevated class 1 ALDH activity is closely correlated with reduction in DNA interstrand cross-linking and lethality. J Biol Chem, 271:11884-11890, 1996.
40. Magni M, Shammah S, Schiró R, *et al.* Induction of cyclophosphamide-resistance by aldehyde-dehydrogenase gene transfer. Blood, 87:1097-1103, 1996.
41. Friedman HS, Colvin OM, Kaufmann SH, *et al.* Cyclophosphamide resistance in medulloblastoma. Cancer Res, 52:5373-5378, 1992.
42. Yoshida A, Dave V, Han H, Scanlon KI. Enhanced transcription of the cytosolic ALDH gene in cyclophosphamide resistant human carcinoma cells. Adv Exp Med Biol, 328:63-72, 1993.
43. Frei E III, Teicher BA, Holden SA, *et al.* Preclinical studies and clinical correlation of the effect of alkylating dose. Cancer Res, 48:6417-6423, 1988.
44. Sreerama L, Sladek NE. Identification and characterization of a novel class 3 aldehyde dehydrogenase overexpressed in a human breast adenocarcinoma cell line exhibiting oxazaphosphorine-specific acquired resistance. Biochem Pharmacol. 45:2487-2505, 1993.
45. Sreerama L, Sladek NE. Overexpression or polycyclic aromatic hydrocarbon-mediated induction of an apparently novel class 3 aldehyde dehydrogenase in human breast adenocarcinoma cells and its relationship to oxazaphosphorine-specific acquired resistance. Adv Exp Med Biol, 328:99-113, 1993.
46. Sladek NE, Sreerama L, Rekha GK. Constitutive and overexpressed human cytosolic class-3 aldehyde dehydrogenases in normal and neoplastic cells/secretions. Adv Exp Med Biol, 372:103-114, 1995.
47. Sreerama L, Sladek NE. Three different stable human breast adenocarcinoma sublines that overexpress ALDH3A1 and certain other enzymes, apparently as a consequence of constitutively upregulated gene transcription mediated by transactivated EpREs (electrophile responsive elements) present in the 5'-upstream regions of these genes. Chem-Biol Interact, 130-132:247-260, 2001.
48. Sreerama L, Sladek NE. Identification of a methylcholanthrene-induced aldehyde dehydrogenase in a human breast adenocarcinoma cell line exhibiting oxazaphosphorine-specific acquired resistance. Cancer Res, 54:2176-2185, 1994.
49. Sreerama L, Rekha GK, Sladek NE. Phenolic antioxidant-induced overexpression of class-3 aldehyde dehydrogenase and oxazaphosphorine-specific resistance. Biochem Pharmacol, 49:669-675, 1995.
50. Rekha GK, Sladek NE. Inhibition of human class 3 aldehyde dehydrogenase, and sensitization of tumor cells that express significant amounts of this enzyme to oxazaphosphorines, by the naturally occurring compound gossypol. Adv Exp Med Biol,

414:133-146, 1997.

51. Rekha GK, Devaraj VR, Sreerama L, *et al.* Inhibition of human class 3 aldehyde dehydrogenase, and sensitization of tumor cells that express significant amounts of this enzyme to oxazaphosphorines, by chlorpropamide analogues. Biochem Pharmacol, 55:465-474, 1998.
52. Sreerama L, Sladek NE. Human breast adenocarcinoma MCF-7/0 cells electroporated with cytosolic class 3 aldehyde dehydrogenases obtained from tumor cells and a normal tissue exhibit differential sensitivity to mafosfamide. Drug Metab Dispos, 23:1080-1084, 1995.
53. Bunting KD, Lindahl R, Townsend AJ. Oxazaphosphorine-specific resistance in human MCF-7 breast carcinoma cell lines expressing transfected rat class 3 aldehyde dehydrogenase. J Biol Chem, 269:23197-23203, 1994.
54. Bunting KD, Townsend AJ. Protection by transfected rat or human class 3 aldehyde dehydrogenases against the cytotoxic effects of oxazaphosphorine alkylating agents in hamster V79 cell lines. Demonstration of aldophosphamide metabolism by the human cytosolic class 3 isozyme. J Biol Chem, 271:11891-11896, 1996.
55. Sladek NE, Kollander R, Sreerama L, Kiang DT. Cellular levels of aldehyde dehydrogenases (ALDH1A1 and ALDH3A1) as predictors of therapeutic responses to cyclophosphamide-based chemotherapy of breast cancer: a retrospective study. Rational individualization of oxazaphosphorine-based cancer chemotherapeutic regimens. Cancer Chemother Pharmacol, 49:309-321, 2002.
56. Kastan MB, Schlaffer E, Russo JE, *et al.* Direct demonstration of elevated aldehyde dehydrogenase in human hematopoietic progenitor cells. Blood, 75:1947-1950, 1990.
57. Moreb J, Turner C, Sreerama L, *et al.* Interleukin-1 and tumor necrosis factor alpha induce class-1 aldehyde dehydrogenase mRNA and protein in bone marrow cells. Leukemia Lymphoma, 20:77-84, 1995.
58. Helander A. Aldehyde dehydrogenase in blood: distribution, characteristics and possible use as marker of alcohol misuse. Alcohol Alcoholism, 28:135-145, 1993.
59. Dockham PA, Sreerama L, Sladek NE. Relative contribution of human erythrocyte aldehyde dehydrogenase to the systemic detoxification of the oxazaphosphorines. Drug Metab Dispos, 25:1436-1441, 1997.
60. Jones RI, Barber JP, Vala MS, *et al.* Assessment of aldehyde dehydrogenase in viable cells. Blood, 85:2742-2746, 1995.
61. Uckun FM, Chandan-Langlie M, Dockham PA, *et al.* Sensitivity of primary clonogenic blasts from acute lymphoblastic leukemia patients to an activated cyclophosphamide, viz., mafosfamide. Leukemia Lymphoma, 13:417-428, 1994.
62. Miller CB, Zehnbauer BA, Piantadosi S, *et al.* Correlation of occult clonogenic leukemia drug sensitivity with relapse after autologous bone marrow transplantation. Blood, 78:1125-1131, 1991.
63. Sladek NE, Manthey CL, Maid PA, *et al.* Xenobiotic oxidation catalyzed by aldehyde dehydrogenases. Drug Metab Revs, 20:697-720, 1989.
64. Evans WE, Relling MV, Rodman JH, *et al.* Conventional compared with individualized chemotherapy for childhood acute lymphoblastic leukemia. N Engl J Med, 338:499-505, 1998.

Chapter 9

MECHANISMS OF RESISTANCE AGAINST CYCLOPHOSPHAMIDE AND IFOSFAMIDE: CAN THEY BE OVERCOME WITHOUT SACRIFICING SELECTIVITY?

Susan M. Ludeman and Michael P. Gamcsik
Duke Comprehensive Cancer Center and Department of Medicine, Duke University Medical Center, Durham, North Carolina, USA

1. INTRODUCTION

Cyclophosphamide (CP, Cytoxan) is a member of the nitrogen mustard class of alkylating agents and the oxazaphosphorine class of chemical compounds. First synthesized as an anticancer drug four decades ago, it continues to be widely used because of its unique efficacy against a broad range of human cancers[1]. To date, the structural isomer ifosfamide (IF, Ifos) is the most clinically useful CP analog, although its current applications in chemotherapy are somewhat modest relative to those of CP itself. On the other hand, IF appears to have some advantages over CP in potentiating the activity of other drugs[2]. This has led to new investigations of the efficacy of IF in combination therapies, including clinical whole body hyperthermia trials[3].

While the kinetics and enzyme specificities of individual steps may vary[4–6], the overall metabolic conversions of CP and IF are parallel and lead to isomeric metabolites. Resistance mechanisms are known to intervene at various points along this metabolic cascade, with the best described of these being mediation of activity by aldehyde dehydrogenase (ALDH)[7] (see also chapter 8 in this volume by Dr. N. Sladek). Glutathione (GSH) and glutathione-S-transferase (GST) levels, as well as various DNA repair mechanisms, have more recently been identified as additional modulators of CP/IF activity[8–16] (see also chapter 4 in this volume by Dr. D. Hamilton and colleagues).

Understanding each of these resistance mechanisms on a molecular level allows one to propose strategies, including structural modifications to CP and IF, that would circumvent these pathways. However, what may be classified as a mechanism of drug resistance in a cancer cell may also be termed a mechanism of protective selectivity in a normal cell. This chapter will review various therapy designs and their impact on resistance, selectivity, and metabolism.

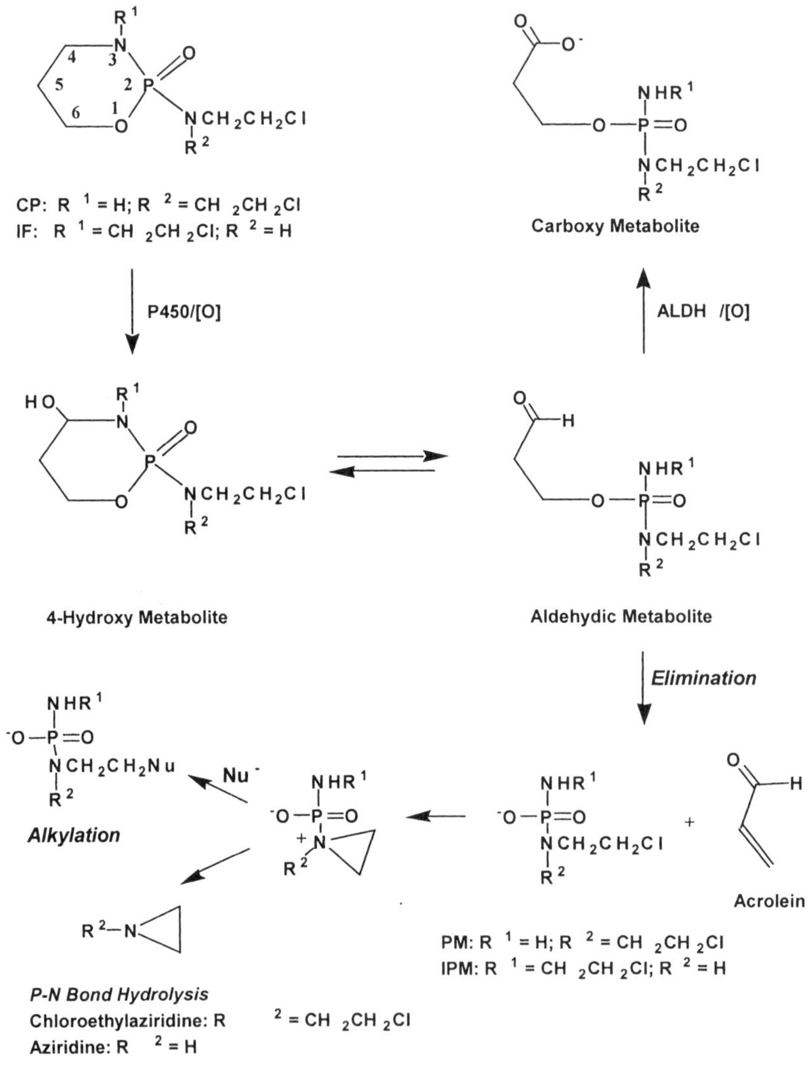

CP: $R^1 = H$; $R^2 = CH_2CH_2Cl$
IF: $R^1 = CH_2CH_2Cl$; $R^2 = H$

P450/[O]

4-Hydroxy Metabolite

Aldehydic Metabolite

ALDH /[O]

Carboxy Metabolite

Elimination

Acrolein

PM: $R^1 = H$; $R^2 = CH_2CH_2Cl$
IPM: $R^1 = CH_2CH_2Cl$; $R^2 = H$

Nu⁻

Alkylation

P-N Bond Hydrolysis
Chloroethylaziridine: $R^2 = CH_2CH_2Cl$
Aziridine: $R^2 = H$

Figure 1. The metabolism of cyclophosphamide (CP) and ifosfamide (IF). [Nu=nucleophile].

2. THE METABOLISM OF CP AND IF

Key features of the metabolism of CP are depicted in Figure 1[4]. Only the initial 'activation' reaction requires enzymatic catalysis; all subsequent steps leading to a DNA crosslinking agent are 'spontaneous' in that no enzymes are necessary. In brief, oxidation by hepatic cytochrome P450 at the C_4 position leads to the formation of 4-hydroxycyclophosphamide (4-HO-CP). 4-HO-CP undergoes facile (and reversible) ring opening to give the aldehydic metabolite aldophosphamide (AP). AP is subject to an irreversible α,β-elimination reaction that provides phosphoramide mustard (PM) and acrolein. PM undergoes an intramolecular cyclization reaction to form a transient aziridinium ion that partitions between alkylation of a nucleophile (e.g., DNA) and P-N bond hydrolysis[17,18]. The chloroethyl group of the mono-alkylated intermediate can form a second aziridinium ion thereby providing for bis-alkylation and DNA crosslinking (see section 4 on DNA Repair). The product of P-N bond scission is another bis-alkylating agent, chloroethylaziridine[16,17]; however, the role, if any, of chloroethylaziridine in the therapeutic efficacy of CP treatment has yet to be determined[19]. Acrolein is most often associated with undesirable side effects such as bladder cystisis; however, there is recent evidence that this metabolite may also contribute to the cytotoxic and/or mutagenic effects of CP[13,14].

The metabolism of IF (Figure 1) is analogous to that of CP, with C_4 oxidation providing 4-hydroxyifosfamide (4-HO-IF) and, subsequently, the tautomer aldoifosfamide (AIF). Fragmentation of AIF leads to the bis-alkylating agent isophosphoramide mustard (IPM) and acrolein. As with PM, IPM also undergoes a sequence of reactions leading to mono- (as shown in Figure 1) and, ultimately, bis-alkylation. The aziridinyl rings derived from IPM are not charged because the nitrogen readily deprotonates at pH 7.4[20]. A competing P-N bond scission reaction gives aziridine which, unlike chloroethylaziridine, is only a mono-alkylator and, therefore, cannot act as a DNA crosslinking agent.

2.1 Aldehyde Dehydrogenase (ALDH)

A major mechanism of resistance to the oxazaphosphorines is the conversion of aldehydic metabolites to carboxylic acids as mediated by ALDH[7]. While multiple pathways of resistance may be operative in any given cell, it has been shown that just the over-expression of human class 1 ALDH is sufficient to confer resistance specific to oxazaphosphorines[21]. Many isozymes of ALDH have been identified in human tissue, but current research supports ALDH1A1 [class 1 (cytosolic) ALDH] and, perhaps, ALDH3A1 [class 3 (cytosolic and microsomal) ALDH] as major determinants of clinically relevant, cellular resistance against CP and IF[7]. Intrinsic and acquired expression of these isoforms varies considerably among and within tissue types, both normal and neoplastic[7].

For CP, detoxification by ALDH specifically involves the oxidation of AP to carboxyphosphamide and for IF, it is the formation of carboxyifosfamide from AIF (Figure 1). Differences in electronic and resonance factors make fragmentation to PM/IPM favorable for AP/AIF but not for the carboxyphosphamides[4]. Thus, AP and AIF play pivotal roles where fragmentation to a phosphoramide mustard leads to cytotoxicity while oxidation through ALDH results in detoxification.

It is not difficult to design analogs of CP and IF that cannot be detoxified through an ALDH-mediated oxidation reaction. More challenging, however, is the task of incorporating these modifications into molecules that will still undergo key facets of oxazaphosphorine metabolism (e.g., activation by P450 and subsequent spontaneous elimination to a phosphoramide mustard). Most challenging is producing an analog or treatment strategy that will overcome ALDH resistance without sacrificing selectivity. The relatively high levels of ALDH in pluripotent and multipotent hematopoietic stem cells are believed to protect these cells from the oxazaphosphorines[7,21]. Thus, while the use of ALDH inhibitors presents a possibility for overcoming resistance[7], systemic administration of such agents would be expected to suppress ALDH-mediated protective mechanisms.

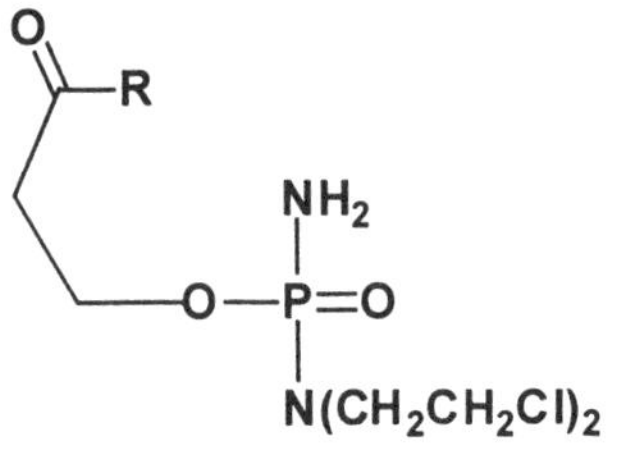

AP: R = H; half-life = 77 min
Methylketophosphamide:
R = CH_3; half-life = 173 min
Phenylketophosphamide:
R = C_6H_5; half-life = 66 min

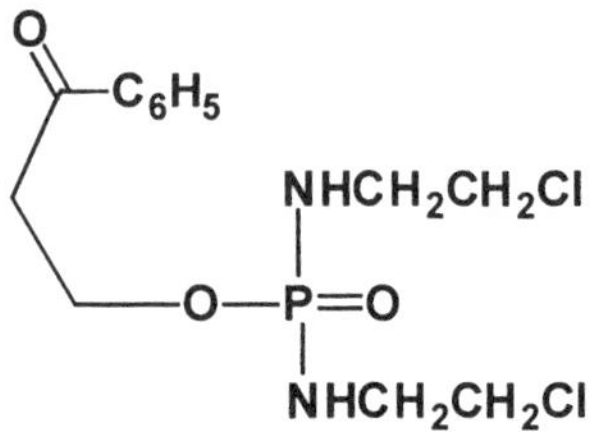

Phenylketoifosfamide :
half-life = 63 min

Figure 2. Ketone analogs of aldehydic metabolites. Half-lives refer to kinetics in solutions of 1 M lutidine-DMSO (8:2), pH 7.4, 37 °C[24].

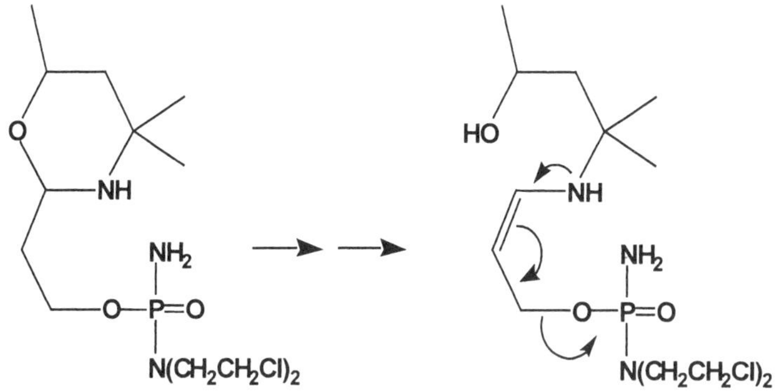

Figure 3. An analog designed to eliminate PM through an enamine[28].

2.2 C_4-Substituted CP/IF and Analogs of AP/AIF

Substitution of an alkyl or aryl group at the C_4 position of CP or IF followed by oxidation and ring opening would yield a ketone metabolite instead of an aldehyde. Unlike aldehydes, ketones are not easily oxidized to carboxylic acids and, therefore, should be resistant to the action of ALDH. Representative analogs of this type which have been studied previously include 4-ethylcyclophosphamide[22] and 4-phenylcyclophosphamide[23]. Both exhibited low therapeutic activities, but these results did not necessarily reflect on the consequences of blocking ALDH intervention; steric constraints associated with substitutions at the C_4 position could have impeded activation by P450. To bypass any factors associated with this initial metabolic step, pre-oxidized analogs were synthesized, as represented in Figure 2 by methylketophosphamide and phenylketophosphamide[24]. These cognates are structurally and functionally analogous to AP in that they spontaneously eliminate PM. Similarly, IPM is formed from the analogous phenyl ketone derivative of AIF, phenylketoifosfamide[24].

Because phenylketophosphamide and phenylketoifosfamide fragmented at rates comparable to that of AP, these compounds were screened for anticancer activity against various cell lines[24–26]. Relative to CP or IF, both ketones generally exhibited greater activity *in vitro* but higher toxicity *in vivo*. The byproduct of fragmentation, the acrolein analog phenylvinylketone [$CH_2{=}CHC(O)C_6H_5$], apparently did not contribute to this toxicity[27]. These results suggested that the phenyl ketones effectively circumvent ALDH-mediated resistance - but at the expense of selectivity. Compounds of this type may still have applications through local delivery. Appropriate modifications to the aromatic ring would allow for coupling reactions to polymers or antibodies designed for uptake by specific tumor cells. Such modifications could also be used to modulate fragmentation times so as to optimize PM/IPM formation at the target site[4].

It is noteworthy that ring-closure of the ketones to give 4-hydroxy tautomers was not observed by NMR spectroscopy[24]. This suggests that the interconversion between cyclic and acyclic metabolites can be markedly perturbed in the direction of the acyclic structure without an attendant loss of activity[4]. Such an observation allows for greater latitude in analog design.

AP analogs of the type shown in Figure 3 were designed to spontaneously eliminate PM through a pathway not involving the intermediacy of an aldehyde[28]. Although the success of the reported compounds was mixed with respect to achieving mechanistic and toxicity goals, this molecular strategy provides opportunities for refinement.

2.3 Stereochemistry

There is a considerable literature[6,29] related to the effects of chirality on the initial P450 oxidations of CP and IF, but the consequences of stereochemistry on the detoxification of AP by ALDH are not well established (asymmetry at phosphorus is maintained in AP but is lost through ring-opening in AIF). One reported study used ^{31}P NMR and cell perfusion techniques to monitor the conversion of the individual enantiomers of AP to carboxyphosphamide in CP-resistant human erythroleukemia K562 cells[30]. While the data indicated that S_P-AP was a slightly (~10-35%) better substrate for ALDH, these results were probably within the experimental error limits of the NMR method used at that time. Enantioselectivity was also studied using conventional cell culture techniques and preactivated R_P- and S_P-CP[30]. Based on the cytotoxicity data, no statistically significant enantioselectivity was found against CP-sensitive or CP-resistant L1210 mouse leukemia cells.

A more thorough investigation of the enantioselectivity of specific ALDH isozymes for AP is warranted. Should, for example, ALDH1A1 show a marked preference for one stereoisomer of AP, then this resistance mechanism could be overcome by treatment with the other, "wrong", isomer. To spare normal cells ordinarily protected by ALDH, targeted delivery of the stereochemically pure AP to cancer cells would presumably be required. Using the aldehydic moiety, AP could be coupled to an appropriate delivery system through a hydrolytically labile bond. Such a strategy has been used to link this metabolite to dextran through a semicarbazone group (Figure 4)[31]. As a precursor to AP, 4-HO-CP offers alternative structural opportunities for binding to macromolecular carriers through, for example, labile sulfhydryl linkages at the C_4 position (Figure 4)[4,32].

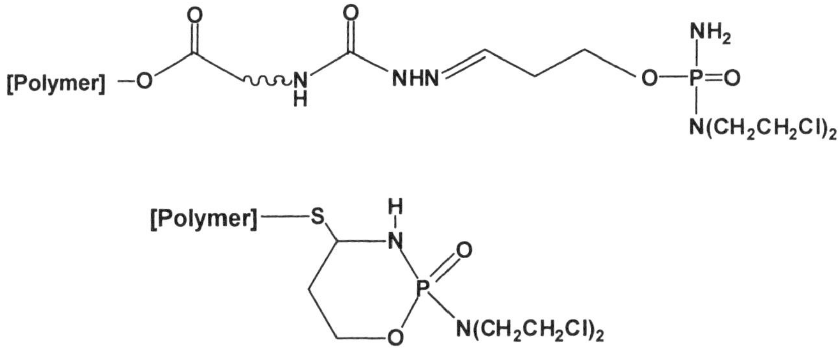

Figure 4. Polymer derivatives of AP (top)[31] and 4-HO-CP (bottom)[32].

2.4 Analogs of PM and IPM

The efficacy of direct treatment with PM or IPM continues to be a subject of some debate. Nevertheless, considerable data has been reported which supports the conclusion that the greatest therapeutic benefits are derived when PM and IPM are generated intracellularly[4,33,34]. At pH 7.4, PM and IPM are anionic and have poor membrane permeability, as has been demonstrated by cell perfusion and ^{31}P NMR techniques[34]. To circumvent the transport issue, prodrugs have recently been designed using strategies of targeted drug delivery and release of a phosphoramide mustard within cancer cells. Such analogs have promise in overcoming resistance to ALDH while at the same time sparing stem cell toxicity.

As represented in Figure 5, nitrothiophene and nitrofuran analogs of PM were investigated as prodrugs wherein elimination of a phosphoramide mustard would be electronically favorable upon reduction of the nitro group[35]. This activating reduction was expected to occur preferentially in hypoxic cells, the presence of which in many refractory solid tumors is well established. Proof of principle was established in that PM release was observed upon reduction, and the analogs in general were very cytotoxic; however, hypoxia-selective activity was only moderate. The authors suggested that activation mechanisms in addition to bioreduction might be operative. It was shown experimentally that such alternative mechanisms were unlikely to include activation by GSH or GST expression. With future refinement, analogs of this type may prove useful against cells resistant to oxazaphosphorines by virtue of ALDH and/or GSH/GST activity (*vide infra*).

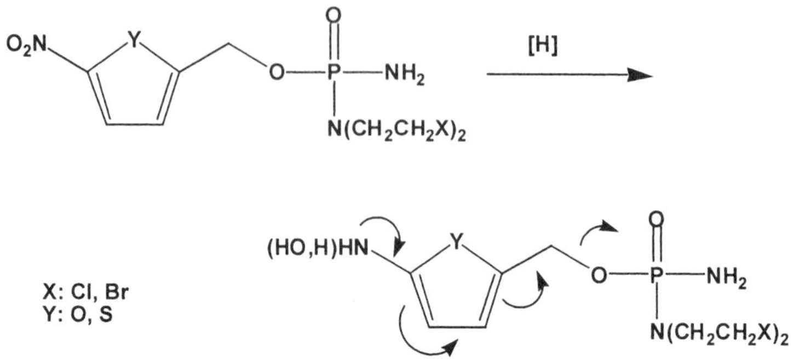

X: Cl, Br
Y: O, S

Figure 5. Nitrothiophenes and nitrofurans designed to eliminate a phosphoramide mustard following bioreduction[35].

An extension of the bioreductive activation strategy has been applied to analogs of the general type shown in Figure 6[36]. These compounds were designed to be reduced by DT-diaphorase, an enzyme that is over-expressed in various solid tumors. As demonstrated experimentally, reduction of the naphthoquinones by human DT-diaphorase triggered the rapid release of phosphoramide mustards. These analogs were uniformly cytotoxic *in vitro*, but the activities did not correlate with cellular levels of DT-diaphorase. This was presumably due to the fact that GSH was found to participate in a competing, enzyme-independent mechanism involving conjugate addition of this nucleophile to the quinone, with subsequent elimination of phosphoramide mustards. Appropriate modifications of the naphthoquinones may yield 'second generation' prodrugs useful against CP- and IF-resistant cancers.

Another IPM prodrug not subject to the action of ALDH is β-D-glucosylisophosphoramide mustard (β-D-Glc-IPM, Figure 7)[37,38]. Its antineoplastic activity *in vitro* is comparable to that of IPM, and *in vivo* it is equivalent to or higher than that of CP and IF. In comparison with the effects of IF, the toxicity of β-D-Glc-IPM to white blood cells, colony forming units and spleen colony forming units is considerably less. It is believed that the selectivity and favorable activity of this prodrug derives from transport into tumor cells by a glucose transporter and intracellular hydrolysis (spontaneously or enzymatically) to IPM. β-D-Glc-IPM is currently in clinical trials and may emerge as a useful alkylator against tumor cells over-expressing ALDH.

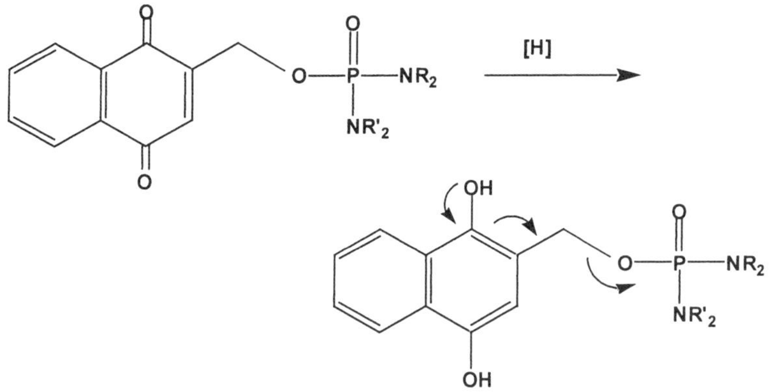

Figure 6. Naphthoquinones designed to eliminate a phosphoramide mustard upon bioreduction[36].

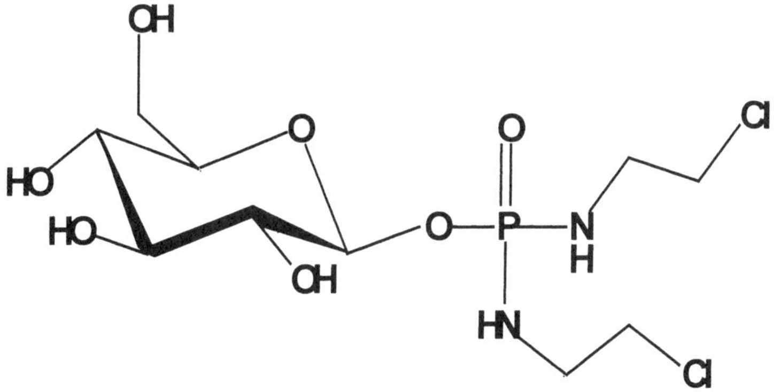

Figure 7. β-D-Glucosylisophosphoramide mustard (β-D-Glc-IPM)[37].

3. GLUTATHIONE AND ITS ASSOCIATED ENZYMES

Biochemical studies have shown that CP and IF or their metabolites can be inactivated by GSH in spontaneous or enzyme-catalyzed reactions[8,17]. That this inactivation may play a role in cellular resistance is supported by studies correlating a reduction in drug toxicity with an increase in the levels of GSH or increases in the activity of associated enzymes such as the GSTs[8]. In some cases, however, pretreatment levels of GSH or enzyme activity have failed to predict response to therapy[39,40], leading to some doubt as to the importance of GSH to CP or IF resistance. Due to the genetic variability of human cancers the latter finding may not be surprising; however, the steady-state levels of GSH or its associated enzymes may not be accurate indicators of response to CP or IF therapy. The ability of the cancer cell to respond to the stress induced by chemotherapy is a key factor in predicting outcome. For example, in a study of tumor samples from twenty patients, Cheng *et al.*[41] found no difference in pre-treatment GSH levels between responders and non-responders to combination therapy including CP. However, the ratio of GSH (and GSTs) taken after therapy to that taken before was increased in non-responders compared to the patients that did respond. Relatively few studies are directed toward monitoring this type of dynamic response to therapy and, therefore, the importance of GSH-mediated resistance may be under appreciated. With this in mind, it seems prudent to include GSH and its associated enzymes in a discussion of methods to circumvent the ability of a cancer cell to resist CP and IF therapy.

3.1 Methods of Circumventing Glutathione-Mediated Resistance

Many of the strategies developed for reversing GSH-mediated resistance have been demonstrated for other alkylating agents but may be just as effective in enhancing the potency of CP and IF. Perhaps the most commonly known method by which to alter GSH metabolism involves the use of the GSH biosynthesis inhibitor buthionine sulfoximine (BSO)[42]. This inhibitor targets γ-glutamylcysteine synthetase, a key enzyme in GSH biosynthesis. Over-expression of this enzyme often correlates with increased GSH levels and resistance to chemotherapy[43]. Exposure of cultured cells to BSO results in depletion of the GSH pool and enhanced activity of CP[8]. Clinical studies of BSO have proceeded in combination with another nitrogen mustard alkylating agent, melphalan, with promising results[44,45]. A similar strategy with CP and IF could be devised; however, animal studies demonstrated only a modest increase in CP efficacy with BSO pretreatment[46]. Another drawback of BSO treatment is its non-selectivity[47], resulting in increased drug toxicity in normal tissue. Selectivity may be improved by exploiting differences in GSH recovery rates between tumor and normal tissues[46,47]. Reversal of resistance through the use of BSO, therefore, is a promising avenue of investigation.

Other agents have been used to acutely deplete GSH[48], including both IF and CP. IF has been shown to be more effective than CP in reducing GSH levels[2,49]. This ability to deplete GSH has spurred interest into using IF in combination regimens to potentiate the activity of a number of drugs[2,50,51]. *In vitro* studies have also suggested that IF metabolites may inhibit the activity of GST[49]; however, clinical studies have not detected significant inhibition[52].

As mentioned previously, methods that deplete GSH may not offer high specificity for tumor tissue. Potentiation of drug activity through targeting of the GSTs may offer more selectivity since elevated levels of these enzymes are often observed in tumor as compared to normal tissue[53]. In addition, the expression of certain isozymes of the GSTs is an important indicator of drug response[54] (see also chapter 4 in this volume by Hamilton and colleagues).

Inhibitors of the GSTs have been effective in increasing the potency of alkylating agents[55]. However, since metabolites of CP[4,17,56] and IF[15] can react spontaneously with GSH, do the transferases play a significant role in resistance to these drugs? This appears likely since CP itself, although inactive, can be a substrate for (rat) liver enzymes to form a GSH conjugate[57]. Even for the more reactive metabolites of CP and IF, the GSTs can accelerate conjugation with GSH[15,58]. In cell studies, an inhibitor of GST, ethacrynic acid, potentiated the cytotoxicity of activated CP and melphalan in previously resistant cell lines[59,60]. The promising results with ethacrynic acid have spurred preliminary clinical testing of this inhibitor[61]. The drawback of this reagent is that it is not isozyme specific and exhibits other pharmacological effects[55,62,63]. In light of this, selective inhibition of isozymes of GST has been achieved with a number of GSH analogs[55,64,65]. Pretreatment of cells with many of these analogs has enhanced the cytotoxicity of alkylating agents and other drugs and offers additional weapons in combating GSH-mediated drug resistance[55,63].

In addition to over-expression of γ-glutamylcysteine synthetase and GST, resistance to alkylating agents can be linked to over-expression of another GSH-associated enzyme, glutathione reductase[12,66,67]. This enzyme catalyzes the reduction of oxidized glutathione disulfide and is critical to maintaining the redox balance in the cell. Inhibition of this enzyme by a non-alkylating nitrosourea depleted GSH and potentiated the activity of 4-hydroperoxycyclophosphamide (4HC, pre-activated CP) in human leukemia cells[68]. This avenue of combating resistance has not been investigated extensively.

These studies with enzyme inhibitors illustrate how resistance can be circumvented by directly confronting the cellular defenses. Another approach is to turn these same defenses against the cell and utilize the high levels of metabolites or enzymes inherent in the drug resistant cell in the activation of prodrugs. Several examples of this approach are presented below.

Based on the effectiveness of GSH analog inhibitors of GST, novel latent alkylating agents were designed which are activated by this enzyme[69,70].

These agents release phosphoramide mustards in a process catalyzed by the P1-1 and A1-1 isozymes of human GST (Figure 8). For example, the activity of one of these agents, TER286, correlates with the levels of GST in cell lines and xenografts[71]. TER286 showed increased cytotoxicity against a 4HC-resistant MCF-7 line compared to the parental line, thereby demonstrating how these novel agents may be used to circumvent resistance.

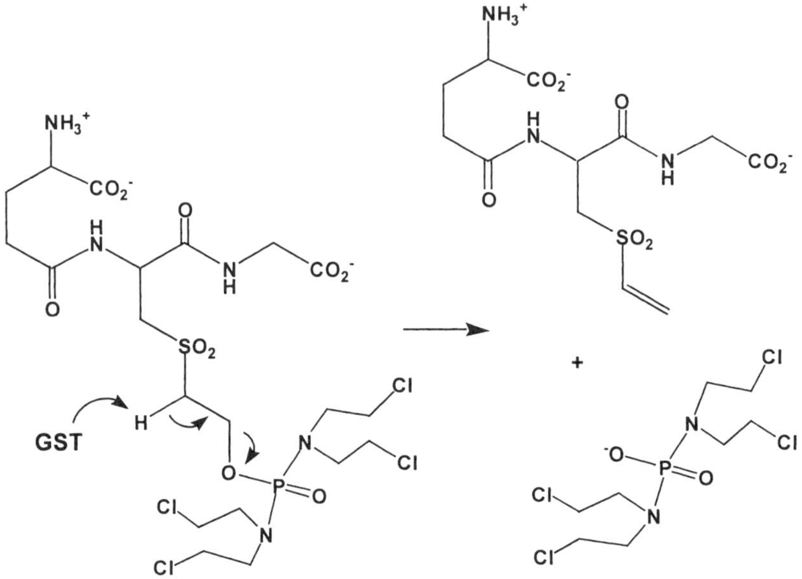

Figure 8. Glutathione S-transferase (GST) activation of TER286. [Adapted from Satyam *et al.*[70]].

In another example of utilizing cellular defenses to enhance therapy, the increased GSH content in resistant cells may be exploited to activate prodrugs. This is demonstrated with a disulfide analog of the alkylating agent mitomycin C that relies on increased GSH levels to generate the cytotoxic metabolite[72]. An analog of CP or IF may be developed with this same strategy in mind.

4. DNA REPAIR

There is increasing evidence that DNA repair mechanisms contribute to cellular resistance against the oxazaphosphorines[8,10,11,13,14] (see also chapter 7 in this volume by Dr. D. Murray). Because investigations in this area are relatively new, the full impact of such events on the activity of CP and IF is not known. Moreover, the mechanistic specifics are not clearly defined on a molecular level other than the fact that they must involve the alkylating metabolites of CP and IF (i.e., PM, IPM, chloroethylaziridine, aziridine, and/or acrolein).

5. PM AND IPM

For PM and IPM, the reaction sequence of therapeutic consequence involves two sequential alkylations of complementary strands of DNA resulting predominantly in interstrand crosslinks between the N_7 positions of 5'-GNC-sequences[73,74]. Figure 9 depicts a generalized view of the reactions of PM (through aziridinium ions) with DNA[75]. The known chemistry of PM and its aziridinyl intermediates suggests that P-N bond scission will compete with alkylation[17,18]. For PM, however, this reaction still allows for crosslinking. The sequential reactions of IPM with DNA are expected to parallel those of PM with the exception that any P-N bond hydrolysis would prohibit crosslinking.

There are data to support the preliminary conclusion that repair can be made to mono-alkylated single strands of DNA as well as to interstrand crosslinked DNA[8,10,11,76]. For the purposes of this text, however, an assumption will be made that any modifications to PM and IPM which increase the rate and, therefore, the frequency of crosslink formation are worthy of investigation[75]. In cells that have been treated with PM or pre-activated CP, maximal crosslinking of DNA occurs 4-6 h after drug removal[76,77]. It is reasonable to assume that the relatively slow formation of crosslinks is primarily related to the rate of the second alkylation sequence. If this pathway were accelerated, there would be less time for repair of mono-alkylated DNA and more crosslinks might result.

By replacing one or more of the chlorine atoms in PM or IPM with a different leaving group, one could modulate the rate of each cyclization reaction and, therefore, the overall rate of crosslinking. Through variations in electronic and/or steric effects, such analogs could also be designed to be poor substrates for enzymes that repair mono-adducted strands of DNA. Cognates of PM, IPM and IF with bromine or a mesyl group (OSO_2CH_3) in place of chlorine have shown activity comparable to or better than that of the parent drugs[78–82]. A bromine analog of IPM has specifically been shown to generate more DNA crosslinks[79]. These data warrant more extensive studies of such modified alkylating agents using cells that over-express DNA repair enzymes.

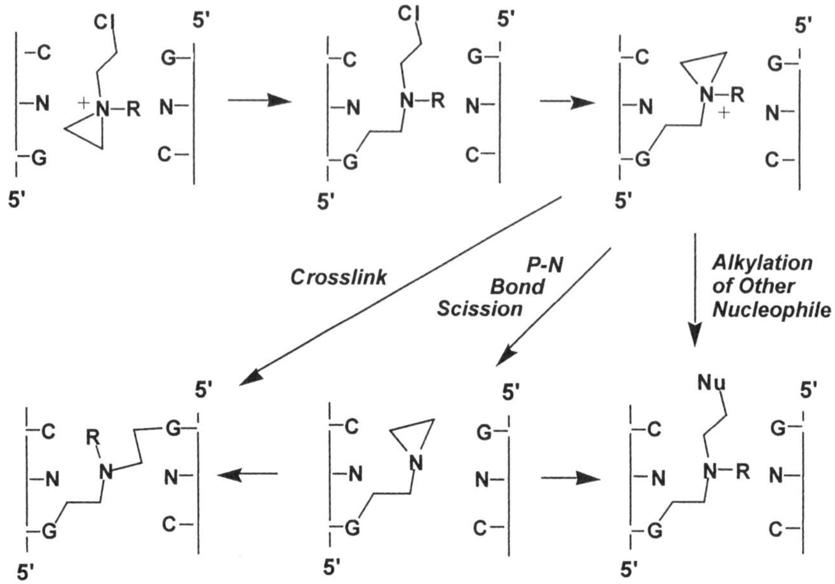

Figure 9. Sequence and possible outcomes from the reaction of phosphoramide mustard with DNA. [Adapted from Colvin *et al.*[75]]. [R = $P(O_2)NH_2$].

Modulations in alkylation kinetics as well as enzyme binding efficiencies could also be achieved by increasing the length of one or both of the carbon chains in PM and IPM. Additional substitutions on the chain or on nitrogen (in IPM) would also affect reactivity both electronically and sterically[36,83].

Assuming that PM/IPM analogs would be generated by metabolism of the corresponding CP/IF cognates, any structural modifications of the type discussed above would be limited to those that would still allow for the facile fragmentation of precursor aldehydic metabolites as well as for the intramolecular cyclization reactions required for bis-alkylation[4,84,85].

Additional strategies for overcoming resistance mechanisms related to DNA repair include inhibiting relevant enzymes such as topoisomerase. In this regard, novobiocin has been found to potentiate the activity of CP both *in vitro* and *in vivo*; however, the clinical significance of this potentiation is uncertain[86].

6. AGT AND ACROLEIN

Recently, it has been suggested that acrolein may contribute to the therapeutic efficacy of CP (and IF) through alkylation of DNA[13]. Furthermore, this alkylation apparently can be repaired through the action of O^6-alkylguanine-DNA alkyltransferase (AGT)[13,14]. As a mechanism of resistance, AGT is perhaps most commonly associated with the nitrosoureas, e.g., BCNU (carmustine). If AGT intervenes to remove the initial O^6-alkylated adduct, the DNA is repaired. The depletion of AGT by an inhibitor such as O^6-benzylguanine (O^6-BG) modulates this resistance and potentiates the cytotoxicity of BCNU[8]. Similarly, O^6-BG could be used to prevent any AGT-mediated repair associated with the alkylation of DNA by acrolein. Interestingly, the use of O^6-BG could serve to simultaneously enhance the activity of PM and IPM. While the mechanism of the interaction has not yet been defined, it has recently been shown that O^6-BG increases the cytotoxic effects of PM and IPM irrespective of AGT content[87].

It is important to establish whether the toxicity shown by acrolein, apparently through O^6-alkylation of guanine, is therapeutically desirable. If so, blocking the AGT repair mechanism would be beneficial. There are other studies, however, which show that the AGT-sensitive acrolein adduct is mutagenic with long-range possibilities of therapy induced leukemias[14]. In the case of acrolein, the repair of DNA by AGT may be more significant as a mechanism of protection than as one of resistance.

CONCLUSION

The inherent or acquired resistance of cancer cells to CP and IF tempers the clinical success of these chemotherapeutics. This chapter has focused on analog design and treatment modifications through the use of small molecules (e.g., inhibitors). There are other strategies, including the current clinical practice of dose escalation. The latter is limited by toxicity to normal cells, but the advantage of increased dosing may be effectively achieved with gene therapy and site specific activation[88,89]. Protection of normal cells by enhancing the expression of, for example, ALDH is another area of recent study[90]. Whether through changes in molecular design, delivery, activation and/or inhibition, the ability to overcome resistance without compromising protective selectivity is predicated on a better understanding of the biochemical and molecular bases of the resistance mechanisms.

ACKNOWLEDGEMENTS

This was supported in part by CA16783 from the National Cancer Institute, Department of Health and Human Services (SML) and DAMD 17-99-1-9175 (MPG).

REFERENCES

1. Colvin OM. An overview of cyclophosphamide development and clinical applications. Curr Pharm Design, 5:555-560, 1999.
2. Vanhoefer U, Schleucher N, Klaassen U, *et al.* Ifosfamide-based drug combinations: Preclinical evaluation of drug interactions and translation into the clinic. Semin Oncol, 27, Suppl 1:8-13, 2000.
3. Kutz ME, Mulkerin DL, Wiedemann GJ, *et al.* In vitro studies of the hyperthermic enhancement of activated ifosfamide (4-hydroperoxy-ifosfamide) and glucose isophosphoramide mustard. Cancer Chemother Pharmacol, 40:167-171, 1997.
4. Ludeman SM. The chemistry of the metabolites of cyclophosphamide. Curr Pharm Design, 5:627-643, 1999.
5. Boal JH, Williamson M, Boyd VL, *et al.* ^{31}P NMR studies of the kinetics of bisalkylation by isophosphoramide mustard: Comparisons with phosphoramide mustard. J Med Chem, 32:1768-1773, 1989.
6. Williams ML, Wainer IW. Cyclophosphamide versus ifosfamide: To use ifosfamide or not to use, that is the three-dimensional question. Curr Pharm Design, 5:665-672, 1999.
7. Sladek NE. Aldehyde dehydrogenase-mediated cellular relative insensitivity to the oxazaphosphorines. Curr Pharm Design, 5:607-625, 1999.
8. Gamcsik MP, Dolan ME, Andersson BS, Murray D. Mechanisms of resistance to the toxicity of cyclophosphamide. Curr Pharm Design, 5:587-605, 1999.
9. Richardson ME, Siemann DW. Tumor cell heterogeneity: Impact on mechanisms of therapeutic drug resistance. Int J Radiat Oncol Biol Phys, 39:789-795, 1997.
10. Andersson BS, Mroue M, Britten RA, Murray D. The role of DNA damage in the resistance of human chronic myeloid leukemia cells to cyclophosphamide analogues. Cancer Res, 54:5394-5400, 1994.
11. Dong Q, Bullock N, Ali-Osman F, *et al.* Repair analysis of 4-hydroperoxycyclophosphamide-induced DNA interstrand crosslinking in the c-myc gene in 4-hydroperoxycyclophosphamide-sensitive and -resistant medulloblastoma cell lines. Cancer Chemother Pharmacol, 37:242-246, 1996.
12. Chen G, Teicher BA, Frei E III. Biochemical characterization of in vivo alkylating agent resistance of a murine EMT-6 mammary carcinoma. Implication for systemic involvement in the resistance phenotype. Cancer Biochem Biophys, 16:139-155, 1998.
13. Friedman HS, Pegg AE, Johnson S, *et al.* Modulation of cyclophosphamide activity by O6-alkylguanine-DNA alkyltransferase. Cancer Chemother Pharmacol, 43:80-85, 1999.
14. Cai Y, Wu MH, Ludeman SM, *et al.* Role of O^6-alkylguanine-DNA alkyltransferase in protecting against cyclophosphamide-induced toxicity and mutagenicity. Cancer Res,

59:3059-3063, 1999.

15. Dirven HAAM, Megens L, Oudshoorn MJ, *et al.* Glutathione conjugation of the cytostatic drug ifosfamide and the role of human glutathione S-transferases. Chem Res Toxicol, 8:979-986, 1995.
16. Giai M, Biglia N, Sismondi P. Chemoresistance in breast tumors. Eur J Gynaecol Oncol, 12:359-373, 1991.
17. Shulman-Roskes EM, Noe DA, Gamcsik MP, *et al.* The partitioning of phosphoramide mustard and its aziridinium ions among alkylation and P-N bond hydrolysis reactions. J Med Chem, 41:515-529, 1998.
18. Lu H, Chan KK. Gas chromatographic-mass spectrometric assay for N-2-chloroethylaziridine, a volatile cytotoxic metabolite of cyclophosphamide in rat plasma. J Chromatogr B Biomed Appl, 678:219-225, 1996.
19. Flowers JL, Ludeman SM, Gamcsik MP, *et al.* Evidence for a role of chloroethylaziridine in the cytotoxicity of cyclophosphamide. Cancer Chemother Pharmacol, 45:335-344, 2000.
20. Millis KK, Colvin ME, Shulman-Roskes EM, *et al.* Comparison of the protonation of isophosphoramide mustard and phosphoramide mustard. J Med Chem, 38:2166-2175, 1995.
21. Bunting KD, Townsend AJ. De novo expression of transfected human class 1 aldehyde dehydrogenase (ALDH) causes resistance to oxazaphosphorine anti-cancer alkylating agents in hamster V79 cell lines. Elevated class 1 ALDH activity is closely correlated with reduction in DNA interstrand cross-linking and lethality. J Biol Chem, 271:11884-11890, 1996.
22. Struck RF, Thorpe MC, Coburn WC Jr, Kirk MC. Isolation of cis- and trans-4-methylcyclophosphamide and antitumor evaluation in vivo. Cancer Res, 35:3160-3163, 1975.
23. Boyd VL, Himes HL, Stalick JK, *et al.* Synthesis and antitumor activity of cyclophosphamide analogues. 3. Preparation, molecular structure determination and anticancer screening of racemic cis- and trans-4-phenylcyclophosphamide. J Med Chem 23:372-375, 1980.
24. Ludeman SM, Boyd VL, Regan JB, *et al.* Synthesis and antitumor activity of cyclophosphamide analogues. 4. Preparation, kinetic studies, and anticancer screening of "phenylketophosphamide" and similar compounds related to the cyclophosphamide metabolite aldophosphamide. J Med Chem, 29:716-727, 1986.
25. Friedman HS, Colvin OM, Ludeman SM, *et al.* Experimental chemotherapy of human medulloblastoma with classical alkylators. Cancer Res, 46:2827-2833, 1986.
26. Friedman HS, Colvin OM, Skapek SX, *et al.* Experimental chemotherapy of human medulloblastoma cell lines and transplantable xenografts with bifunctional alkylating agents. Cancer Res, 48:4189-4195, 1988.
27. Hales BF, Ludeman SM, Boyd VL. Embryotoxicity of phenyl ketone analogs of cyclophosphamide. Teratol, 39:31-37, 1989.

28. Borch RF, Valente RR. Synthesis, activation, and cytotoxicity of aldophosphamide analogues. J Med Chem, 34:3052-3058, 1991.
29. Kusnierczyk H, Radzikowski C, Paprocka M, *et al.* Antitumor activity of optical isomers of cyclophosphamide, ifosfamide and trofosfamide as compared to clinically used racemates. Immunopharmacol, 8:455-480, 1986.
30. Habib AD, Boal JH, Hilton J, *et al.* Effect of stereochemistry on the oxidative metabolism of the cyclophosphamide metabolite aldophosphamide. Biochem Pharmacol, 50:429-433, 1995.
31. Ludeman SM, Chang YH, Roskes ES, *et al.* Polymeric carriers of cyclophosphamide metabolites. Proc Amer Assoc Cancer Res, 38:259: #1738, 1997.
32. Ramonas LM, Erickson LC, Klesse W, *et al.* Differential cytotoxicity and DNA cross-linking produced by polymeric and monomeric activated analogues of cyclophosphamide in mouse L1210 leukemia cells. Mol Pharmacol, 19:331-336, 1981.
33. Colvin M, Chabner BA. Alkylating agents. *In*: Cancer Chemotherapy: Principles and Practice. BA Chabner, JM Collins (eds.), JB Lippincott, Philadelphia, PA, 276-313, 1991.
34. Boal JH, Ludeman SM, Ho CK, *et al.* Direct detection of the intracellular formation of carboxyphosphamides using nuclear magnetic resonance spectroscopy. Arzneim-Forsch/Drug Res, 44:84-93, 1994.
35. Borch RF, Liu J, Schmidt JP, *et al.* Synthesis and evaluation of nitroheterocyclic phosphoramidates as hypoxia-selective alkylating agents. J Med Chem, 43:2258-2265, 2000.
36. Flader C, Liu J, Borch RF. Development of novel quinone phosphorodiamidate prodrugs targeted to DT-diaphorase. J Med Chem, 43:3157-3167, 2000.
37. Pohl J, Bertram B, Hilgard P, *et al.* D-19575 - A sugar-linked isophosphoramide mustard derivative exploiting transmembrane glucose transport. Cancer Chemother Pharmacol, 35:364-370, 1995.
38. Veyhl M, Wagner K, Volk C, *et al.* Transport of the new chemotherapeutic agent beta-D-glucosylisophosphoramide mustard (D-19575) into tumor cells is mediated by the Na+-D-glucose cotransporter SAAT1. Proc Natl Acad Sci USA, 95:2914-2919, 1998.
39. Boven E, Pinedo HM, van Hattum AH, *et al.* Characterization of human soft-tissue sarcoma xenografts for use in secondary drug screening. Br J Cancer, 78:1586-1593, 1998.
40. D'Incalci A, Bonfanti M, Pifferi A, *et al.* The antitumour activity of alkylating agents is not correlated with the levels of glutathione, glutathione transferase and O6-alkylguanine-DNA-alkyltransferase of human tumor xenografts. Eur J Cancer, 34:1749-1755, 1998.
41. Cheng X, Kigawa J, Minigawa Y, *et al.* Glutathione S-transferase-pi expression and glutathione concentration in ovarian carcinoma before and after chemotherapy. Cancer, 79:521-527, 1997.
42. Griffith OW, Meister A. Potent and specific inhibition of glutathione synthesis by buthionine sulfoximine (S-n-butyl homocysteine sulfoximine). J Biol Chem, 254:7558-7560, 1979.
43. Bailey HH, Gipp JJ, Ripple M, *et al.* Increase in γ-glutamylcysteine synthetase activity and steady-state messenger RNA levels in melphalan resistant DU-145 human prostate carcinoma cells expressing elevated glutathione levels. Cancer Res, 52:5115-5118, 1992.
44. Bailey HH. L-S,R-buthionine sulfoximine: Historical development and clinical issues. Chem-Biol Interact, 111-112:239-254, 1998.
45. Calvert P, Yao KS, Hamilton TC, O'Dwyer PJ. Clinical studies of reversal of drug

resistance based on glutathione. Chem-Biol Interact, 111-112:213-224, 1998.

46. Siemann DW, Beyers KL. In vivo therapeutic potential of combination thiol depletion and alkylating chemotherapy. Br J Cancer, 68:1071-1079, 1993.
47. Lee FYF, Allalunis-Turner MJ, Siemann DW. Depletion of tumour versus normal tissue glutathione by buthionine sulfoximine. Br J Cancer, 56:33-38, 1987.
48. Boyland E, Chasseaud LF. The effect of some carbonyl compounds on rat liver glutathione levels. Biochem Pharmacol, 19:1526-1528, 1970.
49. Lind MJ, McGown AT, Hadfield JA, *et al.* The effect of ifosfamide and its metabolites on intracellular glutathione levels in vitro and in vivo. Biochem Pharmacol, 38:1835-1840, 1989.
50. Malik IA, Mehboobali N, Iqbal MP. Effect of ifosfamide on intracellular glutathione levels in peripheral blood lymphocytes and its correlation with therapeutic response in patients with advanced ovarian cancer. Cancer Chemother Pharmacol, 39:561-565, 1997.
51. Millward MJ, Harris AL, Cantwell BM. Phase II study of doxorubicin plus ifosfamide/mesna in patients with advanced breast cancer. Cancer, 65:2421-2425, 1990.
52. Mulders TM, Keizer HJ, Ouwerkerk J, *et al.* Effect of ifosfamide treatment on glutathione and glutathione conjugation activity in patients with advanced cancers. Clin Cancer Res, 1:1525-1536, 1995.
53. Howie A, Forrester L, Glancey M, *et al.* Glutathione S-transferase and glutathione peroxidase expression in normal and tumour human tissues. Carcinogenesis, 11:451-458, 1990.
54. Tew KD. Glutathione-associated enzymes in anticancer drug resistance. Cancer Res, 54:4313-4320, 1994.
55. Mulder GJ, Ouwerkerk-Mahadevan S. Modulation of glutathione conjugation in vivo: How to decrease glutathione conjugation in vivo or in intact cellular systems in vitro. Chem-Biol Interact, 105:17-34, 1997.
56. Dirven HAAM, Venekamp JC, van Ommen B, van Bladeren PJ. The interaction of glutathione with 4-hydroxycyclophosphamide and phosphoramide mustard, studied by P-31 nuclear magnetic resonance spectroscopy. Chem-Biol Interact, 93:185-196, 1994.
57. Yuan ZM, Smith PB, Brundrett RB, *et al.* Glutathione conjugation with phosphoramide mustard and cyclophosphamide. A mechanistic study using tandem mass spectrometry. Drug Metab Dispos, 19:625-629, 1991.
58. Dirven HAAM, van Ommen B, van Bladeren PJ. Involvement of human glutathione S-transferase isoenzymes in the conjugation of cyclophosphamide metabolites with glutathione. Cancer Res, 54:6215-6220, 1994.
59. Chen GA, Waxman DJ. Identification of glutathione S-transferase as a determinant of 4-hydroperoxycyclophosphamide resistance in human breast cancer cells. Biochem Pharmacol, 49:1691-1701, 1995.
60. Tew KD, Bomber AM, Hoffman SJ. Ethacrynic acid and piripost as enhancers of cytotoxicity in drug resistant and sensitive cell lines. Cancer Res, 48:3622-3625, 1988.
61. LaCreta FP, Brennan JM, Nash SL, *et al.* Pharmacokinetics and bioavailability study of

ethacrynic acid as a modulator of drug resistance in patients with cancer. J Pharmacol Exp Ther, 270:1186-1191, 1994.
62. Ciaccio PJ, Shen H, Kruh GD, Tew KD. Effects of chronic ethacrynic acid exposure on glutathione conjugation and MRP expression in human colon tumor cells. Biochem Biophys Res Commun, 222:111-115, 1996.
63. Morgan AS, Ciaccio PJ, Tew KD, Kauvar LM. Isozyme-specific glutathione S-transferase inhibitors potentiate drug sensitivity in cultured human tumor cell lines. Cancer Chemother Pharmacol, 37:353-370, 1996.
63. Flatgaard JE, Bauer KE, Kauvar LM. Isozyme specificity of novel glutathione-S-transferase inhibitors. Cancer Chemother Pharmacol, 33:63-70, 1993.
65. Adang AEP, Brussee J, van der Gen A, Mulder GJ. Inhibition of rat liver glutathione S-transferase isoenzymes by peptides stabilized against degradation by γ-glutamyltranspeptidase. J Biol Chem, 266:830-836, 1991.
66. Kolfschoten GM, Pinedo HM, Scheffer PG, *et al.* Development of a panel of 15 human ovarian cancer xenografts for drug screening and determination of the role of the glutathione detoxification system. Gynecol Oncol, 76:362-368, 2000.
67. Richardson ME, Siemann DW. Thiol-related mechanisms of resistance in a murine tumor model. Int J Radiat Oncol Biol Phys, 29:387-392, 1994.
68. Chresta CM, Crook TR, Souhami RL. Depletion of cellular glutathione by N,N'-bis(trans-4-hydroxycyclohexyl)-N'-nitrosourea as a determinant of sensitivity of K562 human leukemia cells to 4-hydroperoxycyclophosphamide. Cancer Res, 50:4067-4071, 1990.
69. Lyttle MH, Satyam A, Hocker MD, *et al.* Glutathione S-transferase activates novel alkylating agents. J Med Chem, 37:1501-1507, 1994.
70. Satyam A, Hocker MD, Kane-Maguire KA, *et al.* Design, synthesis, and evaluation of latent alkylating agents activated by glutathione S-transferase. J Med Chem, 39:1736-1747, 1996.
71. Morgan AS, Sanderson PE, Borch RF, *et al.* Tumor efficacy and bone marrow-sparing properties of TER286, a cytotoxin activated by glutathione S-transferase. Cancer Res, 58:2568-2575, 1998.
72. Ishida T, Nishio K, Kurokawa H, *et al.* Circumvention of glutathione-mediated mitomycin C resistance by a novel mitomycin C analogue, KW-2149. Int J Cancer, 72:865-870, 1997.
73. Dong Q, Barsky D, Colvin ME, *et al.* A structural basis for a phosphoramide mustard-induced DNA interstrand cross-link at 5'-d(GAC). Proc Natl Acad Sci USA, 92:12170-12174, 1995.
74. Struck RF, Davis RL Jr, Berardini MD, Loechler EL. DNA guanine-guanine crosslinking sequence specificity of isophosphoramide mustard, the alkylating metabolite of the clinical antitumor agent ifosfamide. Cancer Chemother Pharmacol, 45:59-62, 2000.
75. Colvin ME, Sasaki JC, Tran NL. Chemical factors in the action of phosphoramidic mustard alkylating anticancer drugs: Roles for computational chemistry. Curr Pharm Design, 5:645-663, 1999.
76. Crook TR, Souhami RL, McLean AE. Cytotoxicity, DNA cross-linking, and single strand breaks induced by activated cyclophosphamide and acrolein in human leukemia cells. Cancer Res, 46:5029-5034, 1986.
77. Hemminki K. Binding of metabolites of cyclophosphamide to DNA in a rat liver microsomal system and in vivo in mice. Cancer Res, 45:4237-4243, 1985.
78. Struck RF, Schmid SM, Waud WR. Antitumor activity of halogen analogs of

phosphoramide, isophosphoramide, and triphosphoramide mustards, the cytotoxic metabolites of cyclophosphamide, ifosfamide, and trofosfamide. Cancer Chemother Pharmacol, 34:191-196, 1994.

79. Studzian K, Kinas R, Ciesielska E, Szmigiero L. Effects of alkylating metabolites of ifosfamide and its bromo analogues on DNA of HeLa cells. Biochem Pharmacol, 43:937-943, 1992.
80. Glazman-Kusnierczyk H, Matuszyk J, Radzikowski C. Antitumor activity evaluation of bromine-substituted analogues of ifosfamide. I. Stereodifferentiation of biological effects and selection of the most potent compounds. Immunopharmacol Immunotoxicol, 14:883-911, 1992.
81. Takamizawa A, Matsumoto S, Iwata T, *et al.* Synthesis and antitumor activity of preactivated isophosphamide analogues bearing modified alkylating functionalities. J Med Chem, 21:208-214, 1978.
82. Misiura K, Kinas RW, Stec WJ, *et al.* Synthesis and antitumor activity of analogues of ifosfamide modified in the N-(2-chloroethyl) group. J Med Chem, 31:226-230, 1988.
83. Kwon CH, Borch RF. Effects of N-substitution on the activation mechanisms of 4--hydroxycyclophosphamide analogues. J Med Chem, 32:1491-1496, 1989.
84. Springer JB, Colvin ME, Colvin OM, Ludeman SM. Isophosphoramide mustard and its mechanism of bisalkylation. J Org Chem, 63:7218-7222, 1998.
85. Ludeman SM. From nerve agent to anticancer drug: The chemistry of phosphoramide mustard. *In*: Biomedical Chemistry: Applying Chemical Principles to the Understanding and Treatment of Disease. PF Torrence (ed.), John Wiley and Sons, New York, NY, 163-187, 2000.
86. Kennedy MJ, Armstrong DK, Huelskamp AM, *et al.* Phase I and pharmacologic study of the alkylating agent modulator novobiocin in combination with high-dose chemotherapy for the treatment of metastatic breast cancer. J Clin Oncol, 13:1136-1143, 1995.
87. Smith SM, Cai Y, Ludeman SM, Dolan ME. Effect of O^6-benzylguanine (O^6-BG) on ifosfamide-induced cytotoxicity in Chinese hamster ovary (CHO) cells. Proc Amer Assoc Cancer Res, 41:98:#628, 2000.
88. Aghi M, Chou TC, Suling K, *et al.* Multimodal cancer treatment mediated by a replicating oncolytic virus that delivers the oxazaphosphorine/rat cytochrome P450 2B1 and ganciclovir/herpes simplex virus thymidine kinase gene therapies. Cancer Res, 59:3861-3865, 1999.
89. Jounaidi Y, Hecht JE, Waxman DJ. Retroviral transfer of human cytochrome P450 genes for oxazaphosphorine-based cancer gene therapy. Cancer Res, 58:4391-4401, 1998.
90. Giorgianni F, Bridson PK, Sorrentino BP, *et al.* Inactivation of aldophosphamide by human aldehyde dehydrogenase isozyme 3. Biochem Pharmacol, 60:325-338, 2000.

Chapter 10

CELLULAR MECHANISMS OF CYCLOPHOSPHAMIDE RESISTANCE: MODEL STUDIES IN HUMAN MEDULLOBLASTOMA CELL LINES

Henry S. Friedman[1], Stewart P. Johnson[1,2] and O. Michael Colvin[3]
Departments of [1]Neuro-Oncology, [2]Neurosurgery, [3]Medicine, Duke University Comprehensive Cancer Center, Duke University Medical Center, Durham, North Carolina, USA

1. CYCLOPHOSPHAMIDE THERAPY OF MEDULLOBLASTOMA

Cyclophosphamide is extremely active in the treatment of medulloblastoma, the most common malignant tumor arising in the central nervous system of children[1]. Phase 2 trials in children with recurrent and newly diagnosed medulloblastoma have confirmed both clinical and radiographic responses to this alkylating agent[2–5], and a current Children's Oncology Group international Phase 3 trial is comparing a cyclophosphamide-based regimen to a CCNU-based regimen for children with newly diagnosed high-risk medulloblastoma. Unfortunately, patients with medulloblastoma treated with cyclophosphamide frequently fail therapy, confirming the emergence of drug-resistant tumor cells. Although selection of alternative treatment for these patients who relapse is the only option currently available, definition of the mechanism(s) responsible for cyclophosphamide resistance might provide new therapeutic strategies to reverse or even prevent resistance to this alkylator.

2. CYCLOPHOSPHAMIDE METABOLISM

Cyclophosphamide is a prodrug which undergoes cytochrome P450 mixed function oxidase-induced hydroxylation in the liver (Figure 1)[6]. This reaction produces 4-hydroxycyclophosphamide which exists in a tautomeric equilibrium with aldophosphamide. Aldophosphamide is converted to the active alkylating metabolite phosphoramide mustard (PM), which produces DNA interstrand crosslinks (ICLs), the critical cytotoxic lesions[7–9]. Aldehyde dehydrogenase (ALDH)-mediated conversion of aldophosphamide to carboxyphosphamide ameliorates cytotoxic alkylation and is responsible for the relative absence of toxicity to hematopoeitic stem cells and intestinal mucosal cells[10,11].

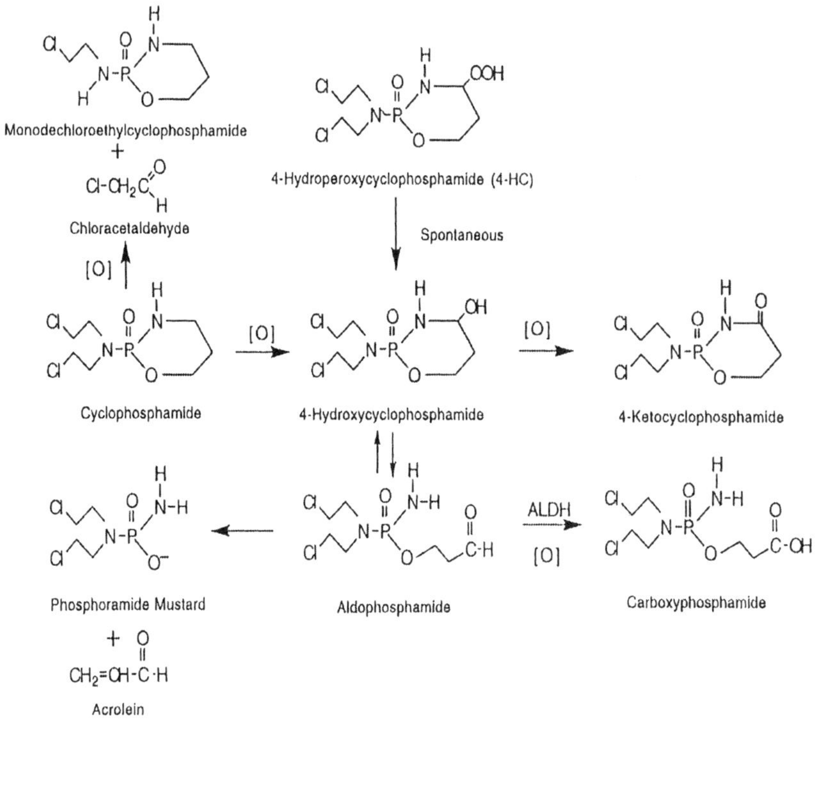

Figure 1. Metabolism of cyclophosphamide.

3. MEDULLOBLASTOMA CELL LINES AS A MODEL FOR THIS TUMOR

We and others have generated a broad panel of cell lines derived from medulloblastoma which has allowed a comprehensive phenotypic and genotypic analysis of this tumor (Table 1)[12–15]. Two cell lines, D341 Med and Daoy, were derived from primary cerebellar tumors at the time of initial diagnosis of a medulloblastoma. D283 Med was derived from the malignant ascites and peritoneal implants of a recurrent medulloblastoma following failure of radiotherapy. D283 Med (4-HCR), D341 Med (4-HCR), and Daoy (4-HCR) were generated by serial pulse treatment with increasing concentrations of 4-hydroperoxycyclophosphamide (4HC). D384 Med was derived from a newly diagnosed medulloblastoma metastatic to the subarachnoid space in a 17-month-old boy who subsequently failed therapy with cyclophosphamide. D425 Med was derived from the primary cerebellar tumor in a 6-year-old boy; D458 Med was derived later from tumor cells in the cerebrospinal fluid of the same patient following failure of radiotherapy plus chemotherapy (cyclophosphamide, vincristine, cisplatin). These cell lines provide the opportunity to evaluate the anti-medulloblastoma activity of cyclophosphamide. Cyclophosphamide is a prodrug which requires activation *in vitro*, a process which can be accomplished using a microsomal preparation. Alternatively, a metabolite distal to the required hydroxylation could be used for *in vitro* studies. Although 4-hydroxycyclophosphamide is too unstable for synthesis and subsequent use, the pre-activated cyclophosphamide derivative, 4HC, is stable and spontaneously converts to 4-hydroxycyclophosphamide and then aldophosphamide when placed in solution[10,16,17]. We used 4HC to demonstrate the cytotoxicity of this agent against a panel of medulloblastoma cell lines. Furthermore, we subsequently established a panel of cell lines resistant to 4HC by serial pulse exposure of parental cell lines to increasing concentrations of 4HC. This, as well as *de novo* establishment of cell lines from cyclophosphamide-resistant primary medulloblastomas, provided the biological reagents to define mechanisms of cyclophosphamide (4HC) resistance in medulloblastoma.

4. MECHANISMS OF CYCLOPHOSPHAMIDE RESISTANCE

Resistance to cyclophosphamide, as is true of all other anti-neoplastic agents, is complex and multifactorial[10,18,19]. These mechanisms may be oxazaphosphorine-specific, such as an increase in ALDH[16,20]. Alternatively, oxazaphosphorine non-specific mechanisms may be responsible, such as elevated glutathione (GSH) or glutathione-S-transferase (GST)[21–24]. Finally, repair of DNA ICLs may mediate resistance to cyclophosphamide and other bifunctional alkylating agents[25].

Table 1. Medulloblastoma-derived cell lines.

Cell Line	Cell Line Derivation	Growth Pattern	Karyotype
D283 Med	Malignant ascites and peritoneal implants from 6-yr-old boy with recurrent medulloblastoma following failure of radiotherapy	Suspension	47,XY,+11,I(17q), $8q^{+}$,$20q^{+}$
D283 Med (4-HCR)	Serial pulse treatment of D283 Med with increasing concentrations of 4HC	Suspension	
D341 Med	Biopsy of cerebellar primary tumor in 4-yr-old boy	Suspension	49,XY,+6,+8,+18,-22,+1p,I(17q), +DMs
D341 Med (4-HCR)	Serial pulse treatment of D341 Med with increasing concentrations of 4HC	Suspension	
Daoy	Biopsy of cerebellar primary tumor in 4-yr-old boy	Adherent	Tetraploid
Daoy (4-HCR)	Serial pulse treatment of Daoy with increasing concentrations of 4HC	Adherent	
D384 Med	Biopsy of cerebellar primary tumor in 17-mo-old boy who subsequently failed initial therapy with cyclophosphamide	Suspension	46,Xy,8,I(17q), +$8q^{+}$,
D425 Med	Biopsy of cerebellar primary tumor in 6-yr-old boy	Suspension	46,XY,I(17q), $0q^{-}$,+DMs
D458 Med	Tumor cells in cerebrospinal fluid following failure of radiotherapy plus chemotherapy (cyclophosphamide, cisplatin, vincristine) in same patient from which D425 Med was derived	Suspension	47,XY,+18,I(17q), $6q^{+}$, $10q^{-}$,+DMs

5. CYCLOPHOSPHAMIDE RESISTANCE IN HUMAN MEDULLOBLASTOMA CELL LINES

We initially reported a panel of medulloblastoma cell lines with cyclophosphamide resistance[22]. Three cell lines, D283 Med (4-HCR), D341 Med (4-HCR), and Daoy (4-HCR), are resistant to 4HC as compared with their respective parental lines (Table 2) and are considered to have *in vitro*-generated resistance. D384 Med, derived from cerebellar primary medulloblastoma and shown to be 4HC resistant, is considered to have *de novo* clinical resistance. D458 Med, isolated following failure of therapy in a patient whose primary tumor was used to establish D425 Med, is considered to have acquired clinical resistance.

Table 2. Derivation of cyclophosphamide-resistant medulloblastoma cell lines.

Cell Line	**Description**	**Etiology of Resistance**	**4HC concentration producing:** 1-log kill (μM)	2-log kill (μM)
D283 Med	Parental		4.7	10.0
D283 Med (4-HCR)	Resistant	*In vitro* selection	37.3	76.1
D341 Med	Parental		6.6	12.9
D341 Med (4-HCR)	Resistant	*In vitro* selection	9.2	18.9
Daoy	Parental		6.1	12.8
Daoy (4-HCR)	Resistant	*In vitro* selection	35.6	66.9
D384 Med	Resistant	Clinical, *de novo*	4.6	12.7
D425 Med	Parental		6.0	11.8
D458 Med	Resistant	Clinical, acquired	7.2	20.4

5.1 ALDH

Most of the cell lines did not display detectable ALDH activity (Table 3). There was a significant ($P<0.5$), albeit small, increase in the ALDH activity in the Daoy (4-HCR) line compared with that of the parental line. A smaller increase was noted in the D283 MED (4-HCR) line compared with D283 MED.

However, quantitation of an increase in ALDH activity does not confirm that there is a role for this enzyme in mediating drug resistance. Therefore, further studies were done with phenylketocyclophosphamide (PKCP), a cyclophosphamide analog that is not metabolized by ALDH. The concentrations of PKCP that produced a one log kill of Daoy and Daoy (4-HCR) were 12.9 ± 2.6 and 22.4 ± 6.5 μM ($P<0.1$), respectively. This demonstrates that Daoy (4-HCR) cells, although displaying ~6 fold resistance to 4HC compared to the parent line, were only ~2 fold resistant to PKCP. This strongly suggests that the elevated ALDH observed in Daoy (4-HCR) cell line does contribute to 4HC resistance. This observation was not true in D283 MED (4-HCR). The concentrations of PKCP that produced a one log kill of D283 MED and D283 MED (4-HCR) were 13.1 ± 3.7 and 65.9 ± 28.3

μM (P<0.01) respectively. Thus D283 MED (4-HCR) cells were cross-resistant to 4HC and PKCP.

Table 3. Biochemical profile of medulloblastoma cell lines.

Cell Line	GSH (nmol/mg protein)	GST (nmol/min/mg protein)	ALDH (nmol/min/mg protein)	γ-GTP (μmol/min/mg protein)
D283 Med	11.1 ± 3.0[a]	273.1 ± 59.2	ND[b]	0.090 ± 0.008
D283 Med (4-HCR)	28.8 ± 4.1[c]	170.6 ± 18.0	0.3	0.129 ± 0.009
D341 Med	15.7 ± 5.4	508.5 ± 24.0	ND	0.002 ± 0.000
D341 Med (4-HCR)	23.8 ± 4.6[c]	154.9 ± 24.0	ND	0.006 ± 0.001[c]
Daoy	7.1 ± 2.7	68.2 ± 14.1	ND	0.012 ± 0.007
Daoy (4-HCR)	13.2 ± 2.1[c]	73.1 ± 17.3	0.8[c]	0.034 ± 0.12[c]
D384 Med	11.4 ± 3.0	50.4 ± 10.2	0.6	ND
D425 Med	28.6 ± 9.4	161.9 ± 52.7	0.8	0.035 ± 0.033
D458 Med	22.5 ± 11.8	143.9 ± 61.3	ND	0.009 ± 0.006

[a] Mean ± SD.

[b] ND, not detected.

[c] Statistically significant (P<0.05) increase as compared with parental line.

5.2 GSH and GST

GSH levels and activities of GST are detailed in Table 3. There was a significant (P<0.05) increase in the GSH content of D283 MED (4-HCR), D341 MED (4-HCR), and Daoy (4-HCR) cells compared with their respective parent lines. No increase in GST activity was noted in any of the resistant cell lines. Furthermore, there was no evidence for the enhanced expression of any specific isoform of GST in the resistant cell lines compared with their sensitive counterparts.

We subsequently treated cell lines with buthionine sulfoximine (BSO) for 24 h which resulted in a marked depletion of GSH content of each of the lines. Cellular GSH contents (nmol/mg protein) were as follows: D283 Med, 2.3 ± 0.6; D283 Med (4-HCR), 1.9 ± 1.3; D341 Med, 4.1 ± 0.9; D341 Med (4-HCR), 3.0 ± 1.0; Daoy, 1.1 ± 0.3; Daoy (4-HCR), 0.9 ± 0.1; D384 Med, 2.0 ± 0.6; D425 Med, 2.2 ± 1.2; and D458 Med, 2.0 ± 0.8. In general, residual GSH in the parental and resistant lines was approximately 17.5 and 10% of controls, respectively.

BSO-mediated depletion of GSH produced a variable enhancement of 4HC cytotoxicity (Table 4). BSO enhanced the 4HC cytotoxicity against D341 MED and D341 MED (4-HCR) with complete restoration of 4HC sensitivity in D341 MED (4-HCR) to parental levels. Similar results were displayed in D425 MED and D4558 MED. However, BSO treatment of Daoy and Daoy (4-HCR) produced some enhancement of 4HC cytotoxicity, particularly in Daoy (4-HCR), but without restoration of sensitivity to parental levels. No effect of BSO on sensitization to 4HC was noted in D283 MED or D283 MED (4-HCR).

Table 4. Modulation of 4HC cytotoxicity by BSO.

Cell Line	**4HC concentration (without BSO) producing**		**4HC concentration (pretreated with BSO) producing**	
	1-log kill (μm)	**2-log kill (μm)**	**1-log kill (μm)**	**2-log kill (μm)**
D283 Med	4.7	10.0	3.9	7.3
D283 Med (4-HCR)	37.3	76.1	39.1	74.8
D341 Med	6.6	12.9	3.0	7.4
D341 Med (4-HCR)	9.2	18.9	4.6	11.6
Daoy	6.1	12.8	4.4	11.1
Daoy (4-HCR)	35.6	66.9	10.1	22.8
D384 Med	4.6	12.7	2.9	8.1
D425 Med	6.0	11.8	3.5	8.5
D458 Med	7.2	20.4	2.4	6.0

The above work revealed explanations for 4HC resistance in all of the cell lines except D283 MED (4-HCR). D283 Med (4-HCR) is ~8 fold resistant to 4HC compared with the parental cell line. It is also ~5 fold resistant to PKCP, an analog that is not affected by ALDH. D283 Med (4-HCR) displays complete resistance to 4HC after depletion of GSH with BSO. These observations suggest that the major mechanism of resistance in D283 MED (4-HCR) does **not** involve either elevated ALDH or GSH. Accordingly, we began a new set of studies designed to define whether the repair of DNA ICLs might be mediating this resistance to 4HC.

5.3 Repair of 4HC-induced DNA Interstrand Crosslinks

We used DNA denaturing/renaturing gel electrophoresis and Southern blot analysis to evaluate the formation and disappearance of 4HC induced DNA ICLs at the *c-myc* gene in D283 Med and D283 Med (4-HCR)[26] (Figure 2).

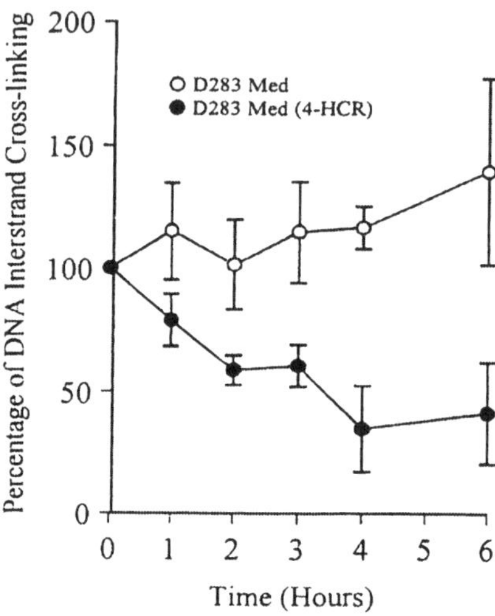

Figure 2. Disappearance of 4HC-induced DNA ICLs in the c-myc gene after 1 h of drug treatment in D283 Med and D283 Med (4-HCR). Drug-sensitive or –resistant cells were treated with 50 μM 4HC for 1 h. Genomic DNA was isolated from cells post-incubated in fresh medium for different lengths of time. The percentage of the crosslinked gene remaining after different post-incubation times was calculated by using the initial amount of crosslinking (at 0 h) of the corresponding line as the reference. [Bars, SEM, n=3].

These results indicate similar 4HC induced DNA ICL formation of *c-myc* genes in D283 MED and D283 MED (4-HCR) but more rapid removal of the DNA ICLs in D283 MED (4-HCR). The precise nature of this enhanced repair remains speculative. A more precise assay was needed for quantitation of DNA ICL repair to allow the definition of the pathways involved in this process.

6. QUANTITATION OF DNA INTERSTRAND CROSSLINK REPAIR

We have developed a novel substrate to assay repair of DNA ICLs. First, PM is reacted with an oligonucleotide duplex which contains a single GNC pair so that the site of crosslinking is defined. As with other N7-alkylguanine sites within DNA, the PM ICL was found to be somewhat unstable, presumably because of the depurination of one of the crosslinked guanosines. We have found that the stability of the PM ICL could be increased if the guanosine in the oligonucleotide is the 2'-O-methylribonucleoside. The crosslinked oligonucleotide is purified and ligated to linear plasmid DNA to produce circular DNA. The plasmid DNA sequence has a FokI recognition site positioned 10 bp from the ICL. This enzyme produces a staggered cut 9 and 13 bp from its recognition site so that the DNA is nicked on each strand on either side of the ICL. When the FokI digested DNA is run on a non-denaturing agarose gel, the presence of the ICL prevents separation of the two fragments and the DNA migrates as uncut DNA. If the ICL is removed, the DNA migrates as two fragments. When the substrate DNA was incubated with HeLa cell nuclear extracts and then digested with FokI, the two smaller DNA fragments were observed following electrophoresis. The removal of the ICL by the HeLa extracts was confirmed by analysis of the DNA products by alkaline agarose gel electrophoresis. Only after incubation with extract was single stranded DNA observed.

CONCLUSION

Mechanisms of resistance to cyclophosphamide in human medulloblastoma are complex and multifactorial. The rationale for identification of these mechanisms is in part the goal of providing strategies to restore sensitivity in patients with cyclophosphamide-resistant tumors. Unfortunately, no mechanisms of resistance to cyclophosphamide identified to date appear specific to medulloblastoma (or indeed, to any other malignancy) compared to normal tissue and organs. Accordingly, attempts to perturb a specific mechanism of cyclophosphamide resistance operational in a medulloblastoma may produce an increase in toxicity produced by the drug. An example is the dramatic and lethal cardiac and skeletal muscle toxicity produced by cyclophosphamide following BSO-induced depletion of GSH[27]. The role of GSH in preventing cardiac toxicity, a well described complication of high-dose cyclophosphamide, was previously unknown. Furthermore, cyclophosphamide had never previously produced skeletal muscle toxicity until GSH depletion facilitated this complication.

Therefore, attempts to restore sensitivity will need to be conducted with rigorous pre-clinical evaluation followed only then by Phase I trials in patients if strategies for reversal of resistance to cyclophosphamide are to be safely and effectively evaluated.

REFERENCES

1. Friedman HS, Oakes WJ, Bigner SH, *et al.* Medulloblastoma: tumor biological and clinical perspectives. J Neurooncol, 11:1-15, 1991.
2. Allen JC, Helson L. High-dose cyclophosphamide chemotherapy for recurrent CNS tumors in children. J Neurosurg, 55:749-756, 1981.
3. Allen JC, Helson L, Jereb B. Preradiation chemotherapy for newly diagnosed childhood brain tumors. A modified phase II trial. Cancer, 52:2001-2006, 1983.
4. Friedman HS, Mahaley MS, Schold SC Jr, *et al.* Efficacy of vincristine and cyclophosphamide in the therapy of recurrent medulloblastoma. Neurosurg, 18:355-340, 1986.
5. Moghrabi A, Fuchs H, Brown M, *et al.* Cyclophosphamide in combination with sargramostim for treatment of recurrent medulloblastoma. Med Pediatr Oncol, 25:190-196, 1995.
6. Colvin M, Hilton J. Pharmacology of cyclophosphamide and metabolites. Cancer Treat Rep, 3:89-95, 1981.
7. Fenselau C, Kan MN, Rao SS. Identification of aldophosphamide as a metabolite of cyclophosphamide in vitro and in vivo in humans. Cancer Res, 37:2538-2543, 1977.
8. Colvin M, Padgett CA, Fenselau C. A biologically active metabolite of cyclophosphamide. Cancer Res, 33:915-918, 1973.
9. Colvin M, Brundrett RB, Kan MN, *et al.* Alkylating properties of phosphoramide mustard. Cancer Res, 36:1121-1126, 1976.
10. Colvin M, Chabner BA. Alkylating agents. *In*: Cancer Chemotherapy Principles and Practice, BA Chabner, JM Collins (eds.), JB Lippincott, Philadelphia, PA, 276-313, 1990.
11. Kastan MB, Schaffer E, Russo JE, *et al.* Direct demonstration of elevated aldehyde dehydrogenase in human hematopoietic progenitor cells. Blood, 75:1947-1950, 1990.
12. Jacobsen PF, Jenkyn DJ, Papadimitriou JM. Establishment of a human medulloblastoma cell line and its heterotransplantation into nude mice. J Neuropathol Exp Neurol, 44:472-485, 1985.
13. Friedman HS, Burger PC, Bigner SH, *et al.* Establishment and characterization of the human medulloblastoma cell line and transplantable xenograft D283 Med. J Neuropathol Exp Neurol, 44:592-605, 1985.
14. Friedman HS, Burger PC, Bigner SH, *et al.* Phenotypic and genotypic analysis of a human medulloblastoma cell line and transplantable xenograft (D341 Med) demonstrating amplification of c-myc. Amer J Pathol, 130:472-484, 1988.
15. Bigner SH, Friedman HS, Vogelstein B, *et al.* Amplification of the c-myc gene in human medulloblastoma cell lines and xenografts. Cancer Res, 50:2347-2350, 1990.
16. Hilton J. Deoxyribonucleic acid crosslinking by 4-hydroperoxycyclophosphamide in cyclophosphamide-sensitive and -resistant L1210 cells. Biochem Pharmacol, 33:1867-1872, 1984.
17. Shulman-Roskes EM, Noe DA, Gamcsik MP, *et al.* The partitioning of phosphoramide mustard and its aziridinium ions among alkylation and P-N bond hydrolysis reactions. J Med Chem, 41:515-529, 1998.
18. Sladek NE. Metabolism of oxazaphosphorines. Pharmacol Ther, 37:301-355, 1988.

19. Sladek NE. Oxazaphosphorine-specific acquired cellular resistance. *In*: Drug Resistance in Oncology, BA Teicher (ed.), Marcel Dekker, New York, NY, 375-411, 1993.
20. Hilton J. Role of aldehyde dehydrogenase in cyclophosphamide-resistant L1210 leukemia. Cancer Res, 44:5156-5160, 1984.
21. Ahmad S, Okine L, Le B, *et al.* Elevation of glutathione in phenylalanine mustard-resistant murine L1210 leukemia cells. J Biol Chem, 262:15048-15053, 1987.
22. Friedman HS, Colvin OM, Kaufmann SH, *et al.* Cyclophosphamide resistance in medulloblastoma. Cancer Res, 52:5373-5378, 1992.
23. McGown AT, Fox BW. A proposed mechanism of resistance to cyclophosphamide and phosphoramide mustard in a Yoshida cell line in vitro. Cancer Chemother Pharmacol, 17:223-226, 1986.
24. Waxman D. Glutathione-S-transferases: role in alkylating agent resistance and possible target for modulation chemotherapy – a review. Cancer Res, 50:6449-6454, 1990.
25. Calsou P, Salles B. Role of DNA repair in the mechanisms of cell resistance to alkylating agents and cisplatin. Cancer Chemother Pharmacol, 32:85-89, 1993.
26. Dong Q, Bullock N, Ali-Osman F, *et al.* Repair analysis of 4-hydroperoxycyclophosphamide induced DNA interstrand crosslinking in the c-myc gene in 4-hydroperoxycyclophosphamide-sensitive and -resistant medulloblastoma cell lines. Cancer Chemother Pharmacol, 37:242-246, 1996.
27. Friedman HS, Colvin OM, Aisaka K, *et al.* Glutathione protects cardiac and skeletal muscle from cyclophosphamide-induced toxicity. Cancer Res, 50:2455-2462, 1990.

Chapter 11

MODEL STUDIES OF CYCLOPHOSPHAMIDE RESISTANCE IN HUMAN MYELOID LEUKEMIA

Borje S. Andersson[1] and David Murray[2]
[1]Department of Blood and Marrow Transplantation, The University of Texas MD Anderson Cancer Center, Houston, Texas, USA
[2]Division of Experimental Oncology, Department of Oncology, University of Alberta and Department of Experimental Oncology, Cross Cancer Institute, Edmonton, Alberta, Canada

1. RESISTANCE TO CYCLOPHOSPHAMIDE ANALOGS IN CANCER TREATMENT

Cyclophosphamide (CP), 4-hydroperoxycyclophosphamide (4HC), mafosfamide, and ifosphamide are antineoplastic alkylating agents collectively referred to as oxazaphosphorines. Oxazaphosphorines are used in the treatment of many types of cancer, including neo-adjuvant, adjuvant and high-dose treatment for breast tumors, salvage chemotherapy for a variety of solid tumors, and high-dose conditioning therapy of patients undergoing hematopoietic stem cell transplantation[1,2]. In the latter context, these drugs are widely used for the treatment of myeloid leukemias, which represent the focus of this chapter.

When chemotherapy fails, it is commonly assumed that the most important factor is tumor-cell "resistance" to the anticancer agent. However, clinical treatment failure, such as that commonly seen after CP therapy, may be the end result of a multitude of contributing factors. In addition to true cellular insensitivity to the anticancer agent itself, this failure may arise from factors such as adverse tumor kinetics or various aspects of sub-optimal drug delivery to the tumor (e.g., see chapter 1 in this volume by Drs. A. Davis and I. Tannock). The latter phenomenon may be related to host factors, such as variable metabolic activity that influences drug pharmacokinetics, which can be important for treatment outcome (see chapters 15 and 16 in this volume by Dr. R. Jones and by Drs. J. McCune and J. Slattery). These mechanisms may help to explain some of the difficulty experienced in correlating a specific cellular resistance mechanism with clinical treatment failure. As outlined in chapter 16 by Drs. McCune and Slattery, the pharmacokinetic optimization of chemotherapy delivery can drastically decrease the fraction of treatment failures related to sub-optimal drug delivery. It is therefore likely that the relevance of treatment failure caused by adverse tumor growth kinetics and by acquired or inherent resistance of the tumor cells to the therapy will become even more important as rational treatment strategies designed to reduce the fraction of clinical failures due to sub-optimal tumor drug delivery are integrated into clinical practice.

Most laboratory studies aimed at improving our understanding of the mechanisms underlying drug resistance have utilized highly drug-resistant tumor models. Many of these models have been informative with respect to specific resistance mechanisms. Indeed, there is now an emerging body of evidence suggesting a correlation between experimentally identified cellular resistance mechanisms, e.g., P-glycoprotein, and clinical treatment outcome[3,4] (see also chapter 3 in this volume by Dr. L. Deng and colleagues). This situation has not yet been convincingly demonstrated for oxazaphosphorine-based chemotherapy (see chapter 8 by Dr. N. Sladek in this volume). As a step towards resolving whether there is a correlation between tumor aldehyde dehydrogenase (ALDH) activity and treatment outcome, Sreerama and Sladek[5] first posed the question of whether primary tumor tissue ALDH levels correlated with those of metastatic lesions. Indeed, they found a high concordance between ALDH levels in primary versus metastatic lesions. Further studies are now needed to elucidate the relationship between ALDH and oxazaphosphorine-based treatment outcome in various tumors.

The underlying hypotheses of studies of oxazaphosphorine resistance performed in our laboratory using chronic myeloid leukemia (CML) cell lines are that: [a] tumor cell drug resistance is an important factor for clinical treatment failure in this disease; and [b] this resistance is complex, including (but not limited to) the known mechanisms such as increased levels of ALDH, glutathione (GSH), glutathione-S-transferase (GST), and DNA repair activity, processes that individually have been found to contribute to CP resistance in experimental model systems. We have also assumed that both known (see above) and novel cellular mechanisms may act in concert to confer a resistant cell phenotype. The clinical reality is that resistance in an individual tumor may be multifactorial and that not all mechanisms will contribute in every case. In correlating cellular resistance factors with clinical resistance, it may therefore be necessary to probe for each of these individual components.

2. THE ROLE OF ALDH IN RESISTANCE TO OXAZAPHOSPHORINES

Intrinsic and/or acquired tumor cell resistance to oxazaphosphorines develops through a number of mechanisms, the best characterized of which is increased activity of the ALDH family of enzymes (see chapter 8 in this volume by Dr. N. Sladek). These enzymes oxidize the important intermediate metabolite aldophosphamide (ALDO) to the relatively non-toxic derivative carboxyphosphamide, thereby suppressing the generation of the active cytotoxic metabolite phosphorodiamidic mustard (PM) as well as of acrolein. Low ALDH levels favor a non-enzymatic elimination reaction that generates PM and acrolein. Elevated ALDH is a major factor in cellular resistance to oxazaphosphorines in numerous CP-resistant murine and human tumor cell lines[6–9] and in a rodent acute myeloid leukemia model[10].

3. THE ROLE OF NON-ALDH MECHANISMS IN RESISTANCE TO OXAZAPHOSPHORINES

Non-ALDH mechanisms of CP resistance are also important in some cell lines[11] (see also chapter 10 in this volume by Dr. H. Friedman and colleagues). Furthermore, ALDH by itself is poorly predictive of responsiveness to oxazaphosphorines in some tumor models[7,12,13] and in clinical tumor samples (see chapter 8 by Dr. N. Sladek in this volume), suggesting the importance of other mechanisms. One such mechanism is increased GSH and/or GST levels/activity, which enables cells to deactivate potentially cytotoxic CP metabolites to non-toxic adducts[11] (see also chapter 4 in this volume by Dr. D. Hamilton and colleagues). Increased GSH levels and/or GST activity have been reported in a variety of cell lines that display resistance to oxazaphosphorines[11]. One 4HC-resistant murine tumor cell line that showed no elevation of ALDH appeared to be resistant primarily because of elevated GSH/GST levels[14].

Another important mechanism of resistance to bifunctional alkylating and platinating agents, such as melphalan and cisplatin, is via the enhanced repair of drug-induced DNA lesions such as interstrand cross-links (ISCs) (see chapter 7 in this volume by Dr. D. Murray). The role of DNA repair in the development of resistance to oxazaphosphorines has received less attention. This may be partly because ALDH elevation in itself provides such an important drug-specific mechanism of resistance that less attention was directed to other factors. It may also be partly because, until recently, the mechanisms by which cells repair these lesions were largely unknown. Chapter 6 in this volume by Drs. R. Legerski and C. Richie deals with the emerging knowledge in this area.

What *is* known in regard to ISC repair and oxazaphosphorines is that certain repair-deficient rodent cells, notably those with defects in the *ERCC1* and *XPF* nucleotide excision repair (NER)/recombinational repair genes, are hypersensitive to activated CP[15] and to 4HC and PM[16]. As more information is published concerning other proteins involved in these recombination-dependent ISC repair pathways, it becomes possible to extend such studies to additional mutants. For example, we have found that rodent mutant cells with defects in the *XRCC2* and *XRCC3* repair genes are as sensitive to PM as are the *ERCC1* and *XPF* mutants (e.g., Figure 1). Thus, like the ERCC1 and XPF enzymes, the RAD51 homologues XRCC2 and XRCC3 appear to be critical for the repair of ISCs induced by oxazaphosphorines.

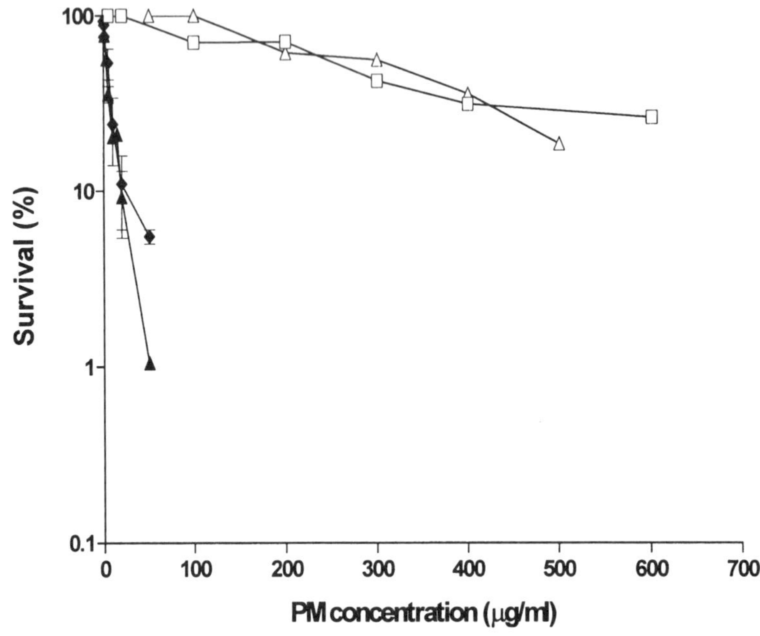

Figure 1. Survival of wild-type V79-4 (Δ) and AA8 (□) cells, and of *XRCC3*-deficient *irs*1 (▲) and *XPF*-deficient UV41 (◆) mutant rodent cells, following exposure to PM for 15 min at 37°C.

We have also examined the sensitivity to PM of several NER-deficient human fibroblast cell lines derived from patients with xeroderma pigmentosum (XP)[17]. Of particular interest is the observation that the human *XPF*-deficient line XP2YOSV was only modestly (~2 fold) sensitive to PM compared with normal fibroblasts. This finding was surprising considering that the rodent *XPF* mutant UV41 line is extremely (~23 fold) sensitive to PM[16] (Figure 1). Clearly, the phenotype of human *XPF*-deficient cells can be quite different from that of their rodent counterparts. To understand why rodent UV41 and human XP2YOSV *XPF*-deficient cells exhibit such different responses, it is important to note two things: (i) unlike rodent cells, *no* human NER mutant to date has been found to exhibit extreme hypersensitivity to drugs that induce ISCs[18]; and (ii) the rodent *XPF* mutants exhibit considerable heterogeneity in their sensitivity to such drugs, with UV41 being among the most sensitive[18,19]. This heterogeneity could reflect: (a) different *XPF* mutations among the cell lines, some of which result in an enzyme that is defective with respect to NER but functional with respect to ISC-repair; (b) differing degrees of leakiness of the mutation in different lines; or (c) the possibility that cells with low residual levels of XPF protein can perform effective ISC repair but not NER[17,19]. These findings indicate that we still have a lot to learn about the response of human cells to these drugs.

As discussed elsewhere in this volume (see chapter 7), mRNA levels of the NER/recombinational repair gene *ERCC1* have been widely studied in the context of predicting clinical response to anticancer drugs such as cisplatin and melphalan. Although such studies have not yet been extended to CP analogs, either in CML or in other tumor types, enhanced recombinational repair *has* been implicated in the development of resistance to the bifunctional alkylator chlorambucil in chronic lymphocytic leukemia[20].

4. A HUMAN MYELOID LEUKEMIA MODEL FOR OXAZAPHOSPHORINE RESISTANCE

The above mechanisms were largely defined using genetic mutants or tumor cell lines with *in vitro*-acquired drug resistance. The latter approach has also been followed in our laboratory, where we have derived a series of variant tumor lines from the KBM-7 human CML cell line that was established from blast cells from a patient in the terminal phase of CML[21,22]. The KBM-7 line was sub-cloned, and one of the sub-clones, KBM-7/B5 (henceforth referred to as B5), was used as the parental strain for the development of a series of variant sub-lines with differing degrees of acquired resistance to CP analogs. The Bcr/Abl-positive B5 and all of these drug-resistant sub-lines carry double copies of the t(9;22) translocation, verified on G-banded metaphase spreads. Our original objective was to use these cell lines to derive a panel of molecular probes that might assist in unraveling the complex problem of CP resistance in CML cells. The expectation was that such probes would subsequently be interfaced with technologies such as flow cytometry and FISH (that are able to report on inter-cellular heterogeneity) to study clinical CML resistance to oxazaphosphorines.

We will here describe the evolution, through almost eight years of study, of our understanding of oxazaphosphorine resistance in these B5-derived sub-lines. First, we will describe the biological characterization of the B5 line and its highly 4HC-resistant variant sub-line, designated B5-180^3. This includes their sensitivity to oxazaphosphorines, pattern of cross-resistance to other DNA-damaging agents, stability of resistance over time, cytogenetic alterations, etc. It also includes the use of a "directed screening" approach for evaluating known or suspected mechanisms of resistance to oxazaphosphorines in these cells. These avenues typically represent the starting point for any characterization of a new laboratory model system.

Because this approach would not be expected to reveal novel or hitherto unrecognized mechanisms of oxazaphosphorine resistance, our studies naturally evolved to embrace newly-emerging technologies such as cDNA arrays and differential display of mRNA (DD-mRNA) that permit the more general identification of genes whose expression is altered in drug-resistant cells. Section 6 will describe our preliminary findings with such methods as they relate to the B5-180^3 phenotype. In the process, we hope to illustrate the enormous potential for utilizing recent advances in genomics and proteomics for studying clinically relevant anticancer drug resistance. The technological aspects of tumor profiling are described in the final chapter of this volume by Drs. S. Damaraju and colleagues.

The latter part of the chapter compares this artificially induced high-grade resistance with a more clinically relevant model of resistance. It describes our studies using additional B5-derived sub-clones that exhibit low-degree resistance to the oxazaphosphorines that can develop after only one or a few exposures of B5 cells to 4HC.

5. PHENOTYPIC/BIOCHEMICAL CHARACTERIZATION OF THE B5-180^3 CML CELL LINE

5.1 Biological Characteristics; Clonogenic Survival

Our initial high-degree oxazaphosphorine resistance model, the B5-180^3 sub-line, was isolated from B5 cultures following exposure to stepwise-incremented concentrations of the *in vitro*-active CP analog 4HC (from 5 to 180 μg/ml)[11,23,24]. B5-180^3 cells displayed ~35 fold resistance to the cytotoxic effects of a short (60 min) "pulse" exposure to 4HC. B5-180^3 cells were ~6 fold cross-resistant to PM (15 min exposure). PM has the same alkylating moiety as 4HC but is not metabolized by ALDH, and its cytotoxic effectiveness does not, therefore, depend on ALDH activity.

B5-180^3 cells also displayed a reduced, but nonetheless significant (~8 fold), resistance to 4HC in the presence of cyanamide, an efficient inhibitor of ALDH[23]. The combined findings that: (i) B5-180^3 cells are more resistant to 4HC than to PM; and (ii) cyanamide only partially restores their sensitivity to 4HC; suggest that resistance to 4HC in these cells is multifactorial in nature, with ALDH probably accounting for about half of this resistance and a second, ALDH-independent, mechanism also being operative in these cells.

5.2 Stability of the B5-180^3 Phenotype

The resistance of the B5-180^3 sub-line is extremely stable in the absence of 4HC selection pressure. B5-180^3 cells examined after almost 2 years in continuous culture retained essentially full resistance to 4HC and cross-resistance to PM, indicating that all mechanisms contributing to this phenotype are genetically stable.

5.3 Cross-resistance to Other DNA-damaging Agents

The cross-resistance pattern of B5-180^3 cells to various other antitumor agents was assessed using a clonogenic survival assay following a continuous exposure in which the drug was added to the soft-agar cultures, rather than the acute exposures referred to above. The first important observation from this study is that the resistance index (RI) of these cells to both 4HC and PM is greatly reduced when the drug exposure is given over an extended time period, rather than acutely (Table 1 versus section 5.1). The clinical implication of this finding is that, rather than giving a single high dose of the oxazaphosphorine, divided doses administered over several days or even as a continuous infusion may improve treatment outcome. This behavior has been exploited in the so-called hyper-CVAD regimen for acute lymphocytic leukemia[25], where the use of fractionated CP reportedly yields an overall improved response compared with the use of single-dose CP in similar patient populations[26].

Table 1. Cross-resistance pattern for B5 and B5-180^3 cells.

Drug	B5 (μg/ml)	B5-180^3 (μg/ml)	RI*
4HC	0.40 ± 0.04	1.65 ± 0.18	4.1
PM	2.35 ± 0.15	6.0 ± 0.4	2.6
IM**	1.5 ± 0.1	4.7 ± 0.1	3.1
AAI**	0.21 ± 0.01	1.65 ± 0.15	7.8
HN_2**	0.28 ± 0.03	2.05 ± 0.07	7.4
Cisplatin	0.30 ± 0.05	1.15 ± 0.05	3.8
Melphalan	0.60 ± 0.04	2.10 ± 0.42	3.5
Busulfan***	54.0 ± 6.0	65 ± 8	1.2
γ-radiation	3.0 Gy	4.0 Gy	1.3
Ara-C**	0.032 ± 0.010	0.010 ± 0.003	0.3
Etoposide	0.115 ± 0.007	0.019 ± 0.008	0.16
Doxorubicin	0.034 ± 0.015	0.008 ± 0.003	0.24

*Resistance Index (RI) was calculated as the ratio of the IC_{90} values for B5-180^3 and B5 cells.

**The abbreviations used are: IM; isophosphoramide mustard, AAI; acetaldoifosphamide, HN_2; nitrogen mustard, Ara-C; cytosine arabinoside.

***Busulfan resistance was assayed after a 60 min exposure only.

Significant cross-resistance was seen to isophosphoramide mustard (IM), cisplatin, melphalan, nitrogen mustard (HN_2) and acetaldoifosphamide (AAI) (which is activated by cellular non-specific esterases)[27] (Table 1). In fact, the RI for AAI and HN_2 actually exceeded that for 4HC and PM. Given the specificity of ALDH for oxazaphosphorines, this latter effect probably reflects the influence of the second, non-ALDH, component of resistance. As discussed below, this component appears to relate to an ability of the resistant cells to tolerate drug-induced ISCs, which may relate in part to the cells' DNA repair capability. There are two important considerations in this regard. First, bifunctional anticancer drugs induce other types of lesions in addition to ISCs (e.g., mono-adducts, intrastrand crosslinks, DNA-protein crosslinks and strand breaks); these lesions are present in varying proportions for different drugs, and are substrates for different DNA repair pathways[28]. Second, different drugs induce chemically distinct ISCs that have different repair-factor requirements[29,30]. Thus, it is not unreasonable that this second component of acquired resistance to 4HC might have even more dramatic effects on the biological response to DNA damage caused by other drugs.

B5-180^3 cells were slightly cross-resistant to busulfan and γ-radiation. Surprisingly, collateral *sensitivity* was detected to cytosine arabinoside, etoposide, and doxorubicin. The reasons for this collateral sensitivity are unclear. However, the gene-array analyses discussed below may provide some clues. For example, we observed the apparent over-expression in B5-180^3 cells of two genes that encode components of the notch signaling pathway that commonly controls cell development via interaction with chromatin remodeling enzymes and components of the transcriptional machinery[31]. This pathway is disrupted in some tumors, including a subset of human T-cell leukemia, leading to disregulated chromatin remodeling and transcription[31,32]. It is therefore of interest that both etoposide and doxorubicin are topoisomerase II-active agents, whereas cytosine arabinoside primarily interacts with DNA replication. It should be noted that topoisomerase II expression was not significantly altered in the resistant cells in the gene-array analysis discussed in section 6.4; similarly, the array data described in section 6.3 indicated that topoisomerase I message was not detectable in either cell line and that topoisomerase IIα was equally expressed in the parental and resistant lines.

5.4 Aldehyde Dehydrogenase

The above-mentioned indirect evidence from studies of cross-resistance to PM and to 4HC plus cyanamide suggest that elevated ALDH activity is an important, although incomplete, factor in the resistance of B5-180^3 cells to 4HC. To confirm this suggestion, cytosolic ALDH activity was assayed in these cells by measuring the rate at which cytosolic fractions catalyzed the oxidation of global or isoform-specific substrates for the enzyme using NAD as the co-factor[33]. Total cytosolic ALDH activity (determined using the global ALDH substrate ALDO) was low in the parental cells but was increased markedly in the B5-180^3 sub-line (Table 2). Similarly, activity of the ALDH-1 isoform (which catalyzes the oxidation of acetaldehyde and

ALDO) was low in B5 cells and greatly increased in the resistant cells (Table 2). Activity of ALDH-3 (which catalyzes the oxidation of benzaldehyde and ALDO) was again low in the parental cells; however, unlike ALDH-1, ALDH-3 activity was only modestly increased in the drug-resistant sub-line.

Table 2. [a]ALDH activity in B5 and B5-180^3 CML cells.

SUBSTRATE/ISOFORM	ALDH ACTIVITY[b]	
	B5	B5-180^3
ALDO/global ALDH	0.5	9.1
Acetaldehyde/ALDH-1	0.4	7.5
Benzaldehyde/ALDH-3	0.4	1.0

[a]:Characterization of altered gene expression in a cyclophosphamide-resistant human myeloid leukemia cell line, KBM-7/B5-180^3. Murray D, Scott A, Sreerama L, Sladek NE, Andersson BS, manuscript in preparation.

[b]:milli-International units of enzyme activity; mean of 4 determinations.

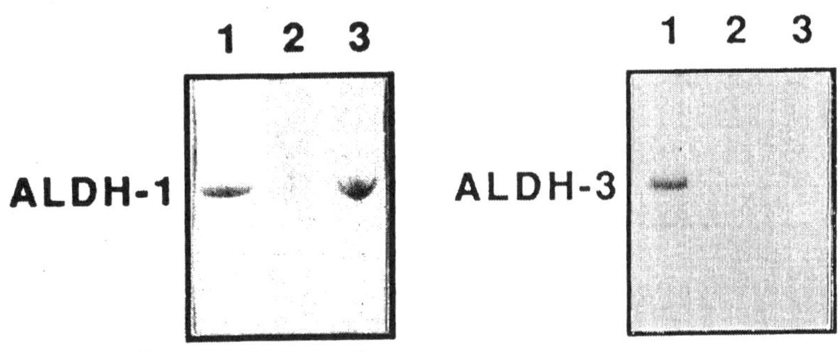

Figure 2. Western blot analysis of ALDH-1 and ALDH-3 in B5 and B5-180^3 cells. 1 µg of purified human ALDH-1 (left panel, lane 1) or ALDH-3 (right panel, lane 1) and soluble protein fractions from B5 (lane 2) and B5-180^3 (lane 3) cells were separated by SDS-polyacrylamide gel electrophoresis, electrotransferred to Immobilon-PVDF membranes, and probed with antibodies against human ALDH-1 and ALDH-3.

ALDH-1 and ALDH-3 protein levels in cytosolic fractions from these cells were assayed by Western blotting. As shown in Figure 2, levels of both the ALDH-1 and ALDH-3 iso-enzymes were very low in the parental cells. The levels of ALDH-1 (but not ALDH-3) were greatly increased in the drug-resistant cells.

To determine whether the increased levels of ALDH-1 protein in B5-180^3 cells could be accounted for by up-regulation of the *ALDH-1* gene and/or message stabilization, we compared the amounts and half-life of *ALDH-1* mRNA in the two cell lines using a pulse-chase technique. Parallel cultures of parental and resistant cells were pulse-labeled with ^{32}P-uridine. At various times thereafter, cells were removed and poly(A)$^+$ RNA was isolated and hybridized to antisense *ALDH-1* cDNA. After RNAse digestion, the *ALDH-1* mRNA/cDNA hybrids were precipitated and quantified by scintillation counting. We found that (i) the total amount of *ALDH-1* mRNA was increased by ≥20 fold in the resistant cells, in general correspondence with the increase in overall ALDH-1 enzyme activity, and (ii) there was no obvious difference in mRNA half-life between the two lines. Thus, the increase in ALDH-1 protein levels appears to be mediated predominantly at the *ALDH-1* gene transcription level.

Table 3. Biological characteristics of B5-180^3 cells compared with parental B5 cells.

CHARACTERISTIC	B5	B5-180^3
Doubling time (h)	24 (22-25)	32 (29-34)
Cloning efficiency (%)	25 ± 8	38 ± 10
Cell cycle distribution		
G_1	48	52
S	36	35
G_2/M	16	13
Cytogenetics	Double Ph$^+$ chromosome.	Double Ph$^+$ chromosome. 5q+, 13q+, 5p– compared with parental line
GST (global) activity, (ng/10^6 cells)	540 ± 141	515 ± 98
GSH (nmol/10^6 cells)	1.3	1.8
p53	wild-type	wild-type

5.5 GST Protein Activity and GSH Levels

Whole cell extracts from B5 and B5-180^3 cells were probed for possible increases in GSH levels (using a fluorometric assay using the dye *o*-phthalicdicarboxaldehyde) and in global GST activity (using a functional assay involving the substrate chlorodinitrobenzene)[34]. GST activity was essentially unaltered, whereas GSH levels were very slightly increased in B5-180^3 relative to B5 cells (Table 3)[35]. To exclude the possibility of a selective up-regulation of GST isoenzymes that might not be apparent when assaying global GST activity, we performed a Western blot using monoclonal antibodies against GST-α, -μ, and -π. The π isoenzyme was present at similar levels in both lines; however, neither the α nor the μ isoenzymes were detectable in either B5 or B5-180^3 cells (Figure 3). Thus, it appears that alterations in GSH and GST levels contribute little to the B5-180^3 phenotype.

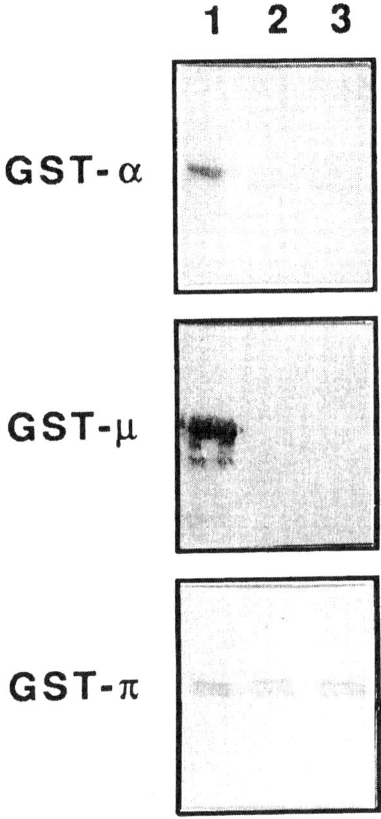

Figure 3. Western blot analysis of GST-α, -μ and -π isoforms in B5 and B5-180^3 cells. Lanes 1, 2 and 3 represent purified human GST-isoenzyme and soluble protein fractions from B5 or B5-180^3 cells, respectively. After separation by SDS-polyacrylamide gel electrophoresis, the protein fractions were electrotransferred to Immobilon-PVDF membranes, and probed with antibodies against the respective human GST-isoenzymes.

5.6 DNA Damage and Repair

The findings described thus far suggest that the enhanced ALDH-dependent metabolism of ALDO can account for approximately half of the total resistance of B5-180^3 cells to 4HC. The mechanism of the remaining non-ALDH component of resistance to 4HC, which also accounts for the cells' cross-resistance to PM and for their residual resistance to 4HC in the presence of cyanamide, is less apparent, but clearly does ***not*** involve GSH or

GST. A significant insight into the nature of the additional mechanism(s) was provided by studies of DNA damage in these cells. It was found that B5-180[3] cells were ~8 fold resistant to 4HC-mediated ISC induction compared with the parental line[23]. In contrast, the variant cells were not appreciably resistant to PM-mediated ISC induction. These findings indicate that a lethal event in the drug-resistant line is associated with ~5 fold higher levels of induced ISCs for both of these drugs. Alternatively viewed, the variant cells have a much greater ability than the parental cells to tolerate ISCs induced by both 4HC and PM.

A potential explanation for this DNA damage-tolerant phenotype would be if the B5-180[3] cells repair ISCs more efficiently than the parental cells. Direct measurements of 4HC-induced ISCs suggest that B5-180[3] cells might repair these lesions somewhat faster than B5 cells[24]. However, extreme caution must be exercised when designing and interpreting such experiments because the cells are necessarily exposed to the drug in order to generate such data. In this specific example[24], we elected to use unequal concentrations of 4HC that would generate similar initial yields of ISCs in the two cell types; naturally, in view of their ~5 fold lower tolerance, this treatment would invoke a much greater cytotoxic response in the parental cells, and this would likely have a significant impact on what is being measured as a cellular response to these lesions. A similar problem would result if drug concentrations were selected to be iso-effective for cell killing. If the experiments were performed using the same drug concentration for both lines, the resistant cells would experience considerably less damage to their genome and undergo virtually no loss of clonogenic potential, unlike the parental cells.

It is of interest to note that in similar investigations into the nature of CP resistance in the D283 Med (4-HCR) human medulloblastoma cell line, resistance to 4HC was also multifactorial[7]. Resistance in this model appeared to involve at least three mechanisms: elevated ALDH, elevated GSH, and an uncharacterized component, which the authors suggested might be related to “temporal” events[7]. Subsequent studies suggested that the increased repair of 4HC-induced ISCs might underlie the latter component[36].

5.7 Cell Cycle Checkpoint Activation

Another cellular response to DNA damage that could contribute to the "tolerance" component of drug resistance is the activation of cell-cycle checkpoints. Cells exposed to anticancer drugs that induce ISCs generally arrest in the G_2 phase, during which time ISCs can be repaired prior to mitosis. An extended G_2 arrest under conditions that are permissive for the repair of DNA damage has been reported in some alkylator-resistant tumor lines[37]. We used flow cytometry to examine the cell-cycle distributions of B5 and B5-180[3] cultures following a 1-h exposure to equi-cytotoxic (IC_{90}) concentrations of 4HC. The data (Figure 4) suggested a slight build-up of *both* lines in S- and G_2-phase, with a concomitant decrease in the G_1 compartment, during the 18-h post-treatment period.

6. GENETIC CHARACTERIZATION OF B5-180^3 CELLS

6.1 Cytogenetics

The B5-180^3 variant cells exhibit several cytogenetic alterations that distinguish them from the parental B5 cells (Table 3). The drug-resistant cells harbor a stable, possibly amplified, region of 5q, where additional chromosomal material has been added or translocated from another genomic region (Figure 5). Similarly, automated comparative genomic hybridization analysis indicated that region 5q is over-represented in B5-180^3 cells (Figure 6). This more sensitive technique also revealed additional changes insofar as the 13q region is over-represented and 5p is under-represented compared with the parental cells (Figure 6). Among other things, these complex cytogenetic changes would be expected to result in significant alterations in gene expression between the two cell lines. More recent methodologies such as microarray-based comparative genomic hybridization should allow more refined mapping of chromosomal alterations in these cell lines[38,39].

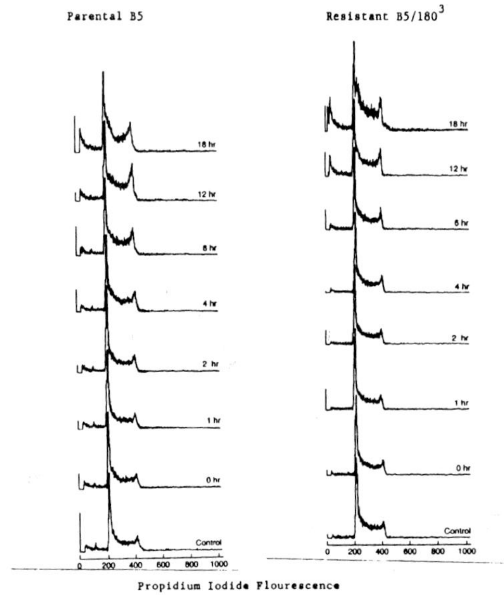

Figure 4. Flow-cytometric analysis of the cell-cycle phase distributions of parental B5 and CP-resistant B5-180^3 cells at various times following a 1-h exposure to equi-cytotoxic (IC_{90}) concentrations of 4HC (2 μg/ml for parental cells and 50 μg/ml for resistant cells). The y axis represents cell number; the x axis represents propidium iodide fluorescence indicating the cells' relative DNA content. The accumulation of cells with G_2 DNA content (right hand peak) is characteristic of the activation of the G_2/M checkpoint.

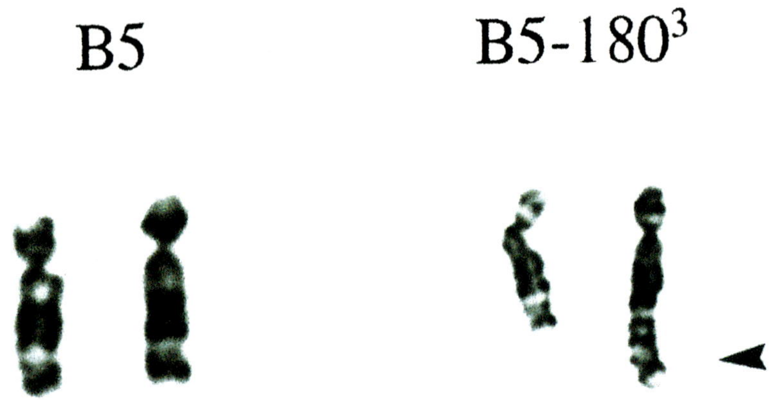

Figure 5. Cytogenetic comparison of chromosome 5 in B5 and B5-180^3 cells. The arrow indicates an over-represented, possibly amplified, region.

Thus, in the B5-180^3 sub-line, an extended arrest in G_2 does not appear to be involved in the damage-tolerance phenotype. However, these types of measurements are subject to many of the design and interpretation problems described above for DNA repair.

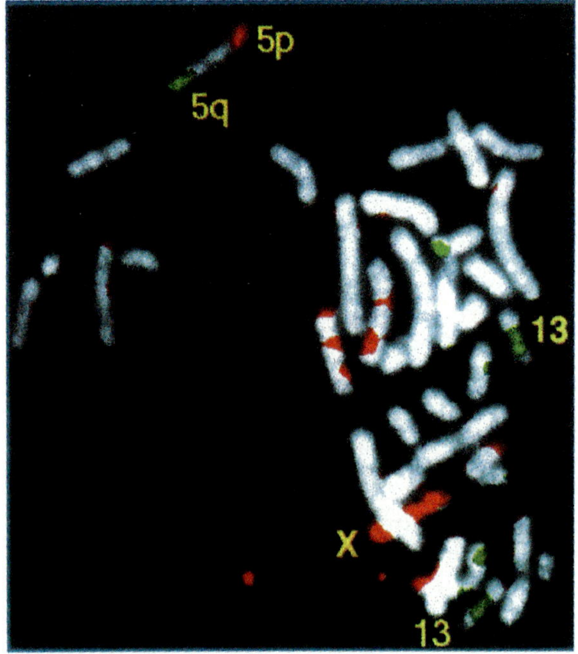

Figure 6. Comparative genomic hybridization analysis of B5 versus B5-180^3 cells. Regions 5q and 13q are over-represented (green), whereas 5p is under-represented (red) relative to the parental B5 line (computer-enhanced representation). [Andersson B, Andreeff M, and Murray D, unpublished data].

6.2 General Approaches to the Assessment of Altered Gene Expression in Drug-resistant Cells

Many factors have been implicated in cellular resistance to DNA-damaging agents. "Directed" screening for changes in the expression of individual candidate genes is therefore an inefficient approach to resolving the non-ALDH (tolerance) component of the B5-180^3 phenotype. In recent years, a number of general strategies, such as subtractive hybridization, DD-mRNA, and cDNA arrays, have been developed for detecting broader alterations in gene expression and for the identification of gene products that may be involved in drug resistance. With each of these methodologies, it is critical that the sequence of interest is confirmed to be differentially expressed by Northern blotting, and preferably by protein analysis, before any major conclusions are drawn. We now describe some of our initial findings using these methods.

6.3 Atlas 7742-1:Human Cancer cDNA Arrays

Figure 7 shows a typical pair of Atlas 7742-1:Human Cancer nylon arrays (588 gene, from Clontech) that were hybridized to ^{32}P-labeled cDNA populations prepared from B5 or B5-180^3 cells. These arrays allow specific groups of genes or pathways to be considered in the context of drug resistance. For example, the 7742-1 array includes various genes that might be involved in the DNA damage-tolerance phenotype, such as DNA repair genes, stress-response genes, and genes involved in regulating the cell cycle and apoptosis.

Many of the genes represented in the 7742-1 array were not strongly expressed in either cell line. Some genes were expressed, but at similar levels in the two lines. A number of genes appeared to be over-expressed in B5-180^3 cells. These included cyclin H, cyclin B1, vimentin, jnk2, patched homolog, c-yes1, and death-associated protein kinase 1. None of the DNA repair genes represented on the array appeared to be strongly differentially expressed. This includes *ERCC1* and *hRAD51*, whose encoded proteins are involved in the homologous recombinational repair of ISCs. The same was true of genes encoding the non-homologous end joining proteins DNA-PK and Ku, the NER proteins XPB, XPG and XPC, and the base excision repair protein XRCC1. Northern blots for *ERCC1* and *XRCC1* mRNA confirmed this lack of differential expression. Thus, altered expression of these particular repair factors does not appear to underlie the DNA damage-tolerance phenotype of B5-180^3 cells.

Another interesting observation is the apparent over-expression in B5-180^3 cells of two genes, jagged 2 and manic fringe, that encode components of the notch signaling pathway. This pathway functions in a variety of processes that regulate tissue development, and may also affect cell proliferation, tumorigenesis, and apoptosis[32,40–43]. For example, a constitutively active intracellular fragment of murine Notch-1 rendered thymomas resistant to glucocorticoid-induced apoptosis[40]. Certainly this finding appears to be worth following up in a more detailed study.

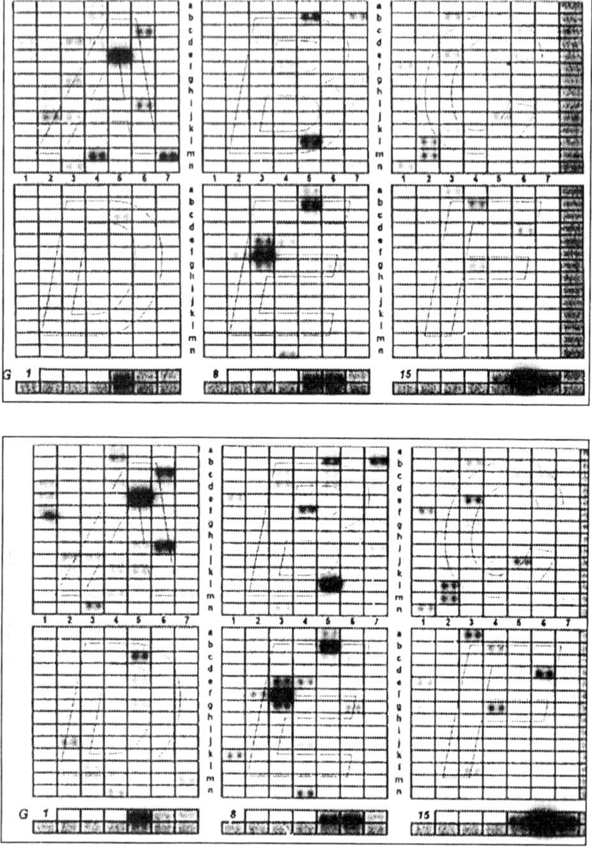

Figure 7. Typical Atlas 7742-1 Human Cancer cDNA Expression Array results comparing the expression of human cancer-related genes in the B5 and B5-180[3] cell lines. Radioactivity was analyzed with a Molecular Imager. Each gene is represented by duplicate spots. The housekeeping genes include GAPDH (array coordinate G12) and β-actin (array coordinate G19). The key to the grid can be found at: http://atlasinfo.clontech.com/atlasinfo/array-info-action.do?catalog_no=7742-1

6.4 Atlas 7850-1:Human 1.2 I cDNA Arrays

In addition to marketing the Atlas kits, Clontech offers microarray analysis for different gene subsets as a service for a fee. The user provides the company with pelleted cell populations of interest. A complete listing of the results for such an analysis of B5 and B5-180[3] cells obtained using the Atlas 7850-1:Human 1.2 I (1176 gene) array has been listed on the website at http://www.cancerboard.ab.ca/davidmurray/. Table 4 presents a sub-set of these data that focuses on certain genes that were common to the Atlas 7850-1 and 7742-1 arrays. To compare these results, we focused on the sub-set of genes that were clearly expressed to a similar degree in both cell lines and that were expressed in both arrays. The reasonable concordance between the two different assays with respect to these ten genes (Table 4) is encouraging given that these assays have many inherent practical pitfalls.

A number of DNA repair genes were represented in the Atlas 7850-1 array. As in the 7742-1 array study, neither *ERCC1* nor *hRAD51* expression was significantly altered in the resistant cells. In contrast *XRCC1* mRNA levels, which were similar in both lines in the 7742-1 array, were ~6 fold higher in the resistant cells in the 7850-1 array analysis. Northern blotting indicated that *XRCC1* was in fact similarly expressed in the two cell lines. Another repair protein, O^6-methylguanine-DNA methyltransferase (MGMT), appeared to be more highly expressed in the parental B5 cells in the 7850-1 data set. MGMT has been implicated in resistance to oxazaphosphorines, with protection presumably being specific for the acrolein metabolite generated upon metabolism of these drugs[11]. However, the observation that the resistance of B5-180^3 cells to 4HC and PM (which do and do not generate acrolein, respectively) is almost identical per induced ISC[23] argues against MGMT being involved in this phenotype[11].

Table 4. Comparison of gene expression patterns in the parent KBM-7/B5 and in 4HC-resistant B5-180^3 sub-line assessed in two independent Clontech gene-array studies.

Gene	**Atlas 7742-1 Human Cancer**[a]		**Atlas 7850-1 Human 1.2 I**[b]	
	B5	**B5-180^3**	**B5**	**B5-180^3**
PCNA	Moderate	Moderate	Moderate	Moderate
GRB-2	Moderate	Moderate	Moderate	Moderate
RhoGDP1	Moderate	Moderate	Moderate	Strong
RFC2	Moderate	Moderate	Moderate	Moderate
ERCC1	Moderate	Moderate	Strong	Strong
RAD23A	Moderate	Moderate	Moderate	Strong
HRAD51	Weak	Weak	Weak	Weak
SOD1	Moderate	Moderate	Moderate	Moderate
IGFBP2	Moderate	Moderate	Strong	Moderate
Topo-II α	Weak	Weak	Weak	Weak

[a]These data were quantitated using an automated image analysis system, and the band intensities were normalized to housekeeping genes.

[b]Gene expression was reported in relative intensity units; the data have been ranked as either weak (≤10 units), moderate (11-99 units), or strong (≥100 units) expression.

6.5 Differential Display of mRNA

DD-mRNA[44] is a PCR-based method for investigating potential differences in gene expression related to drug resistance. Poly(A)$^+$ mRNA was isolated from B5 and B5-180^3 cells and cDNA was prepared by reverse transcription using synthetic 5'-T_{11}MX primers, where M is a mixture of G, A, and C, and X is either G, A, or C. Partial cDNA sequences were amplified using the same 3' primers used for reverse transcription and 5' primers that are arbitrary 10-mer sequences. The resulting PCR products were separated on a sequencing gel. To date, we have recovered a total of 67 cDNAs that appear to be differentially expressed between B5 and B5-180^3 cells. Of these, 42 successfully reamplified into a single band and were radiolabeled and used to probe Northern blots of total RNA from B5 and B5-180^3 cells. Of these, four were clearly differentially expressed in the 4HC-resistant versus parental line.

These four cDNAs were sequenced and compared to known genomic sequences in the Genbank database. Clone 4A showed homology to the human SA hypertension-associated homolog (SAH) mRNA[45]. The Northern blot showed no signal for B5 cells and an intense band for B5-180^3 cells. The deduced protein sequence had slight homology to bacterial acetyl-CoA synthase[46]. Clone 2B was highly homologous to the mRNA for KIAA0603, a protein of unknown function[47]. Interestingly this gene, which encodes a TBC (Tre-2, BUB2, CDC16) domain-containing protein, is one of four candidate genes for the embryonic lethality in mice homozygous for the Ednrb(s-1Acrg) deletion[48]. Clone 4D showed ~2 fold greater expression in B5-180^3 than B5 cells by Northern blotting and limited homology to a novel dual specificity phosphatase, MKP-5, that is elevated by stress stimuli and binds to p38 and SAPK/JNK but not to MAPK/ERK[49]. It also showed homology to a human cDNA, DKFZp434P1735[50]. Clone 7A was ~3 fold more expressed in B5-180^3 than B5 cells by Northern blotting and showed homology to human ADP-ribose pyrophosphatase NUDT9 mRNA which encodes a novel ADP-ribose specific member of the Nudix hydrolase family[51].

One of the earliest clones that we sequenced piqued our interest because it showed limited homology to human alcohol dehydrogenase 5, which is known to catalyze the reduction of ALDO to alcophosphamide[52] and can be viewed as a detoxifying reaction because alcophosphamide is only weakly cytotoxic[53]. However, Northern blots indicated that this gene was in fact only minimally differentially expressed in B5-180^3 versus B5 cells. We have included this example mainly to reiterate the importance of doing Northern blots early in the course of such a study.

6.6 Caveats

In the search for genes responsible for the DNA-damage tolerance phenotype of B5-180^3 cells, various genes encoding proteins related to stress response pathways were identified as being differentially expressed to some degree. As described elsewhere in this volume (see chapter 5 by Dr. S. Grant and colleagues), the activation of stress response pathways is an important component of the ability of cells to tolerate genotoxic damage. Expression of these genes may also depend on the precise conditions under which the cells are cultivated prior to RNA extraction. Thus, it is critical that careful control is exerted over physical and environmental factors that could confuse the interpretation of gene expression changes of relevance to the development of drug resistance. In fact, a rare discrepancy that we noted in comparing the two Atlas array data sets (see above) was for *JNK2*, which the 7850-1 array indicated to be elevated in B5 cells, but which displayed the opposite trend in the 7742-1 array.

Although the B5-180[3] gene expression studies outlined above are at an early stage, this approach clearly represents a potential source of discovering genes of interest in the context of oxazaphosphorine resistance. However, it will be essential in each case to fully define the role of the encoded proteins in drug resistance by suitable modulation of their expression.

Some genes that mediate drug resistance may be induced following genotoxic insult, such that their mRNAs are not appropriately represented until the cells have been challenged with the drug of interest. This issue has not yet been addressed in the context of the B5-180[3] phenotype, but such experiments are clearly critical to completely defining *any* model of drug resistance. This concept has been considered in the context of cisplatin resistance in ovarian cancer[54,55]. It should also be appreciated that the above techniques will only detect differences in steady-state message levels that arise due to alterations at the DNA level or to altered transcription and mRNA stability; they will *not* be informative for alterations at the level of translation, post-translational protein modification, or protein stability. Detecting such changes will require the utilization of the emerging techniques of proteomics and protein-hybridization arrays (see chapter 17 of this volume by Dr. S. Damaraju and colleagues).

7. APOPTOSIS

Many hematological cancer cell lines undergo apoptosis following exposure to oxazaphosphorines[56–61]. For cell lines such as B5-180[3] CML and D283 Med (4-HCR) medulloblastoma[7] whose resistance to 4HC is multifactorial, apoptosis may be involved in several ways. First, those resistance mechanisms such as elevated ALDH that prevent the induction of genotoxic damage (as well as damage to other cellular components) will invariably be associated with a decrease in the triggering of apoptosis, and indeed of all mechanisms responsible for the loss of clonogenic potential that are triggered by genotoxic damage. In this case, the level of apoptosis per induced DNA lesion (such as an ISC) should be similar for the parental and drug-resistant lines.

Another aspect of the modulation of apoptosis in the development of resistance to some anticancer drugs involves the tumor cells switching off pro-apoptotic pathways at some level, such that genotoxic damage fails to activate the apoptotic program.[62–64]. There are two general types of molecular event that might underlie such a response. Either the mechanisms that sense DNA damage and trigger the apoptotic cascade are altered, or the apoptotic effector pathways themselves are blocked at some point. In the case of B5-180^3 cells, such alterations would be expected to contribute to that component of 4HC resistance that has been attributed to DNA damage-tolerance mechanisms.

With respect to damage-sensing mechanisms, the loss of DNA mismatch repair activity has been shown to result in a DNA damage-tolerant phenotype in tumor cells exposed to chemotherapy agents such as cisplatin because of their failure to trigger apoptosis[65]. Information with respect to the oxazaphosphorines in this regard is limited. However, it should be noted that in the Atlas 7742-1 array data set there was no significant difference in the expression of the *hMLH1* mismatch repair gene between the B5 and B5-180^3 cell lines.

With respect to alterations at the level of effector pathways in these CML lines, the cellular expression and function of several such factors was examined by Munker and colleagues[66]. These included Fas (CD95/Apo-1) which, when stimulated by its ligand or by antibodies to the receptor, will trigger apoptosis in sensitive cells, and also members of the bcl-2 family, namely bcl-2, the bcl-x short and long variants, and bax. Surprisingly, B5-180^3 cells showed ~4 fold over-expression of CD95 protein compared with the parental cells. In addition, cellular stimulation with IFN-γ or TNF-α resulted in a further up-regulation of CD95 in both cell lines. However, when the cells were exposed to Fas-ligand, neither line underwent significant levels of apoptosis. A similar situation has been reported for myeloma and certain acute lymphocytic leukemia T-cell blast populations[67,68]. Bcl-2 gene family members were examined by RT-PCR[66]. The parental and resistant cell lines expressed similar levels of bcl-2 transcripts and of bcl-2 protein assessed by antibody staining and flow cytometry. The two CML cell lines also had similar levels of bax and bcl-x_l transcripts. However, levels of bcl-x_s transcript were ~5 fold lower in B5-180^3 cells. This alteration may be significant in 4HC resistance in these cells because over-expression of bcl-x_s has been shown to correlate with sensitization to apoptosis-inducing agents in a breast cancer line[69].

A number of these apoptosis-related genes were also represented in the Atlas arrays described in sections 6.3 and 6.4. These arrays are considerably less sensitive than RT-PCR, so it is not surprising that several of these genes could not be detected by the former assay. Thus, neither Fas nor bcl-2 expression could be detected in either cell line on either the 7742-1 or the 7850-1 arrays. However, the 7850-1 array did indicate that expression of bax was unchanged, while bcl-x expression was significantly increased in the resistant line.

Finally, drug resistance mediated by a repression of apoptotic cell death should result in phenotypic cross-resistance to a number of different drugs, as is clearly the case with B5-180^3 cells (Table 1)[23,24]. It should also be noted that both the B5 and B5-180^3 cell lines express wild-type p53 (Table 3).

8. CLINICALLY-RELEVANT LOW-DEGREE RESISTANCE TO OXAZAPHOSPHORINES IN CML

The usefulness of the highly resistant B5-180^3 variant cell line is that it has enabled the definition of potential resistance mechanisms that can be examined in more clinically relevant low-degree resistance cell lines and, eventually, in clinical material. The induction of low-level drug resistance was studied following a single acute exposure of B5 cells to 4HC. Briefly, 1 x 10^7 B5 cells were exposed for 60 min to 4HC at 60 µg/ml then incubated in soft-agar. Six weeks later, individual colonies were recovered and expanded in suspension. After 2-3 weeks, these "single-step" resistant sub-clones were tested for their sensitivity to 4HC and PM in the clonogenic survival assay. Nine of the seventeen tested sub-clones displayed low-level (1.3 to 3 fold) resistance to 4HC. Three sub-clones having a resistance index of between 1.3 and 1.5 for 4HC (based on IC_{90} values) were passaged in suspension culture without additional drug selection for 6 months before being re-tested for their sensitivity to 4HC and PM. As with the highly resistant B5-180^3 cells, these sub-clones displayed stable resistance characterized by a partial ALDH component, as indicated by their cross-resistance to PM and by direct measurements of their ability to catalyze the metabolism of ALDO (Table 5). Thus, the development of low degree drug resistance appears to be a rapid event that may include multiple components converging in a genetically stable resistance phenotype.

Table 5. Characterization of drug resistance in B5 and single-step 4HC-resistant sub-clones.

		Single-step sub-clone designation number		
	B5	#11	#14	#31
RI [4HC]*	1.0	1.5	1.4	1.3
RI [PM]*	1.0	2.3	2.4	2.3
ALDH-1 activity†	0.6	2.1	2.5	2.6

*RI: Resistance Index based on IC_{90} values after prolonged drug exposure in clonogenic assay as previously described (Table 1).

†based on catalysis of the metabolism of ALDO, using NAD as the cofactor (see Table 2)[33].

ACKNOWLEDGMENTS

This work was supported by operating grant RO1 CA-67270 from the NIH/NCI (USA).

REFERENCES

1. DeVita VT Jr, Hellman S, Rosenberg SA. Cancer: Principles and Practice of Oncology, 6th ed., Lippincott, Williams and Wilkins, Philadelphia, PA, 2001.
2. Holland JF, Frei E III, Cancer Medicine, e.5, Decker B.C., Inc., Hamilton, Ontario, Canada, 2000.
3. List AF, Kopecky KJ, Willman CL, *et al.* Benefit of cyclosporine modulation of drug resistance in patients with poor-risk acute myeloid leukemia: a Southwest Oncology Group study. Blood 98,3212-3220, 2001.
4. Ohno N, Tani A, Chen ZS, *et al.* Prognostic significance of multidrug resistance protein in adult T-cell leukemia. Clin Cancer Res, 10:3120-3126, 2001.
5. Sreerama L, Sladek NE. Primary breast tumor levels of suspected molecular determinants of cellular sensitivity to cyclophosphamide, ifosfamide, and certain other anticancer agents as predictors of paired, metastatic tumor levels of these determinants. Rational individualization of cancer chemotherapeutic regimens. Cancer Chemother Pharmacol, 47:255-262, 2001.
6. Hilton J. Role of aldehyde dehydrogenase in cyclophosphamide-resistant L1210 leukemia. Cancer Res, 44:5156-5160, 1984.
7. Friedman HS, Colvin OM, Kaufmann SH, *et al.* Cyclophosphamide resistance in medulloblastoma. Cancer Res, 52:5373-5378, 1992.
8. Sreerama L, Sladek NE. Identification of a methylcholanthrene-induced aldehyde dehydrogenase in a human breast adenocarcinoma cell line exhibiting oxazaphosphorine-specific acquired resistance. Cancer Res, 54:2176-2185, 1994.
9. Rekha GK, Sreerama L, Sladek NE. Intrinsic cellular resistance to oxazaphosphorines exhibited by a human colon carcinoma cell line expressing relatively large amounts of a class-3 aldehyde dehydrogenase. Biochem Pharmacol, 48:1943-1952, 1994.
10. de Groot CJ, Martens ACM, Hagenbeek A. Aldehyde dehydrogenase involvement in a variant of the brown Norway rat acute myeloid leukaemia (BNML) that acquired cyclophosphamide resistance in vivo. Eur J Cancer, 30A:2137-2143, 1994.
11. Gamcsik MP, Dolan ME, Andersson BS, Murray D. Mechanisms of resistance to the toxicity of cyclophosphamide. Curr Pharm Des, 5:587-605, 1999.
12. Hipkens JH, Struck RF, Gurtoo HL. Role of aldehyde dehydrogenase in the metabolism-dependent biological activity of cyclophosphamide. Cancer Res, 41:3571-3583, 1981.
13. Lin K-H, Lindahl R. Role of aldehyde dehydrogenase activity in cyclophosphamide metabolism in rat hepatoma cell lines. Biochem Pharmacol, 36:3305-3307, 1987.
14. Richardson ME, Siemann DW. Thiol-related mechanisms of resistance in a murine tumor model. Int J Radiat Oncol Biol Phys, 29:387-392, 1994.
15. Hoy CA, Thompson LH, Mooney CL, Salazar EP. Defective DNA cross-link removal in Chinese hamster cell mutants hypersensitive to bifunctional alkylating agents. Cancer Res, 45:1737-1743, 1985.
16. Andersson BS, Sadeghi T, Siciliano MJ, *et al.* Nucleotide excision repair genes as determinants of cellular sensitivity to cyclophosphamide analogs. Cancer Chemother Pharmacol, 38:406-416, 1996.
17. Murray D, Vallee-Lucic L, Rosenberg E, Andersson B. Sensitivity of nucleotide excision repair-deficient human cells to ionizing radiation and cyclophosphamide. Anticancer Res, 22:21-26, 2002.
18. Thompson LH. Nucleotide excision repair. Its relation to human disease. *In*: DNA Damage and Repair, Vol. 2: DNA Repair in Higher Eukaryotes, JA Nickoloff, MF Hoekstra (eds.), Humana Press, Totowa, NJ, 335-393, 1998.

19. Busch DB, van Vuuren H, de Wit J, *et al.* Phenotypic heterogeneity in nucleotide excision repair mutants of rodent complementation groups 1 and 4. Mutat Res, 383:91-106, 1997.
20. Panasci L, Paiement JP, Christodoulopoulos G, *et al.* Chlorambucil drug resistance in chronic lymphocytic leukemia: the emerging role of DNA repair. Clin Cancer Res, 7:454-461, 2001.
21. Andersson BS, Beran M, Pathak S, *et al.* Ph-positive chronic myeloid leukemia with near-haploid conversion in vivo and establishment of a continuously growing cell line with similar cytogenetic pattern. Cancer Genet Cytogenet, 24:335-343, 1987.
22. Andersson BS, Collins VP, Kurzrock R, *et al.* KBM-7, a human myeloid leukemia cell line with double Philadelphia chromosomes lacking normal c-ABL and BCR transcripts. Leukemia, 9:2100-2108, 1995.
23. Andersson BS, Mroue M, Britten R, Murray D. The role of DNA damage in the resistance of human chronic myeloid leukemia cells to cyclophosphamide analogs. Cancer Res, 54:5394-5400, 1994.
24. Andersson BS, Mroue M, Britten RA, *et al.* Mechanisms of cyclophosphamide resistance in a human myeloid leukemia cell line. Acta Oncol, 34:247-251, 1995.
25. Kantarjian HM, O'Brien SO, Smith TL, *et al.* Results of treatment with hyper-CVAD, a dose-intensive regimen, in adult acute lymphocytic leukemia. J Clin Oncol, 18:547-561, 2000.
26. Kantarjian HM, Walters RS, Keating MJ, *et al.* Results of the vincristine, doxorubicin, and dexamethasone regimen in adults with standard- and high-risk acute lymphocytic leukemia. J Clin Oncol, 8:994-1004, 1990.
27. Wang Y, Farquhar D. Aldophosphamide acetal diacetate and structural analogues: Synthesis and cytotoxicity studies. J Med Chem, 34:197-203, 1991.
28. O'Connor PM, Kohn KW. Comparative pharmacokinetics of DNA lesion formation and removal following treatment of L1210 cells with nitrogen mustards. Cancer Commun, 2:387-394, 1990.
29. Caldecott K, Jeggo P. Cross-sensitivity of gamma-ray-sensitive hamster mutants to cross-linking agents. Mutat Res, 255:111-121, 1991.
30. De Silva IU, McHugh PJ, Clingen PH, Hartley JA. Defining the roles of nucleotide excision repair and recombination in the repair of DNA interstrand cross-links in mammalian cells. Mol Cell Biol, 20:7980-7990, 2000.
31. Bresnick EH, Chu J, Christensen HM, *et al.* Linking Notch signaling, chromatin remodeling, and T-cell leukemogenesis. J Cell Biochem Suppl, 35:46-53, 2000.
32. Joutel A, Tournier-Lasserve E. Notch signalling pathway and human diseases. Semin Cell Dev Biol, 9:619-625, 1998.
33. Sreerama L, Sladek NE. Identification and characterization of a novel class 3 aldehyde dehydrogenase overexpressed in a human breast adenocarcinoma cell line exhibiting oxazaphosphorine-specific acquired resistance. Biochem Pharmacol, 45:2487-2505, 1993.
34. Habig WH, Pabst MJ, Jakoby WB. Glutathione S-transferases: The first enzymatic step in mercapturic acid formation. J Biol Chem, 249:7130-7139, 1974.
35. Andersson BS, Bullard C, Farquhar D, Murray D. Mechanisms of acquired resistance to cyclophosphamide analogs in human myeloid leukemia. Proc Amer Assoc Cancer Res, Abstract 2782, 1992.
36. Dong Q, Bullock N, Ali-Osman F, *et al.* Repair analysis of 4-hydroperoxycyclophosphamide-induced DNA interstrand crosslinking of the c-myc gene in 4-hydroperoxycyclophosphamide-sensitive and -resistant medulloblastoma cell lines. Cancer Chemother Pharmacol, 37:242-246, 1996.

37. O'Connor PM, Ferris DK, White GA, *et al.* Relationships between cdc2 kinase, DNA cross-linking, and cell cycle perturbations induced by nitrogen mustard. Cell Growth Differ, 3:43-52, 1992.
38. Pollack JR, Perou CM, Alizadeh AA, *et al.* Genome-wide analysis of DNA copy-number changes using cDNA microarrays. Nature Genet, 23:41-46, 1999.
39. Hui AB, Lo KW, Yin XL, *et al.* Detection of multiple gene amplifications in glioblastoma multiforme using array-based comparative genomic hybridization. Lab Invest, 81:717-723, 2001.
40. Deftos ML, He YW, Ojala EW, Bevan MJ. Correlating notch signaling with thymocyte maturation. Immunity, 9:777-786, 1998.
41. Weinmaster G. Notch signal transduction: a real rip and more. Curr Opin Genet Dev, 10:363-369, 2000.
42. Callahan R, Raafat A. Notch signaling in mammary gland tumorigenesis. J Mammary Gland Biol Neoplasia, 6:23-36, 2001.
43. Frisen J, Lendahl U. Oh no, Notch again! Bioessays, 23:3-7, 2001.
44. Liang P, Pardee AB. Differential display of eukaryotic messenger RNA by means of the polymerase chain reaction. Science, 257:967-971, 1992.
45. Iwai N, Inagami T. Isolation of preferentially expressed genes in the kidneys of hypertensive rats. Hypertension, 17:161-169, 1991.
46. Iwai N, Ohmichi N, Hanai K, *et al.* Human SA gene locus as a candidate locus for essential hypertension. Hypertension, 23:375-380, 1994.
47. Nagase T, Ishikawa K, Miyajima N, *et al.* Prediction of the coding sequences of unidentified human genes. IX. The complete sequences of 100 new cDNA clones from brain which can code for large proteins in vitro. DNA Res, 5:31-39, 1998.
48. Kurihara LJ, Semenova E, Miller W, *et al.* Candidate genes required for embryonic development: a comparative analysis of distal mouse chromosome 14 and human chromosome 13q22. Genomics, 79:154-161, 2002.
49. Tanoue T, Moriguchi T, Nishida E. Molecular cloning and characterization of a novel dual specificity phosphatase, MKP-5. J Biol Chem, 274:19949-19956, 1999.
50. Wiemann S, Weil B, Wellenreuther R, *et al.* Toward a catalog of human genes and proteins: sequencing and analysis of 500 novel complete protein coding human cDNAs. Genome Res, 11:422-435, 2001.
51. Perraud AL, Fleig A, Dunn CA, *et al.* ADP-ribose gating of the calcium-permeable LTRPC2 channel revealed by Nudix motif homology. Nature, 411:595-599, 2001.
52. Domeyer BE, Sladek NE. Metabolism of 4-hydroxycyclophosphamide/aldophosphamide in vitro. Biochem Pharmacol, 29:2903-2912, 1980.
53. Sladek NE. Metabolism and pharmacokinetic behavior of cyclophosphamide and related oxazaphosphorines. *In*: Anticancer Drugs: Reactive Metabolism and Drug Interactions, G Powis (ed.), Pergamon Press, New York, NY, 79-156, 1994.
54. Ferry KV, Ozols RF, Hamilton TC, *et al.* Expression of nucleotide excision repair genes in CDDP-sensitive and resistant human ovarian cancer cell lines. Proc Amer Assoc Cancer Res, Abstract 2492, 1996.
55. Reed E. Ovarian cancer: Molecular abnormalities. *In*: Encyclopedia of Cancer, Vol. II, JR Bertino (ed.), Academic Press, San Diego, CA, 1192-1200, 1997.
56. Davidoff AN, Mendelow BV. Cell-cycle disruptions and apoptosis induced by the cyclophosphamide derivative mafosfamide. Exp Hematol, 21:922-927, 1993.
57. Yamauchi T, Nowak BJ, Keating MJ, Plunkett W. DNA repair initiated in chronic lymphocytic leukemia lymphocytes by 4-hydroperoxycyclophosphamide is inhibited by fludarabine and clofarabine. Clin Cancer Res, 7:3580-3589, 2001.

58. Lopes EC, Garcia MG, Vellon L, *et al.* Correlation between decreased apoptosis and multidrug resistance (MDR) in murine leukemic T cell lines. Leukemia Lymphoma, 42:775-787, 2001.
59. Klein A, Miera O, Bauer O, *et al.* Chemosensitivity of B cell chronic lymphocytic leukemia and correlated expression of proteins regulating apoptosis, cell cycle and DNA repair. Leukemia, 14:40-46, 2000.
60. Skorski T, Nieborowska-Skorska M, Wlodarski P, *et al.* Treatment of Philadelphia leukemia in severe combined immunodeficient mice by combination of cyclophosphamide and bcr/abl antisense oligodeoxynucleotides. J Natl Cancer Inst, 89:124-133, 1997.
61. Bullock G, Tang C, Tourkina E, *et al.* Effect of combined treatment with interleukin-3 and interleukin-6 on 4-hydroperoxycyclophosphamide-induced programmed cell death or apoptosis in human myeloid leukemia cells. Exp Hematol, 21:1640-1647, 1993.
62. Inoue S, Salah-Eldin AE, Omoteyama K. Apoptosis and anticancer drug resistance. Human Cell, 14:211-221, 2001.
63. Makin G, Dive C. Apoptosis and cancer chemotherapy. Trends Cell Biol, 11:S22-26, 2001.
64. Mow BM, Blajeski AL, Chandra J, Kaufmann SH. Apoptosis and the response to anticancer therapy. Curr Opin Oncol, 13:453-462, 2001.
65. Fink D, Aebi S, Howell SB. The role of DNA mismatch repair in drug resistance. Clin Cancer Res, 4:1-6, 1998.
66. Munker R, Zhao S, Jiang S, *et al.* Further characterization of cyclophosphamide resistance: expression of CD95 and of bcl-2 in a CML cell line. Leukemia Res, 22:1073-1077, 1998.
67. Shima Y, Nishimoto N, Ogata A, *et al.* Myeloma cells express Fas antigen (CD95) but only some are sensitive to anti-Fas antibody resulting in apoptosis. Blood, 85:757-764, 1995.
68. Debatin KM, Krammer PH. Resistance to APO-1 (CD95) induced apoptosis in T-ALL is determined by a bcl-2 independent anti-apoptotic program. Leukemia, 9:815-820, 1995.
69. Sumantran VN, Elovega MW, Nunez G, *et al.* Over-expression of Bcl-x_s sensitizes MCF-7 cells to chemotherapy-induced apoptosis. Cancer Res, 55:2507-2510, 1995.

Chapter 12

MECHANISMS OF DRUG RESISTANCE IN AML

Michael Andreeff and Marina Konopleva
Section of Molecular Hematology and Therapy, Department of Blood and Marrow Transplantation, The University of Texas MD Anderson Cancer Center, Houston, Texas, USA

1. INTRODUCTION

The acute myelogenous leukemias (AML) are diverse in their clinical presentation, molecular, biological and immunological characteristics, and response to therapies. They encompass a wide spectrum of clinical features, developing slowly from myelodysplastic syndromes (MDS) or presenting with dramatic clinical features without prior warning, such as high circulating blast count resulting in leucostastis and bleeding, coagulopathies, cutaneous and organ infiltration, sepsis due to neutropenia, and anemia. Morphological classification was initially codified in the French-American-British (FAB) system,[1] and was recently modified in the World Health Organization (WHO) system.[2] The leukemic transformation is believed to occur at an early stem cell level, based on the ability of $CD34^{+}38^{-}$ leukemic cells to repopulate NOD/scid mice,[3] with the exception of acute promyelocytic leukemias (APL) that probably originate in $CD34^{-}33^{+}$ cells. However, leukemic cells were recently reported to reside in the pre-CD34 "side-population" (SP) cell population,[4] suggesting an even more primitive cell of origin.

Immunophenotyping of AML has revealed an abundance of antigens expressed, usually reflecting their origin from myeloid progenitors, with some notable exceptions: T cell antigens such as CD7 can be aberrantly expressed, glycophorin A and myeloid markers are found on erythroleukemic cells (FAB M6), and megakaryocytic markers on megakaryocytic AML (FAB M7). Also, early and late myeloid antigens are regularly co-expressed on AML cells, a constellation not found in normal hematopoiesis.

Cytogenetic and molecular studies have provided important clues to the pathophysiology of AML and are slowly evolving into a molecular classification of AML.[5] In the context of clinical drug resistance, cytogenetic findings have long been used to distinguish between "good" [inversion of chromosome 16, t(8;21), t(15;17)], "intermediate" [diploid, trisomy of chromosome 8], and "poor" prognosis [abnormalities of chromosomes 5, 7, and 11, translocations and deletions]. However, multiple underlying mechanisms of drug resistance have been identified and will be reviewed here. It is the focus on these resistance pathways that is hoped to provide a rationale for the development of more effective therapies. Of note, 5-year survival of adult AML patients was 7% 25 years ago and is now only 11%, as reported in the NIH SEER database. The particular challenge lies in the identification of drug resistance of minimal residual disease in AML, as the initial rates of complete remissions (CR) vary from 30% (poor-prognosis cytogenetics, prior MDS) to over 90% (APL). These remissions are achieved with relatively simple regimens consisting of cytosine arabinoside (Ara-C) and anthracyclines such as daunorubicin or idarubicin. In APL, the introduction of all-trans-retinoic acid (ATRA)[6] dramatically increased the CR rate, suggesting that novel approaches to AML therapy have great promise. The complexity of the resistance mechanisms discussed below suggest that combined approaches will be needed to overcome them.

2. CYTOKINES AND CYTOKINETIC RESISTANCE

Proliferation, survival and maturation of human AML cells *in vitro* is absolutely dependent on the addition of hematopoietic growth factors (HGF). Growth factors are known to exert both proliferative and anti-apoptotic effects. In the bone marrow, they are provided either by direct contact with marrow stroma or secreted by stromal cells into the circulation.

Growth factors are produced either as soluble factors or as transmembrane molecules. Specific receptor-ligand interactions induce a cascade of signal transduction biochemical events. The cytokine receptors can be divided into [1] hematopoietin receptor superfamily that lack intrinsic tyrosine kinase activity, but transmit signals through adaptors, for example through the "Janus kinase" (JAK) family of cytoplasmic tyrosine kinases and STAT (signal transducers and activators of transcription), and [2] receptors with intrinsic tyrosine kinase activity. These membrane-anchored receptors have an extracellular ligand-binding domain and an intracellular catalytic tyrosine kinase domain. They include receptors for stem cell factor (SCF), FLT3, macrophage colony-stimulating factor (M-CSF), and platelet-derived growth factor (PDGF), which are encoded by the genes c-*kit*, *FLT3*, c-*fms*, and *PDGFR* (α and β). Receptor studies indicate that AML cells express CSF receptors at a physiologic density and with physiologic affinity.

JAKs and STATs are involved in the signaling of granulocyte colony-stimulating factor (G-CSF) and granulocyte-macrophage colony-stimulating factor (GM-CSF). In normal cells, expression of JAK/STAT was found to be related to their clonogenic potential, with $CD34^+$ cells having the highest expression levels. Recently, constitutive tyrosine phosphorylation of STAT5 or STAT3 was found in over 70% of AML samples.[7] Another study, however, demonstrated deficiency of at least one JAK in 10 of 25 AML patients.[8] In addition, a deficiency of three JAKs was more common in patients with an abnormal phenotype (inv11q, inv7), and a lack of JAK2 and Tyk2 was strongly associated with FAB M2. These findings could explain the lack of proliferation of AML blasts in response to G-CSF or GM-CSF in a cohort of patients receiving G-CSF *in vivo* (see below).

In addition to the JAK-STAT pathway, many growth factors stimulate MAP kinase signal transduction pathways. MAP kinases (ERK1 and ERK2) are activated in response to IL-3, GM-CSF, erythropoietin and thrombopoietin. A constitutive activation of MAP kinase was demonstrated in 50%[9,10] of AML samples. This may reflect the role of autocrine and paracrine production of colony-stimulating factors in the autonomous growth of leukemic cells.

In most AML patients, proliferation of the leukemic cells can be stimulated *in vitro* by IL-3, GM-CSF, G-CSF and less frequently by M-CSF.[11] G-CSF plays a critical role in granulocyte differentiation of myeloid progenitors. In addition, G-CSF also induces proliferation of stem and progenitor cells of the myeloid lineage. The G-CSF receptor is a type I protein, with singular extracellular, transmembrane, and cytoplasmic domains. However, in the majority of AML, G-CSF is unable to induce differentiation, while inducing proliferation.[12] A recent report by Tweardy *et al.*[13] attributed this to the increased amounts of the class IV isoform of the G-CSF receptor that retains the membrane proximal sequence required for the proliferation signaling, but is deficient in the c-terminal region critical for maturation. This would explain the heterogeneous response of AML cells to G-CSF *in vitro* and perhaps *in vivo*.

Two cytokines, SCF and FLT3 ligand (FL), cause a proliferative response in a high percentage of AML samples.[14–16] SCF, through its receptor c-kit (which possesses tyrosine kinase properties), plays a crucial role in the survival of normal immature hematopoietic progenitors. Expression of the receptor was found in normal stem cells and in myeloid progenitors and in 23% to 87% of AML cases,[17] and more frequently in immature phenotypes.[18] Expression of the SCF in c-kit-positive AML suggests that it could contribute to autonomous growth of leukemic blasts as a result of autocrine production.[14]

FLT3 is a member of the tyrosine kinase class of receptors. Its ligand exists in both membrane-bound and soluble isoforms. FLT3 was found to be expressed in the majority of primary AML samples and in myelo-monocytic cell lines.[19,20] Synergism in inducing proliferation was found for FL and G-CSF, M-CSF, GM-CSF, IL-3 and SCF.[15,16] FL also prevented apoptosis of primary AML cells,[16] presumably through down-regulation of Bax expression.

Recently, a novel somatic mutation of the *FLT3* gene was found in about 20% of AML cases and in patients with leukemic transformation of myelodysplasia to AML.[21] An internal tandem (in frame) duplication of sequences coding for the juxtramembrane domain, leaving the tyrosine kinase domain intact, may induce abnormal proliferation of leukemic cells.

The receptor for the gene product of the obesity gene, leptin (OB-R), was recently reported to be expressed on murine and human hematopoietic progenitor cells.[22] Interestingly, the primary structure of OB-R shows homologies to the signaling subunits of the IL-6-type cytokine receptors, including gp130, and to receptors for the leukemia inhibitory factor and the G-CSF.[23] We observed expression of both the long and short isoforms of OB-R in the majority of samples from AML patients, whereas it was essentially absent in samples of chronic or acute lymphocytic leukemia.[24] In addition, recombinant human leptin alone and in combination with G-CSF, IL-3, and SCF induced proliferation of myeloid leukemic cell lines and of blasts from primary AML and increased colony formation. Intriguingly, leukemic but not normal promyelocytes from newly diagnosed and recurrent APL patients express both isoforms. Hence, it is conceivable that the proliferation of leukemic promyelocytes is driven, in part, by increased leptin levels of obese APL patients who have been reported to have an increased body mass index.[25] Because leptin is produced by adipocytes and stromal cells,[26,27] which make up a significant part of the bone marrow microenvironment, it could stimulate leukemic and normal progenitors in a paracrine fashion.

2.1 Priming Effects of HGF in AML: Cytokinetic Resistance

HGF priming strategies are based on their stimulation of AML blasts *in vitro*, their modulation of cellular Ara-C metabolism and enhancement of clonogenic cell kill by Ara-C.[28] Several clinical trials employing HGF before or simultaneously with chemotherapy were conducted. Recruitment was demonstrated *in vivo* in the majority of 18 patients by bromodeoxyuridine incorporation after 24- to 48-h infusion of GM-CSF before chemotherapy.[29] 83% of the patients achieved CR. Several studies showed a trend toward more remissions and/or survival. A German multicenter randomized trial where four to five courses of growth factor were administered found a reduction in relapses during the first 6 months.[30] In a recent MD Anderson Cancer Center randomized trial, addition of G-CSF ± ATRA to FAI (fludarabine, high-dose Ara-C and idarubicin) improved the CR rate.[31]

The known anti-apoptotic effect of growth factors was implicated in the decreased CR and survival rate described in one study.[32] However, data from a Japanese study demonstrated induction of apoptosis in AML samples *ex vivo* from patients treated with low-dose Ara-C and G-CSF.[33] Similar data were obtained *in vitro*, suggesting that apoptosis plays a role in eradicating leukemic cells by G-CSF/chemotherapy combinations. These somewhat contradictory results have recently been clarified by *in vitro* studies that demonstrate that AML samples from patients with good-prognosis cytogenetics have autocrine cytokine production, high "spontaneous" proliferation, and respond poorly to exogenous cytokines, while the opposite was found for poor-cytogenetic AML. These results are consistent with the numerous positive reports obtained with "FLAG" or "FLAG-Ida" protocols in poor-prognosis patients.

No major toxicity from growth factor-priming regimens was noted, and there is no evidence for G-CSF-induced chemoresistance of leukemic cells. Because improved survival was observed in several studies, growth factor priming strategy remains an interesting therapeutic approach in AML that may be more effective in a multiple course design. This concept is presently being re-assessed in large randomized German and Italian studies.

2.2 Angiogenic Growth Factors in AML

Vascular endothelial growth factor (VEGF) is a homodimeric multifunctional cytokine that is known to stimulate angiogenesis[34]. The effect of VEGF is mediated by three specific receptors with intrinsic tyrosine kinase activity: Flt-1 (fms-like tyrosine kinase-1 receptor), KDR/Flk-1 (kinase-insert-domain-containing receptor) and a recently described Flt-4[35].

Murine embryos with inactivating *FLK-1* mutations remain "bloodless" suggesting that VEGF may play an important role in the development of stem cells. This effect could be mediated either by a primary stem cell defect or by impaired vascularization and blood island development.[36,37] In favor of the first hypothesis are two recent reports. Kennedy *et al.*[38] reported that VEGF and SCF stimulate the development of common precursors for primitive and definitive murine haemopoiesis. In another study, pluripotent HSCs but not lineage-committed stem cells expressed VEGFR2, also known as KDR, suggesting that KDR is a positive functional marker for stem cells.[39]

Two recent reports demonstrated that Flt-1 but not KDR is frequently expressed in primary AML cells, and that leukemic cells secrete much more VEGF than their normal counterparts.[40,41] In addition, VEGF co-stimulated the growth of CFU-GM in 15% of AML patients. These data support the hypothesis of autocrine stimulation of the leukemic cell growth mediated by VEGF production. In addition, a secretion of VEGF may serve as a signal for angiogenesis and growth of blood vessels that might in turn induce secretion of different paracrine growth factors.[35] In support of the functional role for the proliferation of endothelial cells and developing angiogenesis is the data demonstrating the formation of new vessels in the bone marrow of ALL patients.[42] In a recent study conducted at the MD Anderson Cancer Center, a positive correlation between increasing VEGF levels and shorter survival (P=0.01), as well as shorter disease-free survival, was found in 99 patients with newly diagnosed AML by radioimmunoassay.[43] These results point to the potential role of VEGF-stimulated angiogenesis in AML and suggest that abrogation of its function may be of therapeutic importance. Clinical trials are underway to inhibit angiogenesis in AML.

2.3 Chemokines in AML

Chemokines are cytokines that stimulate pro-inflammatory activity by eliciting the chemotactic migration of leukocytes and their adhesion to the endothelial cells.[44] In α-chemokines, the first two cysteines are separated by one amino acid (C-X-C motif) while β-chemokines are characterized by two contiguous cysteines (C-C motif). A member of the β-chemokine group, MIP-1α, besides its chemotactic activity, inhibits primitive bone marrow progenitors, and MIP-1β prevents the inhibitory activity of MIP-1α.[45]

Stromal-derived factor-1 (SDF-1), a member of the CXC subfamily of chemokines, is produced by stromal cells and is a chemotactic factor for T cells, monocytes and $CD34^+$ progenitors. CXCR4 is expressed in normal and AML $CD34^+$ cells, including $CD34^+38^-$.[46] SDF-1/CXCR4 knockout mice die perinatally with virtual absence of hematopoiesis in the bone marrow, indicating the pivotal role of SDF-1/CXCR4 for the establishment of normal hematopoiesis.[47,48] Moreover, SDF-1/CXCR4 interactions are critical for the engraftment of human progenitors in NOD/*scid* mice (see below).

Recently, two new human β-chemokines were isolated.[49] MPIF-1 is homologous to MIP-1α, is chemotactic for resting T-lymphocytes and monocytes, and is a potent suppressor of CFU-Mix and CFU-GM. MPIF-2 exhibits similarity to MCP-3 and MIP-1α. MPIF-2 strongly suppressed the colony formation by normal high proliferative potential colony-forming cells (HPP-CFC), which represent a multipotential hematopoietic progenitor. The inhibitory effect of MPIF-1 and -2 on normal stem cells suggests that these novel chemokines may protect hematopoietic progenitors from the cytotoxic effects of chemotherapeutic drugs.

3. LEUKEMIC/STROMAL CELL INTERACTIONS IN AML

Growth and differentiation of most types of hematopoietic cells *in vivo* requires direct contact with stromal cells.[50] However, the molecular mechanisms of the interaction between stromal and hematopoietic cells are not fully defined. It has been shown that stromal cells produce a variety of growth factors, and in some cellular systems, that direct cell-cell contact is needed for cell growth and differentiation to occur.[51] Furthermore, β1 and β2 integrins[52] as well as adhesion receptors CD31[53] and c-kit[54] were shown to be involved in the homing of leukemic cells to the bone marrow niches.

Since leukemic cells originate from their normal counterparts and reside within the bone marrow microenvironment, it is likely that stromal cells influence the proliferation and apoptosis of leukemic cells. Studies have suggested that stromal cells can prevent serum-deprivation-induced and chemotherapy-induced apoptosis of leukemic cells *in vitro*.[51,55] In a prospective study of 70 childhood B-ALL cases, the high recovery of ALL blasts in stroma-supported cultures was noted to predict a lower 4-year event-free survival rate (50% vs. 91%).[56] This study further suggested that protective signals within the stromal microenvironment maintain residual leukemic cells, which eventually results in recurrence of the disease. Our experiments demonstrated that anti-apoptotic Bcl-2 expression was consistently higher in Ara-C-exposed AML cells growing *in vitro* in the presence of stromal cells, especially in patients resistant to systemic chemotherapy.[57] This suggests that in a subset of patients, stromal/hematopoietic interactions favor the outgrowth of the leukemic progenitors with high Bcl-2 levels that survive induction chemotherapy and give rise to a relapse. Agents that target Bcl-2, such as ATRA[58] and anti-Bcl-2 oligodeoxynucleotides,[59,60] could therefore be useful adjuncts to currently available chemotherapeutic drugs.

4. STEM CELLS IN AML

4.1 NOD/*scid* Model: A Novel Functional Stem Cell Phenotype

Quantitative analyses of human stem cells have been limited to *in vitro* assays where the proliferative potential of the progenitors is evaluated in the presence of various combinations of cytokines. They include the colony-forming blast (CFU-blast), HPP-CFC assays, and several stromal-based assays, including the long-term culture-initiating cell assay (LTC-IC) and cobblestone-area-forming assays.[61] None of these assays, however, reflects the true properties of human pluripotent stem cells. The best characterized *in vivo* assays have utilized murine model systems. These assays measure the capacity of stem cells to engraft myeloablated recipients and sustain long-term multi-lineage hematopoiesis *in vivo*.

The majority of experiments that allow investigation of human leukemic cell biology were performed in immunodeficient *scid* mutant mice. The murine *scid* mutation interrupts T and B lymphocyte development, thereby allowing mice to accept a variety of xenografts without specific rejection. In limiting dilution experiments, the frequency of leukemia-initiating cells in the peripheral blood of AML patients was 1/250,000 cells.[3] These cells were enriched in the $CD34^{+}38^{-}$ subset. In a recent publication, 61 AML samples of various subtypes were studied in NOD/*scid* mice.[62] The average engraftment was 13% AML cells, with 70% of samples capable of engrafting. Poor prognosis cytogenetics and cytokine-independent CFU-L growth correlated with higher engraftment. The frequency of leukemia "stem cells" as determined by limiting dilution assay varied from 0.7 to $45/10^7$ cells.

Recently, Lapidot *et al.*[63] have demonstrated that CXCR4, the receptor for the SDF-1 chemokine, is critical for the engraftment of normal hematopoietic cells in NOD/*scid* mice, presumably due to the ability of CXCR4-expressing normal progenitors to home to the bone marrow microenvironment. Our preliminary studies in AML indicate relatively low levels of the receptor,[64] which is consistent with the heterogeneity of receptor expression in AML described by Mohle and colleagues.[46] Studies are underway to investigate whether CXCR4/SDF-1 interactions in AML are the determining factors in the engrafting capabilities of *scid*-repopulating leukemic cells.

Wulf *et al.*[4] have recently investigated the penetration of SP cells in AML. SP cells have the intrinsic ability to efflux the fluorescent dye Hoechst 33342. Using molecular cytogenetics and the NOD/*scid* model, Wulf *et al.*[4] reported that clonal leukemic cells are frequent in the SP population in AML. They were also able to grow these cells in the NOD/*scid* model in selected cases. These cells possess intrinsic resistance to certain chemotherapeutic agents (e.g., mitoxantrone), which may be related to over-expression of the ABC transporters MDR1 or BCRP.[65]

In conclusion, the NOD/*scid* model is a valuable tool to elucidate mechanisms of homing and survival of leukemic stem cells. Recognition of the factors influencing the engraftment of leukemia-initiating cells would allow use of the NOD/*scid* AML model for pre-clinical drug testing *in vivo*.

5. SURFACE ANTIGENS AS THERAPEUTIC TARGETS IN AML

5.1 Antibody-targeted Therapy for AML

Since the advent of monoclonal antibody technology, there has been hope to develop a selective approach to killing cancer cells. Studies performed to date have investigated three types of monoclonal antibodies: naked antibody, drug-antibody conjugates, and radiolabeled antibodies. CD33 antigen is an attractive target for AML treatment because it is expressed in the majority of AML cases but not in normal stem cells.[66] Anti-CD33 antibody has rapid access to bone marrow and spleen due to high vascularization.

Several studies have been conducted at Memorial Sloan-Kettering Cancer Center, first using murine antibody[67] and then humanized M195 antibody[68] reactive with CD33 antigen. In pre-clinical studies, antibody treatment destroyed leukemic clonal cells, restored normal myeloid colonies,[69] and eliminated leukemic cells in a murine HL-60 xenograft model. However, results from clinical trials using unmodified antibody in AML therapy have been disappointing. Despite a decreased in blast count, few CRs were obtained.[68] The likely reason for the failure is the rapid internalization of the antibody and perhaps the inability to elicit an immune response.

In contrast, use of the cold humanized M195 antibody proved to be effective in eliminating minimal residual disease cells in patients with APL. In a study performed at the Memorial Sloan-Kettering Cancer Center, only 1 of 15 APL patients was found to be PCR-negative after ATRA induction and before antibody administration. Following treatment with M195, four more patients became PCR-negative.[70] This suggests that this anti-CD33 antibody may have utility in reducing residual leukemic cells in APL.

The observation that anti-CD33 antibody is rapidly internalized by the target cells led to the development of antibody-targeted chemotherapy consisting of an engineered human anti-CD33 antibody linked with the potent antitumor antibiotic calicheamicin gamma. When internalized, calicheamicin generates an active radical species that binds to DNA and causes double-strand breaks. *In vitro* studies revealed that this conjugate selectively inhibits growth of leukemic cell lines and primary AML clonogenic cells. Furthermore, in a mouse model of the HL-60 xenograft, the conjugate induced complete tumor regression.[71]

In a Phase I dose-escalation trial, 40 patients with relapsed or refractory AML received CMA-676 as a therapeutic agent.[72] 13% of patients achieved CR. Interestingly, response correlated with both antigen saturation and low drug efflux rate. In a Phase II study, 3 of 23 patients in first relapse achieved CR, and in seven patients complete elimination of the leukemic blasts was achieved.[73] Thus, the overall response rate was 43%. In addition, CMA-676 was well tolerated and reportedly less toxic than standard chemotherapy.

Another type of immunoconjugate are radiolabeled antibodies aiming at delivery of high doses of radiation to target organs, such as marrow or spleen. A study in advanced AML was conducted at the Fred Hutchinson Cancer Research Center using ^{131}I-labeled anti-CD33 (p67) antibody. Patients with favorable (predominantly in hematopoietic organs) antibody biodistribution received a therapeutic dose of the antibody combined with cyclophosphamide followed by total body irradiation (TBI) and bone marrow transplantation (BMT).[74] This led to prolonged severe pancytopenia in many patients, due to detrimental effects of unbound antibody on normal stem cells.

To overcome the limitations of ^{131}I-labeled anti-CD33 antibody, investigators at the Memorial Sloan-Kettering Cancer Center used ^{213}bismuth (Bi)-labeled humanized M195 antibody.[75] Unlike ^{131}I, ^{213}Bi emits a high linear energy transfer α-particle with a short path length (5-8 μm) and has a very short plasma elimination half-life (46 minutes). The ^{213}Bi-labeled antibody was evaluated in a Phase I trial in relapsed or refractory AML patients. Decrease in bone marrow and peripheral blood blasts were observed in the majority of patients, with myelosuppression that lasted 8-21 days.

Researchers at the Fred Hutchinson Cancer Research Center conducted clinical trials using ^{131}I-labeled anti-CD45 antibody combined with conventional preparative regimens followed by BMT. CD45 is expressed at very high levels in hematopoietic tissues, and does not internalize after antibody binding. In contrast to TBI, which induces a general effect, the radiolabeled anti-CD45 antibody concentrates irradiation on the hematopoietic organs without significant increase in toxicity as demonstrated in a Phase I trial.[76] In an ongoing Phase II clinical trial in AML patients in first remission who received BMT following a standard busulfan/cyclophosphamide regimen and ^{131}I-labeled anti-CD45, 22 of the 25 are in remission.[71]

In summary, encouraging results were obtained in AML patients using unmodified antibody or immunotoxin- or radionuclide-conjugated antibodies to the commonly expressed antigens. The role of these antibodies in AML therapy is now being carefully investigated in Phase I/II clinical trials.

6. MULTIDRUG RESISTANCE IN AML

6.1 MDR1

One molecular mechanism of pleiotropic drug resistance, typical multidrug resistance (MDR), has been recognized as an independent prognostic factor in AML. The spectrum of drugs affected by this form of resistance typically includes the anthracyclines, vinca alkaloids and epipodophyllotoxins. Multidrug resistance is known to be conferred by two different membrane proteins, the 170-kDa P-glycoprotein (P-gp)[77] and the 190-kDa multidrug resistance-associated protein (MRP).[78] P-gp and MRP belong to the ATP-binding cassette (ABC) superfamily of transport proteins and confer resistance to a similar profile of chemotherapeutic drugs despite low structural similarity. The recently described breast cancer resistance protein (BCRP) is a novel member of the ABC family of transport proteins.[79] Other proteins have been associated with drug resistance *in vitro*, including the p110 lung resistance-related protein, LRP, which was identified as the major vault protein,[80] enzymes in the glutathione (GSH) metabolic pathways,[81] and the DNA topoisomerases.[82]

P-gp is localized at the plasma membrane, can be induced by analogues of anthracyclines *in vitro*, and was shown by us to be over-expressed in *ex vivo* samples from AML patients undergoing chemotherapy.[83] Recent data demonstrate that the MDR phenotype may be acquired as a result of *MDR1* promoter methylation changes.[84]

It is now apparent that P-gp also plays a specific anti-apoptotic function that protects MDR1-expressing cells from cell death.[85,86] Cells expressing P-gp were resistant to Fas-mediated apoptosis and UV irradiation due to decreased production of active caspase-3, but retained sensitivity to caspase-independent cell death mediated by pore-forming proteins and granzyme B. The resistance to Fas-mediated apoptosis can be reversed by P-gp inhibitors. The mechanism of this anti-apoptotic function of P-gp is unknown, but may involve intracellular alkalinization that is reversed by MDR1 modulators.

P-gp has also been found in normal cells, and its physiological functions awaits further elucidation. High expression of MDR1 in the apical surface of secretory epithelial cells (e.g., intestinal, renal, liver) suggests a general protective role in the excretion of xenobiotics, and possibly endogenous metabolites, in these tissues. P-gp is also expressed in normal hematopoietic progenitor cells. The efflux pump was shown to protect rhodamine dull (RhoD) cells from anthracycline toxicity, and the P-gp inhibitor verapamil restored sensitivity to anthracyclines. With this in mind, reinfusion of MDR1 transfected stem cells has been suggested, and was utilized in a clinical Phase I trial at MD Anderson to protect against Taxol myelotoxicity in patients with breast and ovarian cancers. No direct protective effect could be demonstrated, perhaps due to low transduction frequencies, but the clinical results were encouraging nevertheless.[87] However, the development of a myeloproliferative disorder in mice transplanted with expanded MDR1-transduced stem cells suggests that this strategy can have adverse consequences.[88]

MRP can confer a multidrug resistance phenotype that, *in vitro*, is similar to that of P-gp, although there are some differences. For example, MRP confers only low levels of resistance to paclitaxel, colchicine and arsenic.[89] High levels of MRP mRNA have been detected in a variety of tumor cell lines, including leukemias, fibrosarcoma, lung, breast, cervix, prostate, and bladder carcinomas. MRP appears to transport drugs conjugated to GSH and also unmodified cytostatic agents in the presence of GSH.[90]

MDR1 is frequently expressed in AML and is associated with lower CR rate and/or survival.[91,92] An analysis of MDR1 expression in 211 elderly AML patients in a SWOG trial found MDR1 expression in more than 70% of the patients.[91] In this study, MDR1 expression was associated with a significantly poorer CR rate, secondary AML, and unfavorable cytogenetics. Strikingly, *de novo* patients with favorable or intermediate cytogenetics and absence of MDR1 expression had a CR rate of 81%, whereas only 12% of patients with MDR1$^+$ secondary AML and unfavorable cytogenetics achieved CR.

A retrospective study of 352 newly diagnosed younger AML patients confirmed the association between MDR1 expression and both CR rate and resistant disease.[93] In contrast, the expression of the MDR-associated proteins MRP1 or LRP did not correlate with outcome. MRP was found to be expressed in only 10% of AML cases. The absence of correlations between MRP expression and clinical outcome was also reported in other studies.[94,95] In contrast, LRP was expressed in 43% of AML and increased significantly with increasing white count. While no correlation between LRP expression and clinical outcome was found in this study and in the paper by Legrand *et al.*[96], both List *et al.*[97] and Filipits[98] found correlations between LRP expression and a poor outcome. Whether these discrepancies reflect merely the methodologies used (flow cytometry versus immunohistochemistry) or differences in the patient population remains to be seen.

The deletion of a part of one MRP allele has been reported in some cases of FAB M4Eo, reported to be associated with prolonged duration of disease-free survival.[99] It is tempting to speculate that a reduction of MRP may increase the sensitivity to daunomycin, frequently used in AML therapy.

A new stem cell compartment was recently discovered based on the ability of small progenitor/stem cell populations to eliminate the DNA-binding dye Hoechst 33342.[100] These "SP" cells may also have unexpected plasticity and are able to differentiate into cells residing in other organs.[101] Blockade of Hoechst 33342 efflux can be achieved with verapamil and PSC833, suggesting a role for MDR1 and perhaps other ABC transporters in these cells. We have recently demonstrated that AML stem cells can reside in this compartment[4] and that commonly used anti-leukemic agents such as doxorubicin and mitoxantrone are eliminated from SP cells. Sorrentino and co-workers[102] have recently suggested that BCRP over-expression confers the "SP" phenotype. In a recent report, expression of BCRP was found in 4/14 AML patients with resistant leukemia and unfavorable cytogenetics. These studies are ongoing and important, as they have the potential to identify intrinsically drug resistant, functionally defined normal and leukemic stem cells.

6.2 MDR Modulators

Elucidation of the functional role of MDR1 in the resistance of tumor cells has led to the development of a variety of approaches to overcome these protective mechanisms. Modifications of the anthracycline structure or formulation may partially restore the sensitivity of tumor cells to MDR-substrate drugs. Thus, liposome-incapsulated daunorubicin (Daunoxome) appears to be partially protected from P-gp, at least *in vitro*.[103] The new anthracycline, Annamycin, has reduced cardiotoxicity but is more effective in inhibiting the growth of the MDR^+ cells compared to Adriamycin.[104] We are presently conducting a Phase I clinical trial in refractory AML patients.[105]

A variety of MDR inhibitors have been employed, including calcium antagonists, calmodulin inhibitors and cyclosporins.[106] Most of these MDR-reversing agents interfere with drug binding to P-gp, and some of them are the substrates for P-gp-mediated transport. Some MDR modulators, including verapamil, quinidine, cyclosporin A (CsA) and its analog SDZ PSC833,[107] are now in Phase I/II clinical trials. Recently, several new, less toxic P-gp inhibitors have been described, including GF120918,[108] MS-209,[109] dexniguldipine,[110] PAK-104P,[111] RS-33295-198[112] and a novel non-macrocyclic ligand of FKBP12, VX-710.[113]

PSC833 was tested by us in a Phase I study in patients with relapsed/refractory leukemias,[114] in combination with mitoxantrone and etoposide. Mucositis was the dose-limiting toxicity, with no responses being observed.

In a multicenter Phase II clinical trial, 37 patients with refractory or relapsed AML were treated with PSC833 (Valspodar; Novartis) in combination with mitoxantrone, etoposide, and cytarabine (PSC-MEC).[115] Pharmacokinetic (PK) studies showed a 57% decrease in etoposide clearance and a 1.8-fold longer half-life for mitoxantrone. The doses of these drugs were reduced to compensate for these PK changes that correlated with enhanced toxicity. Overall, PSC-MEC was relatively well tolerated in these patients with poor prognosis, with 32% of patients achieving CR and 11% partial response. ECOG is currently testing this regimen versus standard MEC chemotherapy in a Phase III trial. Recent studies suggest that delivery of anticancer drugs using liposomal carriers, may avoid exacerbation of the toxicity of the anticancer drugs by PSC833 co-administration and enhance the therapeutic efficacy in resistant tumors when combined with PSC833.[116]

Encouraging results were obtained in a randomized trial in high-risk AML patients who received the MDR1 modulator cyclosporine A.[117] Both overall survival (OS) and relapse-free survival (RFS) were significantly better: 3-year

OS was 22% among CsA-treated patients compared with 6% among the control group, while RFS was at 43% compared with 10%.

Alternative approaches were developed to directly influence *MDR1* expression levels, including anti-*MDR1* hammerhead ribozymes.[118] Retroviral transduction of *MDR1*-expressing leukemia cell lines decreased the expression of *MDR1*, P-gp and drug efflux and restored sensitivity to vincristine. *MDR1* antisense oligonucleotides decreased the percentage of AML blasts expressing P-gp and significantly increased chemosensitivity to Daunorubicin[119], suggesting the validity of this approach to overcoming multidrug resistance in leukemia.

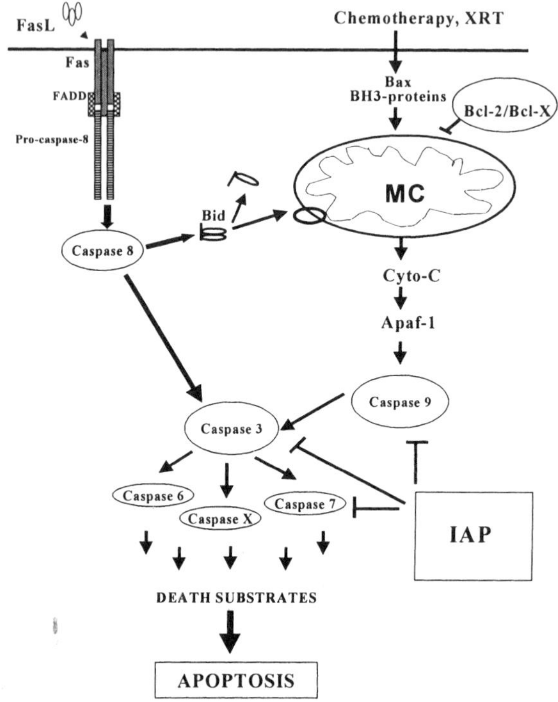

Figure 1. The apoptotic cascade.

7. APOPTOSIS

The last few years have seen a dramatic increase in our knowledge of apoptotic pathways. Apoptosis is a genetically determined process that is evolutionarily conserved from yeast to the nematode C. elegans and to mammalian cells. The apoptotic cascade can be divided into several stages

(Figure 1). First, multiple signaling pathways lead from death-triggering extracellular or intracellular agents to a central control and an execution stage.

In this stage, the activation of CED3/caspases occurs, which leads to the acquisition of the apoptotic phenotype. Two regulatory pathways have been elucidated. The death receptor pathway, triggered by members of the tumor necrosis factor (TNF) family, is mediated by recruitment of the proximal regulator caspase 8 to the death receptor complex. The activated initiator caspases in turn activate the effector caspases 3, 6 and 7. The mitochondrial apoptotic pathway is controlled by the release of cytochrome c from the mitochondria and the subsequent activation of Apaf-1, caspase 9 and the cleavage of the effector caspases. In a clinical context, these shared pathways provide an explanation for the frequently observed resistance of tumors to multiple drugs and even to different treatment modalities. A hallmark of all apoptotic pathways is the extensive interaction between pro- and anti-apoptotic proteins.[120,121]

7.1 Role of Apoptosis Regulators in AML

The Fas ligand (FasL, CD95) is a type II membrane protein that is predominantly expressed in activated T cells. Fas/FasL can be induced by many cytotoxic drugs, and it has been postulated to be one of the mechanisms by which anticancer drugs kill cells.[122] Resistance to chemotherapy was associated with downregulation of CD95.[123] Downstream regulatory factors can suppress Fas/FasL death signaling, including FLIP (for FLICE-inhibitory proteins), toso, and FAIM (Fas inhibitory molecule). However, in two separate reports, Fas-resistant Jurkat and 8226 cells were equally susceptible to anticancer drugs that activated caspase 8 and caspase 3.[124,125]

Numerous studies have evaluated the expression of Fas or FasL in normal and malignant hematopoiesis and the sensitivity of the cells to FasL. In primary AML samples, FAB-M1 cases had lower Fas expression compared to M2, 4, and 5 cases.[126] The induction of apoptosis by the anti-Fas antibody[126] or by FasL[127] was reported. However, Fas ligation in AML resulted in apoptosis of only a few leukemic cells, supporting the notion of impaired Fas signaling in AML.

TRAIL ("TNF-related apoptosis inducing ligand" or APO2-L)[128] is a molecule that binds to a different family of death-inducing receptors DR3, DR4, DR5, and DR6. Subsequently, non-signaling decoy receptors that lack functional death domains (DcR1, DcR2) were identified in normal human tissues, but not in most cancer cell lines examined. Their recognition of TRAIL may prevent TRAIL from binding to functional TRAIL receptors, thereby blocking and not transducing the cell death signal. At this time, the definitive role of TRAIL in apoptosis remains to be determined, since the presence of "decoy" TRAIL receptors does not correspond to resistance to TRAIL-mediated apoptosis in some systems.[129] The fact that DR4 and DR5 are expressed in many tumors while DcR1 and DcR2 are expressed predominantly in normal tissues suggests that TRAIL can differentially induce apoptosis in tumor cells, but exceptions to this paradigm have already been observed.

Discovery of the apoptosis-inducing ligands Fas and TRAIL has created great interest in the potential efficacy of administering exogenous versions of either for the treatment of various tumor types, including hematological malignancies. The enthusiasm for the clinical use of Fas as a target was dampened, however, by the observation that anti-FAS antibody leads to the rapid death of mice from fulminant hepatic toxicity.[130] As a consequence, no trials in humans are underway. TRAIL has also been evaluated as a possible therapeutic agent and appears to have more promise than Fas. We reported that recombinant soluble TRAIL induced significant apoptosis in 4 of 10 myeloid and 4 of 11 lymphoid cell lines, but >25% decrease in viability was observed in only 4 of 22 samples from patients with hematological malignancies.[131] Taken together, these results suggest that TRAIL and FasL have only limited capacity of inducing apoptosis in AML and are consistent with the Weissman model implicating dysfunctional Fas in the pathogenesis of AML.

Apoptosis normally eliminates cells with damaged DNA or an aberrant cell cycle, that is, those most likely to undergo neoplastic transformation. With the discovery of the anti-apoptotic function of Bcl-2, the concept emerged that inhibition of apoptosis represents a central step in tumorigenesis. The oncogenic function of the Bcl-2 over-expressing translocation t(14;18), found in most follicular lymphomas, was verified in Bcl-2-transgenic mice.[132] In this model, deregulated expression of Bcl-2 coupled to additional mutations such as enforced expression of c-Myc can rapidly lead to the transformation of cells of the B lymphoid lineage. Fifteen percent of Fas-deficient mice constitutively expressing Bcl-2 in myeloid cells develop a myeloproliferative disease similar to human AML (FAB M2).[133] This *in vivo* murine model suggests that deregulated expression of Bcl-2 and loss of Fas function may be crucial events in a transformation resulting in myeloid leukemias. Although Bcl-2 levels can become elevated as a result of the t(14;18) translocations, high levels of Bcl-2 protein expression were documented in the vast majority of AML cases without any structural alterations in the Bcl-2 gene.

Cell-cycle inhibitory effects of Bcl-2 may have evolved to reduce the oncogenic potential of Bcl-2. An inverse correlation between Bcl-2 expression and proliferative activity was found in non-Hodgkin's lymphomas, colon carcinomas, and breast cancer. The inhibitory effect of Bcl-2 on entry into the cell cycle ($G_0 \rightarrow G_1$) may contribute to the indolent nature of hematopoietic malignancies associated with Bcl-2 over-expression. Likewise, patients with "poor prognosis" AML defined by certain cytogenetic abnormalities had significantly extended survival when high levels of Bcl-2 were found at diagnosis.[134] Delayed cell cycle entry could result in longer times to relapse. However, the opposite was true for AML with "good prognosis" cytogenetics. Since most chemotherapeutic drugs target dividing cells, malignant cells expressing Bcl-2 are "doubly" protected: they are refractory to apoptosis and more likely to be quiescent.[135]

Far less is known about the expression of other members of the bcl-2 family in AML. Elevated expression of Mcl-1 was found at the time of leukemic relapse in AML and ALL.[136] Caspases 2 and 3 were found to be prognostic factors in AML.[137]

A new family of proteins known as IAPs (Inhibitors of Apoptosis Proteins) was identified through their homology with the baculovirus IAP gene. Several human cellular homologs have been isolated recently: IAP-1, IAP-2, NAIP (neuronal apoptosis inhibitory protein), XIAP (X-linked protein) and survivin. IAPs directly inhibit caspase-3 and caspase-7, which are involved in the distal portion of the protease cascade of apoptosis. Therefore, IAPs may confer resistance to tumor cells independently from the regulatory control of the more "upstream" survival proteins Bcl-2 and Bcl-X_L.

Survivin, the smallest IAP, is expressed in fetal but not in adult differentiated tissue. In contrast, it is present in most common human cancers of lung, colon, breast, pancreas and prostate and found frequently in high-grade but not in low-grade non-Hodgkin lymphomas. Moreover, high levels of survivin are associated with an inferior clinical outcome in patients with neuroblastoma, colon cancer, and gastric cancer.[138–140] Survivin is also involved in cell cycle control. Survivin is the first apoptosis inhibitor selectively expressed in the G_2-M cell cycle phase and directly associates with mitotic spindle microtubules.[141] Therefore, survivin appears to regulate apoptosis during cell proliferation, and over-expression of survivin may favor aberrant progression of cancer cells through mitosis.

One means of regulating apoptosis is through phosphorylation of key regulatory proteins. Growth factor-regulated protein kinase phosphorylation of Bad was proposed as a possible mechanism for growth factor-induced cell survival due to loss of the ability of Bad to heterodimerize with the survival proteins Bcl-2 and Bcl-X_L.[142] It has been shown that phosphorylation of Bad at Ser-136 is mediated by the serine/threonine protein kinase Akt which is downstream of phosphatidylinositol 3-kinase (PI3-K).[143] While phosphorylation at either of two sites of Bad results in loss of function, some data suggest that phosphorylation on Ser-112 is dependent on the activation of the mitogen-activated protein kinase (MAPK) pathway.[144] Hence, survival factors can suppress apoptosis by activating the serine/threonine kinases AKT and MAP-kinase ERK, which then phosphorylate and inactivate components of the apoptotic machinery. The elucidation of the molecular mechanisms of apoptosis may therefore create the basis to manipulate the physiological cell death pathway and to interfere in diseases associated with hyper- or hypo-apoptosis.

7.2 Modulation of Apoptosis as a Strategy in Cancer Treatment

Although the precise contribution of apoptotic pathways to the pathophysiology and the resistance to drugs and radiation in many human tumors remains to be defined, major efforts are underway to modulate them. While anti-apoptotic strategies aim at reducing tissue damage in autoimmune diseases, stroke, myocardial infarction and hepatitis, to name a few, mostly by interfering with caspase activation, pro-apoptotic interventions have already been employed in cancer therapy. Because Bcl-2 has been extensively investigated, it has become the target of many attempts to modulate its expression and function. Bcl-2 antisense oligonucleotides[60] are able to induce apoptosis in leukemia cell lines and primary samples, and enhance chemotherapy-induced apoptosis. This approach was already successfully implemented in a recent Phase I study in lymphoma patients.[145] ATRA downregulates Bcl-2 and Bcl-X_L mRNA, phosphorylates Bcl-2 with resulting loss of protective function, and enhances the effect of Ara-C when administrated after, but not before, Ara-C.[58,83] Ribozyme directed against Bcl-2,[146] intracellular anti-Bcl-2 single chain antibody (sFv),[147] Bax and Bcl-X_S inactivate the anti-apoptotic function of Bcl-2. The apoptotic action of 16-residue BH3 peptides provides a new field for pharmacological intervention.[148] Bryostatin, Taxol and the retinoid-analog 4-HPR phosphorylate Bcl-2, but their precise modulation of apoptotic pathways remains to be determined.

IAPs function by blocking caspase activation and may contribute to the chemoresistance of leukemic cells that have escaped the regulatory control of upstream Bcl-2 proteins. Therefore, agents targeting these inhibitory proteins would potentially induce apoptosis in resistant leukemic cells. Finally, interference with the major signaling pathways (Akt, MAPK) utilizing specific kinase inhibitors could exhibit substantial antileukemic activity, in part due to inhibition of Bad phosphorylation. Preliminary data suggest that agents targeting the apoptosis pathways will have antileukemia activity; however, they may exert maximal effect only in combination with each other and with already established chemotherapeutics.

REFERENCES

1. Bennett JM, Catovsky D, Daniel MT, *et al.* Proposals for the classification of the acute leukemias. French-American-British (FAB) co-operative group. Br J Haematol, 33:451-458, 1976.
2. Heaney ML, Golde DW. Critical evaluation of the World Health Organization classification of myelodysplasia and acute myeloid leukemia. Curr Oncol Rep, 2:140-143, 2000.
3. Bonnet D, Dick JE. Human acute myeloid leukemia is organized as a hierarchy that originates from a primitive hematopoietic cell. Nature Med, 3:730-737, 1997.
4. Wulf GG, Wang RY, Kuehnle I, *et al.* A leukemic stem cell with intrinsic drug efflux capacity in acute myeloid leukemia. Blood, 98:1166-1173, 2001.
5. Gilliland DG. Molecular genetics of human leukemia. Leukemia, 12:S7-12, 1998.
6. Warrell RP Jr, Frankel SR, Miller WH Jr, *et al.* Differentiation therapy of acute promyelocytic leukemia with tretinoin (all-trans-retinoic acid). N Engl J Med, 324:1385-1393, 1991.
7. Hayakawa F, Towatari M, Iida H, *et al.* Differential constitutive activation between STAT-related proteins and MAP kinase in primary acute myelogenous leukaemia. Br J Haematol, 101:521-528, 1998.
8. Biethahn S, Alves F, Wilde S, *et al.* Expression of granulocyte colony-stimulating factor- and granulocyte-macrophage colony-stimulating factor-associated signal transduction proteins of the JAK/STAT pathway in normal granulopoiesis and in blast cells of acute myelogenous leukemia. Exp Hematol, 27:885-894, 1999.
9. Kim SC, Hahn JS, Min YH, *et al.* Constitutive activation of extracellular signal-regulated kinase in human acute leukemias: combined role of activation of MEK, hyperexpression of extracellular signal-regulated kinase, and downregulation of a phosphatase, PAC1. Blood, 93:3893-3899, 1999.
10. Milella M, Kornblau SM, Estrov Z, *et al.* Therapeutic targeting of the MEK/MAPK signal transduction module in acute myeloid leukemia. J Clin Invest, 108:851-859, 2001.
11. Delwel R, Salem M, Pellens C, *et al.* Growth regulation of human acute myeloid leukemia: effects of five recombinant hematopoietic factors in a serum-free culture system. Blood, 72:1944-1949, 1988.
12. Park LS, Waldron PE, Friend D, *et al.* Interleukin-3, GM-CSF, and G-CSF receptor expression on cell lines and primary leukemia cells: receptor heterogeneity and relationship to growth factor responsiveness. Blood, 74:56-65, 1989.
13. White SM, Ball ED, Ehmann WC, *et al.* Increased expression of the differentiation-defective granulocyte colony-stimulating factor receptor mRNA isoform in acute myelogenous leukemia. Leukemia, 12:899-906, 1998.
14. Pietsch T, Kyas U, Steffens U, *et al.* Effects of human stem cell factor (c-kit ligand) on proliferation of myeloid leukemia cells: heterogeneity in response and synergy with other hematopoietic growth factors. Blood, 80:1199-1206, 1992.
15. Piacibello W, Fubini L, Sanavio F, *et al.* Effects of human FLT3 ligand on myeloid leukemia cell growth: heterogeneity in response and synergy with other hematopoietic growth factors. Blood, 86:4105-4114, 1995.
16. Lisovsky M, Estrov Z, Zhang X, *et al.* Flt3 ligand stimulates proliferation and inhibits apoptosis of acute myeloid leukemia cells: regulation of Bcl-2 and Bax. Blood, 88:3987-3997, 1996.
17. Muroi K, Amemiya Y, Miura Y. Specificity of CD117 expression in the diagnosis of acute myeloid leukemia. Leukemia, 10:1048,1996.

18. Di Noto R, Lo PC, Schiavone EM, *et al.* Stem cell factor receptor (c-kit, CD117) is expressed on blast cells from most immature types of acute myeloid mallignancies but is also a characteristic of a subset of acute promyelocytic leukaemia. Br J Haematol, 92:562-564, 1996.
19. Birg F, Courcoul M, Rosnet O, *et al.* Expression of the FMS/KIT-like gene FLT3 in human acute leukemias of the myeloid and lymphoid lineages. Blood, 80:2584-2593, 1992.
20. Carow CE, Levenstein M, Kaufmann SH, *et al.* Expression of the hematopoietic growth factor receptor FLT3 (STK-1/Flk2) in human leukemias. Blood, 87:1089-1096, 1996.
21. Yokota S, Kiyoi H, Nakao M, *et al.* Internal tandem duplication of the FLT3 gene is preferentially seen in acute myeloid leukemia and myelodysplastic syndrome among various hematological malignancies. A study on a large series of patients and cell lines. Leukemia, 11:1605-1609, 1997.
22. Cioffi JA, Shafer AW, Zupancic TJ, *et al.* Novel B219/OB receptor isoforms: possible role of leptin in hematopoiesis and reproduction. Nature Med, 2:585-589, 1996.
23. Tartaglia LA, Dembski M, Weng X, *et al.* Identification and expression cloning of a leptin receptor, OB-R. Cell, 83:1263-1271, 1995.
24. Konopleva M, Mikhail A, Estrov Z, *et al.* Expression and function of leptin receptor isoforms in myeloid leukemia and myelodysplastic syndromes: proliferative and anti-apoptotic activities. Blood, 93:1668-1676, 1999.
25. Estey E, Thall P, Kantarjian H, *et al.* Association between increased body mass index and a diagnosis of acute promyelocytic leukemia in patients with acute myeloid leukemia. Leukemia, 11:1661-1664, 1997.
26. Bennett BD, Solar GP, Yuan JQ, *et al.* A role for leptin and its cognate receptor in hematopoiesis. Curr Biol, 6:1170-1180, 1996.
27. Laharrague P, Larrouy D, Fontanilles AM, *et al.* High expression of leptin by human bone marrow adipocytes in primary culture. FASEB J, 12:747-752, 1998.
28. Griffin JD, Young D, Herrmann F, *et al.* Effects of recombinant human GM-CSF on proliferation of clonogenic cells in acute myeloblastic leukemia. Blood, 67:1448-1453, 1986.
29. Bettelheim P, Valent P, Andreeff M, *et al.* Recombinant human granulocyte-macrophage colony-stimulating factor in combination with standard induction chemotherapy in de novo acute myeloid leukemia. Blood, 77:700-711, 1991.
30. Buchner T, Hiddemann W, Wormann B, *et al.* The role of GM-CSF in the treatment of acute myeloid leukemia. Leukemia Lymph, 11:21-24, 1993.
31. Estey EH, Thall PF, Pierce S, *et al.* Randomized phase II study of fludarabine + cytosine arabinoside + idarubicin +/- all-trans retinoic acid +/- granulocyte colony-stimulating factor in poor prognosis newly diagnosed acute myeloid leukemia and myelodysplastic syndrome. Blood, 93:2478-2484, 1999.
32. Estey E, Thall PF, Kantarjian H, *et al.* Treatment of newly diagnosed acute myelogenous leukemia with granulocyte-macrophage colony-stimulating factor (GM-CSF) before and during continuous-infusion high-dose ara-C + daunorubicin: comparison to patients treated without GM-CSF. Blood, 79:2246-2255, 1992.
33. Bai A, Kojima H, Hori M, *et al.* Priming with G-CSF effectively enhances low-dose Ara-C-induced in vivo apoptosis in myeloid leukemia cells. Exp Hematol, 27:259-265, 1999.
34. Fong GH, Rossant J, Gertsenstein M, *et al.* Role of the Flt-1 receptor tyrosine kinase in regulating the assembly of vascular endothelium. Nature, 376:66-70, 1995.
35. Fiedler W, Graeven U, Ergun S, *et al.* Vascular endothelial growth factor, a possible paracrine growth factor in human acute myeloid leukemia. Blood, 89:1870-1875, 1997.

36. Shalaby F, Rossant J, Yamaguchi TP, *et al.* Failure of blood-island formation and vasculogenesis in Flk-1-deficient mice. Nature, 376:62-66, 1995.
37. Shalaby F, Ho J, Stanford WL, *et al.* A requirement for Flk1 in primitive and definitive hematopoiesis and vasculogenesis. Cell, 89:981-990, 1997.
38. Kennedy M, Firpo M, Choi K, *et al.* A common precursor for primitive erythropoiesis and definitive haematopoiesis. Nature, 386:488-493, 1997.
39. Ziegler BL, Valtieri M, Porada GA, *et al.* KDR receptor: a key marker defining hematopoietic stem cells. Science, 285:1553-1558, 1999.
40. Fielder W, Graeven U, Ergun S, *et al.* Expression of FLT4 and its ligand VEGF-C in acute myeloid leukemia. Leukemia, 11:1234-1237, 1997.
41. Ratajczak MZ, Ratajczak J, Machalinski B, *et al.* Role of vascular endothelial growth factor (VEGF) and placenta-derived growth factor (PlGF) in regulating human haemopoietic cell growth. Br J Haematol, 103:969-979, 1998.
42. Perez-Atayde AR, Sallan SE, Tedrow U, *et al.* Spectrum of tumor angiogenesis in the bone marrow of children with acute lymphoblastic leukemia. Amer J Pathol, 150:815-821, 1997.
43. Aguayo A, Estey E, Kantarjian H, *et al.* Cellular vascular endothelial growth factor is a predictor of outcome in patients with acute myeloid leukemia. Blood, 94:3717-3721, 1999.
44. Campbell JJ, Qin S, Bacon KB, *et al.* Biology of chemokine and classical chemoattractant receptors: differential requirements for adhesion-triggering versus chemotactic responses in lymphoid cells. J Cell Biol, 134:255-266, 1996.
45. Graham GJ, Wright EG, Hewick R, *et al.* Identification and characterization of an inhibitor of haemopoietic stem cell proliferation. Nature, 344:442-444, 1990.
46. Mohle R, Bautz F, Rafii S, *et al.* The chemokine receptor CXCR-4 is expressed on CD34+ hematopoietic progenitors and leukemic cells and mediates transendothelial migration induced by stromal cell-derived factor-1. Blood, 91:4523-4530, 1998.
47. Nagasawa T, Hirota S, Tachibana K, *et al.* Defects of B-cell lymphopoiesis and bone-marrow myelopoiesis in mice lacking the CXC chemokine PBSF/SDF-1. Nature, 382:635-638, 1996.
48. Ma Q, Jones D, Borghesani PR, *et al.* Impaired B-lymphopoiesis, myelopoiesis, and derailed cerebellar neuron migration in CXCR4- and SDF-1-deficient mice. Proc Natl Acad Sci USA, 95:9448-9453, 1998.
49. Patel VP, Kreider BL, Li Y, *et al.* Molecular and functional characterization of two novel human C-C chemokines as inhibitors of two distinct classes of myeloid progenitors. J Exp Med, 185:1163-1172, 1997.
50. Dexter TM. Regulation of hemopoietic cell growth and development: experimental and clinical studies. Leukemia, 7:469-474, 1989.
51. Bendall LJ, Daniel A, Kortlepel K, *et al.* Bone marrow adherent layers inhibit apoptosis of acute myeloid leukemia cells. Exp Hematol, 22:1252-1260, 1994.
52. Bendall LJ, Kortlepel K, Gottlieb DJ. Human acute myeloid leukemia cells bind to bone marrow stroma via a combination of beta-1 and beta-2 integrin mechanisms. Blood, 82:3125-3132, 1993.
53. Tanaka Y, Albelda SM, Horgan KJ, *et al.* CD31 expressed on distinctive T cell subsets is a preferential amplifier of beta 1 integrin-mediated adhesion. J Exp Med, 176:245-253, 1992.
54. Kinashi T, Springer TA. Steel factor and c-kit regulate cell-matrix adhesion. Blood, 83:1033-1038, 1994.
55. Manabe A, Coustan-Smith E, Behm FG, *et al.* Bone marrow-derived stromal cells prevent apoptotic cell death in B-lineage acute lymphoblastic leukemia. Blood, 79:2370-2377, 1992.

56. Kumagai M, Manabe A, Pui CH, *et al.* Stroma-supported culture in childhood B-lineage acute lymphoblastic leukemia cells predicts treatment outcome. J Clin Invest, 97:755-760, 1996.
57. Konopleva M, Konoplev S, Hu W, *et al.* Stroma cells prevent apoptosis of AML cells by upregulation of anti-apoptotic proteins. Leukemia, In Press, 2002.
58. Hu ZB, Minden MD, McCulloch EA. Phosphorylation of BCL-2 after exposure of human leukemic cells to retinoic acid. Blood, 92:1768-1775, 1998.
59. Campos L, Sabido O, Rouault JP, *et al.* Effects of BCL-2 antisense oligodeoxynucleotides on in vitro proliferation and survival of normal marrow progenitors and leukemic cells. Blood, 84:595-600, 1994.
60. Konopleva M, Tari A, Estrov Z, *et al.* Liposomal Bcl-2 antisense oligonucleotides enhance proliferation, sensitize AML to cytosine-arabinoside, and induce apoptosis independent of other anti-apoptotic proteins. Blood, 95:3929-3938, 2000.
61. McNiece IK, Stewart FM, Deacon DM, *et al.* Detection of a human CFC with a high proliferative potential. Blood, 74:609-612, 1989.
62. Ailles LE, Gerhard B, Kawagoe H, *et al.* Growth characteristics of acute myelogenous leukemia progenitors that initiate malignant hematopoiesis in nonobese diabetic/severe combined immunodeficient mice. Blood, 94:1761-1772, 1999.
63. Peled A, Petit I, Kollet O, *et al.* Dependence of human stem cell engraftment and repopulation of NOD/SCID mice on CXCR4. Science, 283:845-848, 1999.
64. Konopleva M, Monaco G, Zhao S, *et al.* Engraftment potential of AML progenitors into NOD/*scid* mice is dependent on baseline CXCR4 expression. Blood, 94:165b, 1999.
65. Zhou S, Schuetz JD, Bunting KD, *et al.* The ABC transporter Bcrp1/ABCG2 is expressed in a wide variety of stem cells and is a molecular determinant of the side-population phenotype. Nature Med, 7:1028-1034, 2001.
66. Matthews DC. Immunotherapy in acute myelogenous leukemia and myelodysplastic syndrome. Leukemia, 12:S33, 1998.
67. Multani PS, Grossbard ML. Monoclonal antibody-based therapies for hematologic malignancies. J Clin Oncol, 16:3691-3710, 1998.
68. Caron PC, Dumont L, Scheinberg DA. Supersaturating infusional humanized anti-CD33 monoclonal antibody HuM195 in myelogenous leukemia. Clin Cancer Res, 4:1421-1428, 1998.
69. Bernstein ID, Singer JW, Andrews RG, *et al.* Treatment of acute myeloid leukemia cells in vitro with a monoclonal antibody recognizing a myeloid differentiation antigen allows normal progenitor cells to be expressed. J Clin Invest, 79:1153-1159, 1987.
70. Jurcic JG, DeBlasio A, Dumont L, *et al.* Molecular remission induction without relapse after anti-CD33 monoclonal antibody HuM195 in acute promyelocytic leukemia. Blood, 90:416a, 1997.
71. Appelbaum FR. Antibody-targeted therapy for myeloid leukemia. Semin Hematol, 36:2-8, 1999.
72. Sievers EL, Appelbaum FR, Spielberger RT, *et al.* Selective ablation of acute myeloid leukemia using antibody-targeted chemotherapy: a phase I study of an anti-CD33 calicheamicin immunoconjugate. Blood, 93:3678-3684, 1999.
73. Sievers E, Larson RA, Estey E, *et al.* Interim analysis of the efficacy and safety of CMA-676 in patients with AML in first relapse. Blood, 96:613a, 1998.
74. Wilder RB, DeNardo GL, DeNardo SJ. Radioimmunotherapy: recent results and future directions. J Clin Oncol, 14:1383-1400, 1996.
75. Jurcic JG, McDevitt MR, Sgouros G, *et al.* Targeted alpha-particle therapy for myeloid leukemias: A phase I trial of bismuth-21-HuM195 (anti-CD33). Blood, 90:504a, 1997.

76. Mathews DC, Appelbaum FR, Eary JF, *et al.* Phase I study of 131I-anti-CD45 antibody plus cyclophosphamide and total body irradiation for advanced acute leukemias and myelodysplastic syndrome. Blood, 90:417a, 1997.
77. Gros P, Ben Neriah YB, Croop JM, *et al.* Isolation and expression of a complementary DNA that confers multidrug resistance. Nature, 323:728-731, 1986.
78. Cole SP, Bhardwaj G, Gerlach JH, *et al.* Overexpression of a transporter gene in a multidrug-resistant human lung cancer cell line. Science, 258:1650-1654, 1992.
79. Doyle LA, Yang W, Abruzzo LV, *et al.* A multidrug resistance transporter from human MCF-7 breast cancer cells. Proc Natl Acad Sci USA, 95:15665-15670, 1998.
80. Scheffer GL, Wijngaard PL, Flens MJ, *et al.* The drug resistance-related protein LRP is the human major vault protein. Nature Med, 1:578-582, 1995.
81. O'Brien ML, Tew KD. Glutathione and related enzymes in multidrug resistance. Eur J Cancer, 32A:967-978, 1996.
82. Nitiss JL, Beck WT. Antitopoisomerase drug action and resistance. Eur J Cancer, 32A:958-966, 1996.
83. Andreeff M, Jiang S, Zhang X, *et al.* Expression of bcl-2-related genes in normal and AML progenitors: Changes induced by chemotherapy and retinoic acid. Leukemia, 13:1881-1892, 1999.
84. Kantharidis P, El Osta A, deSilva M, *et al.* Altered methylation of the human MDR1 promoter is associated with acquired multidrug resistance. Clin Cancer Res, 3:2025-2032, 1997.
85. Smyth MJ, Krasovskis E, Sutton VR, *et al.* The drug efflux protein, P-glycoprotein, additionally protects drug-resistant tumor cells from multiple forms of caspase-dependent apoptosis. Proc Natl Acad Sci USA, 95:7024-7029, 1998.
86. Johnstone RW, Cretney E, Smyth MJ. P-glycoprotein protects leukemia cells against caspase-dependent, but not caspase-independent, cell death. Blood, 93:1075-1085, 1999.
87. Rahman Z, Kavanagh J, Champlin R, *et al.* Chemotherapy immediately following autologous stem-cell transplantation in patients with advanced breast cancer. Clin Cancer Res, 4:2717-2721, 1998.
88. Bunting KD, Galipeau J, Topham D, *et al.* Transduction of murine bone marrow cells with an MDR1 vector enables ex vivo stem cell expansion, but these expanded grafts cause a myeloproliferative syndrome in transplanted mice. Blood, 92:2269-2279, 1998.
89. Cole SP, Sparks KE, Fraser K, *et al.* Pharmacological characterization of multidrug resistant MRP-transfected human tumor cells. Cancer Res, 54:5902-5910, 1994.
90. Loe DW, Almquist KC, Deeley RG, *et al.* Multidrug resistance protein (MRP)-mediated transport of leukotriene C4 and chemotherapeutic agents in membrane vesicles. Demonstration of glutathione-dependent vincristine transport. J Biol Chem, 271:9675-9682, 1996.
91. Leith CP, Kopecky KJ, Godwin J, *et al.* Acute myeloid leukemia in the elderly: assessment of multidrug resistance (MDR1) and cytogenetics distinguishes biologic subgroups with remarkably distinct responses to standard chemotherapy. A Southwest Oncology Group study. Blood, 89:3323-3329, 1997.
92. Campos L, Guyotat D, Archimbaud E, *et al.* Clinical significance of multidrug resistance P-glycoprotein expression on acute nonlymphoblastic leukemia cells at diagnosis. Blood, 79:473-476, 1992.
93. Leith CP, Kopecky KJ, Chen IM, *et al.* Frequency and clinical significance of the expression of the multidrug resistance proteins MDR1/P-glycoprotein, MRP1, and LRP in acute myeloid leukemia: a Southwest Oncology Group study. Blood, 94:1086-1099, 1999.

94. Filipits M, Suchomel RW, Zochbauer S, *et al.* Multidrug resistance-associated protein in acute myeloid leukemia: No impact on treatment outcome. Clin Cancer Res, 3:1419-1425, 1997.
95. Ross DD, Doyle LA, Schiffer CA, *et al.* Expression of multidrug resistance-associated protein (MRP) mRNA in blast cells from acute myeloid leukemia (AML) patients. Leukemia, 10:48-55, 1996.
96. Legrand O, Simonin G, Perrot JY, *et al.* Pgp and MRP activities using calcein-AM are prognostic factors in adult acute myeloid leukemia patients. Blood, 91:4480-4488, 1998.
97. List AF, Spier CS, Grogan TM, *et al.* Overexpression of the major vault transporter protein lung-resistance protein predicts treatment outcome in acute myeloid leukemia. Blood, 87:2464-2469, 1996.
98. Filipits M, Pohl G, Stranzl T, *et al.* Expression of the lung resistance protein predicts poor outcome in de novo acute myeloid leukemia. Blood, 91:1508-1513, 1998.
99. Kuss BJ, Deeley RG, Cole SP, *et al.* Deletion of gene for multidrug resistance in acute myeloid leukaemia with inversion in chromosome 16: prognostic implications. Lancet, 343:1531-1534, 1994.
100. Goodell MA, Rosenzweig M, Kim H, *et al.* Dye efflux studies suggest that hematopoietic stem cells expressing low or undetectable levels of CD34 antigen exist in multiple species. Nature Med, 3:1337-1345, 1997.
101. Jackson KA, Mi T, Goodell MA. Hematopoietic potential of stem cells isolated from murine skeletal muscle. Proc Natl Acad Sci USA, 96:14482-14486, 1999.
102. Ross DD, Karp JE, Chen TT, *et al.* Expression of breast cancer resistance protein in blast cells from patients with acute leukemia. Blood, 96:365-368, 2000.
103. Michieli M, Damiani D, Ermacora A, *et al.* Liposome-encapsulated daunorubicin for PGP-related multidrug resistance. Br J Haematol, 106:92-99, 1999.
104. Kolonias D, Podona T, Savaraj N, *et al.* Comparison of annamycin to adriamycin in cardiac and MDR tumor cell systems. Anticancer Res, 19:1277-1283, 1999.
105. Andreeff M, Giles R, Sanchez-Williams G, *et al.* Phase I study of Annamycin: A novel MDR-1 independent anthracycline in relapsed/refractory AML. Blood, 94:225b, 1999.
106. Ford JM. Experimental reversal of P-glycoprotein-mediated multidrug resistance by pharmacological chemosensitisers. Eur J Cancer, 32A:991-1001, 1996.
107. Boesch D, Muller K, Pourtier-Manzanedo A, *et al.* Restoration of daunomycin retention in multidrug-resistant P388 cells by submicromolar concentrations of SDZ PSC 833, a nonimmunosuppressive cyclosporin derivative. Exp Cell Res, 196:26-32, 1991.
108. Hyafil F, Vergely C, Du VP, *et al.* In vitro and in vivo reversal of multidrug resistance by GF120918, an acridonecarboxamide derivative. Cancer Res, 53:4595-4602, 1993.
109. Sato W, Fukazawa N, Nakanishi O, *et al.* Reversal of multidrug resistance by a novel quinoline derivative, MS-209. Cancer Chemother Pharmacol, 35:271-277, 1995.
110. Hofmann J, Gekeler V, Ise W, *et al.* Mechanism of action of dexniguldipine-HCl (B8509-035), a new potent modulator of multidrug resistance. Biochem Pharmacol, 49:603-609, 1995.
111. Shudo N, Mizoguchi T, Kiyosue T, *et al.* Two pyridine analogues with more effective ability to reverse multidrug resistance and with lower calcium channel blocking activity than their dihydropyridine counterparts. Cancer Res, 50:3055-3061, 1990.
112. Slate DL, Bruno NA, Casey SM, *et al.* RS-33295-198: a novel, potent modulator of P-glycoprotein-mediated multidrug resistance. Anticancer Res, 15:811-814, 1995.
113. Germann UA, Shlyakhter D, Mason VS, *et al.* Cellular and biochemical characterization of VX-710 as a chemosensitizer: reversal of P-glycoprotein-mediated multidrug resistance in vitro. Anticancer Drugs, 8:125-140, 1997.

114. Kornblau SM, Estey E, Madden T, *et al.* Phase I study of mitoxantrone plus etoposide with multidrug blockade by SDZ PSC-833 in relapsed or refractory acute myelogenous leukemia. J Clin Oncol, 15:1796-1802, 1997.
115. Advani R, Saba HI, Tallman MS, *et al.* Treatment of refractory and relapsed acute myelogenous leukemia with combination chemotherapy plus the multidrug resistance modulator PSC 833 (Valspodar). Blood, 93:787-795, 1999.
116. Krishna R, Mayer LD. Liposomal doxorubicin circumvents PSC 833-free drug interactions, resulting in effective therapy of multidrug-resistant solid tumors. Cancer Res, 57:5246-5253, 1997.
117. List AF, Kopecky KJ, Willman CL, *et al.* Benefit of cyclosporine (CsA) modulation of anthracycline resistance in high-risk AML: A Southwest Oncology Group (SWOG) study. Blood, 92:321a, 1999.
118. Kobayashi H, Takemura Y, Wang FS, *et al.* Retrovirus-mediated transfer of anti-MDR1 hammerhead ribozymes into multidrug-resistant human leukemia cells: screening for effective target sites. Int J Cancer, 81:944-950, 1999.
119. Motomura S, Motoji T, Takanashi M, *et al.* Inhibition of P-glycoprotein and recovery of drug sensitivity of human acute leukemic blast cells by multidrug resistance gene (mdr1) antisense oligonucleotides. Blood, 91:3163-3171, 1998.
120. Konopleva M, Andreeff M. Regulatory pathways in programmed cell death. Cancer Mol Biol, 6:1229-1260, 1999.
121. Kornblau S, Konopleva M, Andreeff M. Apoptosis regulating proteins as targets of therapy for hematological malignancies. Expert Opin Invest Drugs, 8:2027-2057, 1999.
122. Friesen C, Herr I, Krammer PH, *et al.* Involvement of the CD95 (APO-1/FAS) receptor/ligand system in drug-induced apoptosis in leukemia cells. Nature Med, 2:574-577, 1996.
123. Friesen C, Fulda S, Debatin KM. Deficient activation of the CD95 (APO-1/Fas) system in drug-resistant cells. Leukemia, 11:1833-1841, 1997.
124. Eischen CM, Kottke TJ, Martins LM, *et al.* Comparison of apoptosis in wild-type and Fas-resistant cells: chemotherapy-induced apoptosis is not dependent on Fas/Fas ligand interactions. Blood, 90:935-943, 1997.
125. Wesselborg S, Engels IH, Rossmann E, *et al.* Anticancer drugs induce caspase-8/FLICE activation and apoptosis in the absence of CD95 receptor/ligand interaction. Blood, 93:3053-3063, 1999.
126. Iijima N, Miyamura K, Itou T, *et al.* Functional expression of Fas (CD95) in acute myeloid leukemia cells in the context of CD34 and CD38 expression: Possible correlation with sensitivity to chemotherapy. Blood, 90:4901-4909, 1997.
127. Snell V, Clodi K, Zhao S, *et al.* Activity of TNF-related apoptosis-inducing ligand (TRAIL) in haematological malignancies. Br J Haematol, 99:618-624, 1997.
128. Golstein P. Cell death: TRAIL and its receptors. Curr Biol, 7:R750-R753, 1997.
129. Griffith TS, Chin WA, Jackson GC, *et al.* Intracellular regulation of TRAIL-induced apoptosis in human melanoma cells. J Immunol, 161:2833-2840, 1998.
130. Ogasawara J, Watanabe-Fukunaga R, Adachi M, *et al.* Lethal effect of the anti-fas antibody in mice. Nature, 364:806-809, 1993.
131. Snell V, Clodi K, Zhao S, *et al.* Activity of TNF-related apoptosis-inducing ligand (TRAIL) in haematological malignancies. Br J Cancer, 99:624,1997.
132. Vaux DL, Cory S, Adams JM. Bcl-2 gene promotes haemopoietic cell survival and cooperates with c-myc to immortalize pre-B cells. Nature, 335:440-442, 1988.
133. Traver D, Akashi K, Weissman IL, *et al.* Mice defective in two apoptosis pathways in the myeloid lineage develop acute myeloblastic leukemia. Immunity, 9:47-57, 1998.

134. Kornblau SM, Thall P, Estrov Z, *et al.* The prognostic impact of bcl2 protein expression in acute myelogenous leukemia varies with cytogenetics. Clin Cancer Res, 5:1758-1766, 1999.
135. Konopleva M, Zhao S, Hu W, *et al.* The antiapoptotic genes Bcl-X_L and Bcl-2 are overexpressed and contribute to chemoresistance of nonproliferating leukemic $CD34^+$ cells. Br J Haematol, In Press, 2002.
136. Kaufmann SH, Karp JE, Svingen PA, *et al.* Elevated expression of the apoptotic regulator Mcl-1 at the time of leukemic relapse. Blood, 91:991-1000, 1998.
137. Estrov Z, Thall PF, Talpaz M, *et al.* Caspase 2 and caspase 3 protein levels as predictors of survival in acute myelogenous leukemia. Blood, 92:3090-3097, 1998.
138. Adida C, Berrebi D, Peuchmaur M, *et al.* Anti-apoptosis gene, survivin, and prognosis of neuroblastoma. Lancet, 351:882-883, 1998.
139. Lu CD, Altieri DC, Tanigawa N. Expression of a novel antiapoptosis gene, survivin, correlated with tumor cell apoptosis and p53 accumulation in gastric carcinomas. Cancer Res, 58:1808-1812, 1998.
140. Kawasaki H, Altieri DC, Lu CD, *et al.* Inhibition of apoptosis by survivin predicts shorter survival rates in colorectal cancer. Cancer Res, 58:5071-5074, 1998.
141. Li F, Ambrosini G, Chu EY, *et al.* Control of apoptosis and mitotic spindle checkpoint by survivin. Nature, 396:580-584, 1998.
142. Zha J, Harada H, Yang E, *et al.* Serine phosphorylation of death agonist BAD in response to survival factor results in binding to 14-3-3 not Bcl-X. Cell, 87:619-628, 1996.
143. del Peso L, Gonzalez-Garcia M, Page C, *et al.* Interleukin-3-induced phosphorylation of BAD through the protein kinase Akt. Science, 278:687-689, 1997.
144. Scheid MP, Duronio V. Dissociation of cytokine-induced phosphorylation of Bad and activation of PKB/akt: involvement of MEK upstream of Bad phosphorylation. Proc Natl Acad Sci USA, 95:7439-7444, 1998.
145. Webb A, Cunningham D, Cotter F, *et al.* BCL-2 antisense therapy in patients with non-Hodgkin lymphoma. Lancet, 349:1137-1141, 1997.
146. Dorai T, Goluboff ET, Olsson CA, *et al.* Development of a hammerhead ribozyme against BCL-2. II. Ribozyme treatment sensitizes hormone-resistant prostate cancer cells to apoptotic agents. Anticancer Res, 17:3307-3312, 1997.
147. Piche A, Grim J, Rancourt C, *et al.* Modulation of Bcl-2 protein levels by an intracellular anti-Bcl-2 single-chain antibody increases drug-induced cytotoxicity in the breast cancer cell line MCF-7. Cancer Res, 58:2134-2140, 1998.
148. Cosulich SC, Worrall V, Hedge PJ, *et al.* Regulation of apoptosis by BH3 domains in a cell-free system. Curr Biol, 7:913-920, 1997.

Chapter 13

BIOCHEMICAL AND MOLECULAR MECHANISMS OF CISPLATIN RESISTANCE

Zahid H. Siddik
Department of Experimental Therapeutics, The University of Texas MD Anderson Cancer Center, Houston, Texas, USA

1. INTRODUCTION

According to the DISCOVERY Anticancer Drug Screen of the National Cancer Institute in the USA, the inorganic antitumor agent cisplatin (*cis*-diammine-dichloro-platinum(II); Figure 1) and its analogs fall into at least 13 clustered regions, each reflecting a distinct mechanism of action[1]. Many of these analogs have not been investigated in depth to unravel their fundamental mechanism of action. Indeed, almost 30 years after its clinical acceptance as a potent antitumor drug, which has dramatically changed the course of treatment of ovarian, testicular and head and neck cancers[2], we are still searching for answers to explain how cisplatin works. There is no doubt, however, that DNA is the primary target of cisplatin[3], but understanding how signals emanating from the damaged DNA are relayed to the apoptotic or cell death machinery is still a subject of much debate. An understanding of this process can be an important step toward defining mechanisms of resistance, which continues to impede the curative use of cisplatin in the clinic. This impediment can be gleaned from the knowledge that in ovarian cancer, for instance, the initial response rate of up to 70% leads to a 5-year survival rate of only 15-20%[4]. Indeed, the majority (80-85%) of patients relapse and fail to respond to further treatment with cisplatin as a result of acquired drug resistance. Similarly, in patients with small cell lung cancer, the relapse rate can be as high as 95%[5].

Knowledge of resistance mechanisms, which are either intrinsic to the tumor or acquired following drug exposure, is also of paramount importance in defining targets for the rational design of analogs. So far, however, analogs of interest have been identified largely through painstaking empirical efforts involving synthesis and screening exercises.

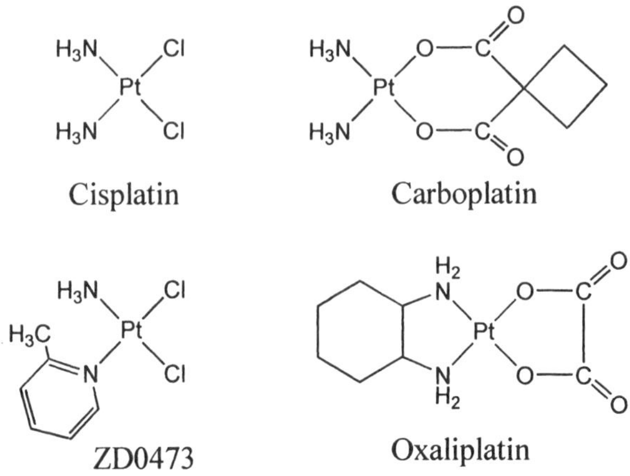

Figure 1. Structure of cisplatin and selected analogs.

These exercises, however, are not necessarily futile. The selection of the clinically active analog carboplatin, for instance, involved an initial examination of over 300 congeners[6]. Although carboplatin represents an important advancement in overcoming the irreversible nephrotoxicity and peripheral neuropathy associated with cisplatin use in patients, it is, however, fully cross-resistant with the parent molecule[7,8]. In the last two decades, greater effort has been devoted to analogs capable of circumventing cisplatin resistance, and a number of them have been introduced into clinical trials with various degrees of success[6]. The 1,2-diaminocyclohexane (DACH) complex oxaliplatin (Figure 1) is fulfilling its potential against specific refractory cancers[9], but the underlying basis for its activity is still to be defined. Indeed, this and other analogs, such as ZD0473[6], are still under active clinical investigations and once resistance to these agents is recognised, defining the associated mechanisms will become important. For this reason, this chapter will focus on mechanisms of resistance induced by cisplatin. However, it is useful to first review our present understanding relating to the mode of action of cisplatin.

2. DNA AS A TARGET OF CISPLATIN ACTION

Cisplatin is a square planar inorganic complex which needs to pass from the extracellular environment through the cell and into the nucleus and then interact with DNA to induce cell cycle arrest and/or cell death. The programmed form of cell death, also referred to as apoptosis, occurs via a series of signal transduction pathways, which are activated as a net effect of the ability of tumor cells to recognise, repair and tolerate the DNA damage. Cell death can also occur through an effect on the cell cycle, and recent data suggest an involvement of the G_2/M phase kinase complex (Cdc2-cyclin A or

B) in this process[10,11]. This is consistent with published reports that abrogation of the G_2/M checkpoint with specific agents can enhance the cytotoxicity of cisplatin[12].

For interaction to occur with DNA, however, the neutral cisplatin has to first transform to an active state. This activation is spontaneous and is caused by sequential aquation reactions involving the replacement of the chloro-ligands of cisplatin with aqua species[13,14]. The chloro-monoaquo form (Figure 2), which carries a single positive charge, has a very short life and is the major 'alkylating' species at physiological pH. In an activated state, cisplatin can also interact non-specifically with many endogenous nucleophilic molecules and macromolecules, such as glutathione (GSH), methionine, metallothionein and protein. Thus, when cisplatin enters cells through a predominantly non-saturable passive diffusion process[14], it is potentially vulnerable to cytoplasmic inactivation by these intracellular components.

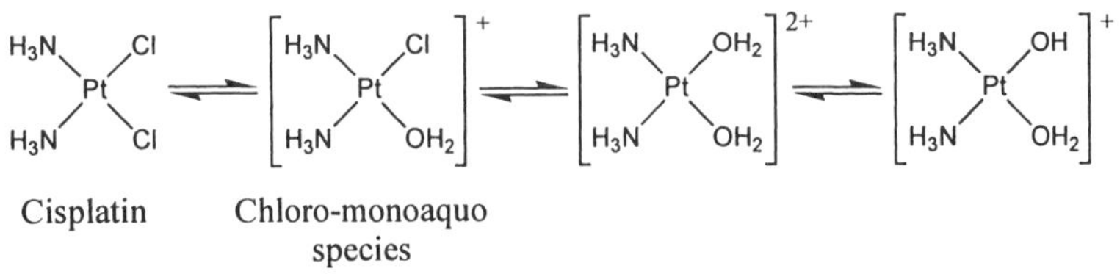

Cisplatin   Chloro-monoaquo species

Figure 2. Formation of the active chloro-monoaquo species following aquation of cisplatin.

It is not known in which chemical form cisplatin enters the nucleus, but once inside, cisplatin can interact with purine bases in DNA in a bifunctional manner to form DNA-DNA cross-links[15]. Although cisplatin can form several types of cross-links (Figure 3), there is uncertainty whether the interstrand (between opposing DNA strands) or intrastrand (on the same DNA strand) crosslinks are the critical cytotoxic lesions[16]. Evidence, however, suggests that intrastrand adducts provide the strongest basis for the cytotoxic action of cisplatin[17]. Interstrand cross-links, on the other hand, have also been directly correlated to cytotoxicity[16] and continue to be of interest. The preponderance of interest in intrastrand cross-links is consistent with the knowledge that 1,2-intrastrand ApG and GpG cross-links account for the bulk (about 85-90%) of total DNA adducts[18]. In contrast, the 1,3-intrastrand GpXpG (X = any nucleotide) cross-links, interstrand G-G cross-links, and monofunctional adducts each make up about 2-6% of the platinum bound to DNA. The ApXpG adduct, on the other hand, is a minor product of cross-link reactions. The high intrastrand:interstrand ratio may be due in part to the reported conversion of the unstable interstrand cross-links to the more stable intrastrand form, with a half-life of about 29 h[19,20]. Similar distribution of adducts has also been reported for the analog DACH-sulfato-platinum(II) in an *in vitro* system[21]. Since cells resistant to cisplatin have only a low level of cross-resistance to this and other similar analogs[22], it follows that the difference in the mode of action between platinum complexes must arise after the formation of analog-specific, structurally-distinct adducts.

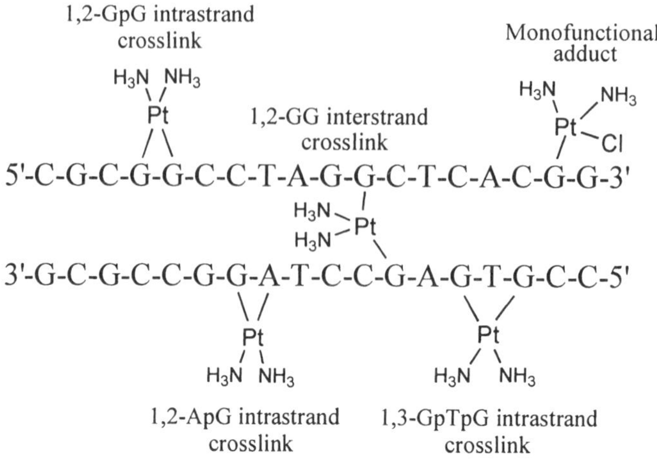

Figure 3. Nature of DNA cross-links induced by cisplatin.

It is widely understood that cross-linked adducts induced by cisplatin disrupt replication and transcriptional processes, but such biological changes do not necessarily correlate directly with cytotoxic effects. Therefore, formation of cross-link lesions should merely be considered as the initial step toward further biological processing, which can involve protecting adducts from repair to activating signal transduction pathways that ultimately lead to cell cycle arrest or apoptosis. To understand this complex process, it is essential to appreciate the effects of cross-links on DNA structure and the role of proteins that recognise DNA damage. Both interstrand and intrastrand cross-links induce local unwinding and bending in the DNA double helix. The ApG, GpG and GpXpG intrastrand adducts unwind DNA by 13-23° and bend the double helix by 32-34°[23]. Interstrand cross-links, on the other hand, induce much greater effects: unwinding of 79° and greater, and bends of 45-47° have been reported[20]. Proteins with damage recognition properties bind to these distortions in the DNA and thereby affect cellular events, such as cell cycle arrest and apoptosis. Damage recognition proteins also may have a role in the nucleotide excision repair (NER) pathway[24]. Over 20 damage recognition proteins have been identified, and there appears to be some specificity for the individual DNA adduct. The mismatch repair (MMR) complex and human upstream binding factor (hUBF) proteins, for instance, bind to DNA adducts of cisplatin with much greater affinity than to those induced by oxaliplatin[25]. Although the high mobility group 1 (HMG1) protein can recognize adducts of both cisplatin and oxaliplatin[26], the relative affinity appears to be greater for adducts of cisplatin[25]. In contrast, the TATA binding protein (TBP) recognises adducts of both platinum agents[25]. It is possible that adducts of oxaliplatin, and perhaps other analogs, may be preferentially recognised by alternative damage recognition proteins, but this needs to be fully investigated. The possibility exists that recognition proteins dictate biological effects and may explain differences in the mode of actions between platinum analogs.

How the damage recognition proteins determine the fate of the cell is not entirely clear. On the one hand, they have been implicated in shielding DNA adducts from repair, and this is consistent with the report that over-expression of HMG1 by estrogen sensitized breast tumor cells to cisplatin and carboplatin[27]. On the other hand, they may have a role in transducing signalling processes, which can include post-translational activation of the tumor suppressor p53[28–30]. When p53 is activated by DNA damaging agents, it can transcriptionally activate DNA in a sequence-specific manner to eventually give rise to proteins such as $p21^{Waf1/Cip1}$ or bax that can facilitate cell cycle arrest or cell death, respectively[31]. That p53 is an important protein in these processes comes from the realisation that about 50% of all cancers have mutated p53, which has lost normal functions[28,32–34]. It is not surprising, therefore, that the presence of mutant p53 in tumors correlates with poor prognosis[35]. However, several reports have demonstrated that cell cycle arrest and cell death can occur in a p53-independent manner[36–39], which is presently not well understood. Indeed, under certain conditions, inactivation of p53 can enhance cytotoxic sensitivity to cisplatin and other selected agents[40,41].

3. MECHANISMS OF CISPLATIN RESISTANCE

Although the level of cisplatin resistance in patients is difficult to define, at least a 2-fold resistance is recognised as inferred from re-induction of responses in some patients by doubling the standard clinical dose of cisplatin[42–44]. Literature data, however, appear to suggest that resistance up to 5 fold can be encountered in patients[45,46]. This is supported by the clinical study of Jodrell *et al.*[47] who indicated that at least a 4-fold resistance can be acquired from the therapeutic use of the cross-resistant analog carboplatin. In practice, it seems that greater levels of resistance likely exist as judged from the high IC_{50}s that have been reported for cisplatin in cell lines established from clinically-refractory tumors[48]. From this study, resistance factors up to 40 to 45 fold can be ascertained for the OVCAR-10 and OVCA-433 human ovarian tumor models when compared to the most sensitive A2780 model, which was drug-naïve at the time of its establishment (Figure 4). Similarly, 86 and 115 fold differences in the IC_{50} have been reported between the most sensitive and the most resistant ovarian tumor model in a panel of human ovarian tumor cell lines[49,50]. It is critical to exercise caution in interpreting these *in vitro* data as comparison of IC_{50} is not necessarily between isogenic cell lines derived from the same patient before and after therapy.

It should be borne in mind that mechanisms of cisplatin resistance have largely been derived from differences between parental tumor cells and variant isogenic lines having cisplatin resistance acquired through intermittent or continuous exposure to progressively increasing concentrations of the drug. However, there is some evidence to indicate that these mechanisms are in concordance with the clinical understanding[5]. Indeed, cell lines established from refractory tumors of a patient following relapse confirm this conjecture[51]. However, it is possible that in few cases the level of resistance derived in model systems may not apply to the clinical situation. The reason for this is inherent in the definition of resistance, which is derived from the ratio of drug concentration that causes 50% reduction in numbers of resistant cells (that is, an IC_{50} concentration) to that causing an equivalent effect in the sensitive line. It is, therefore, possible that drug doses in patients may result in plasma concentrations that may exceed the *in vitro* IC_{50} level, in which case a robust clinical response may be observed even though the tumor has silently acquired resistance with increasing cycles of therapy. Conversely, if the dose is severely limited by side effects, then the plasma concentration achieved will be insufficient to affect the patient's tumor. In this case, no responses will be observed leading to the conclusion that the tumor is drug resistant, although it may appear sensitive if characterised *in vitro*. It is easy to understand, therefore, that tumors could be misclassified as resistant from *in vivo* data, and, if established as a model, could lead to erroneous conclusions on resistance mechanisms and in the selection of novel designer platinum-based therapeutics targeted against the refractory disease.

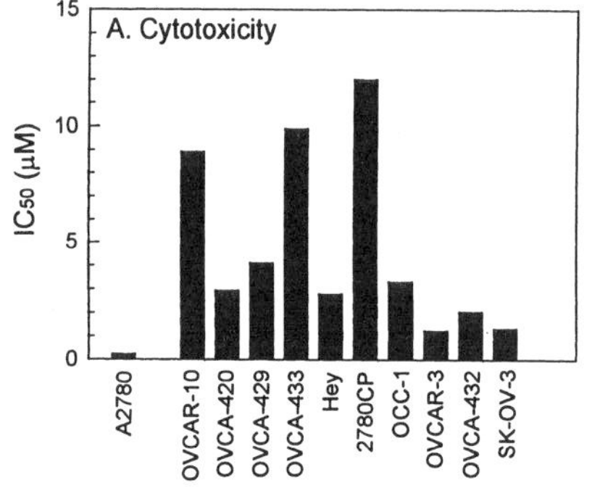

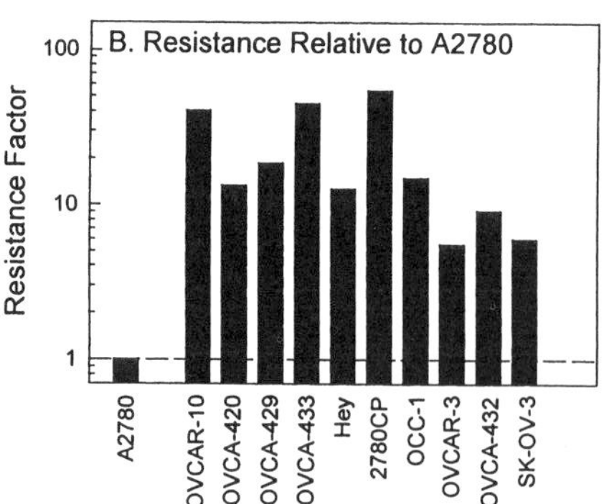

Figure 4. Activity of cisplatin, expressed as the IC_{50} concentration causing 50% cell kill, against a panel of human ovarian tumor models (A) and resistance of tumor models to cisplatin relative to sensitive A2780 cells (B). [Adapted from Siddik *et al.*[134]].

With the knowledge that cytotoxic effects of cisplatin require a complex process from the initial drug entry into cells to the final stages of apoptosis, it follows that any interference of this well orchestrated sequence of events will lead to drug resistance. Thus, resistance mechanisms can arise as a consequence of changes in either the biochemical or molecular process within the cell. A single mechanism of resistance in a cell line is possible[52], but in practice resistance is usually multifactorial[53–55]. Furthermore, the profile of multifactorial resistance varies among cell lines, and some mechanisms may be absent in specific resistant models[18] and expressed in others only when the tumor is grown *in vivo*[56]. Both biochemical and molecular mechanisms may co-exist to give a high net level of resistance[57].

3.1 Biochemical Mechanisms of Resistance

The biochemical aspects of cisplatin resistance relate to drug accumulation, intracellular thiol levels, DNA adduct repair and relative ability to tolerate DNA damage, as depicted in Figure 5. There is already substantial evidence that the level and persistence of adducts will dictate cytotoxic outcome[58], and, therefore, resistance will arise due to changes in the biochemical pharmacology of the agent.

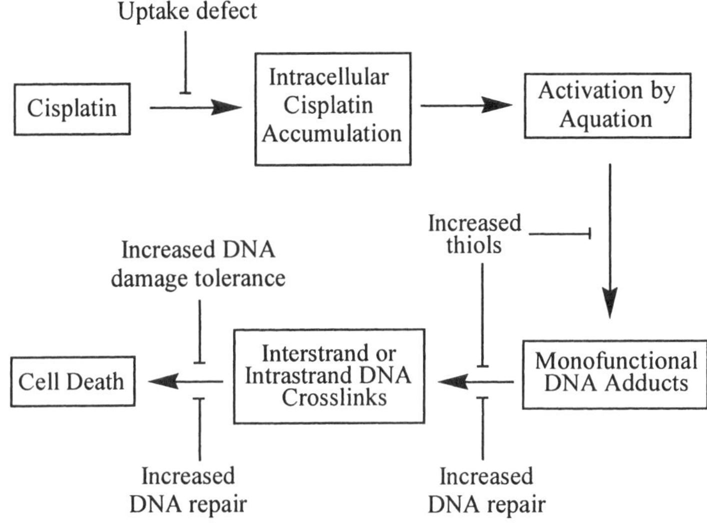

Figure 5. Biochemical pharmacologic reactions of cisplatin leading to cell death and inhibition of the sequence of events by biochemical resistance mechanisms.

3.1.1 Drug accumulation

Many reports point to reduced drug accumulation as a significant mechanism of cisplatin resistance. Reductions in the range 20-70% have been documented in cell lines, which were resistant by a factor of 3-40 fold[18]. Reduction in drug accumulation, however, was not proportional to the level of resistance among a heterogeneous mix of tumor types (Figure 6). This lack of correlation has also been demonstrated in a panel of ovarian tumor cell lines[59]. These data suggest that the mechanism of resistance relating to drug uptake is not present in a fixed proportion to total resistance. Indeed, the resistance profile of a given cell line may not include a defect in drug accumulation as a mechanism[52,60]. It is noteworthy that in cell lines exhibiting diminished intracellular drug accumulation, this is a major mechanism at low levels of drug resistance. Thus, decreases in uptake of ~2-5 fold represents a substantial component of overall resistance in tumors displaying <8-fold resistance (Figure 6). More specifically, in PC-9 non-small cell lung cancer (NSCLC) and 41M ovarian cancer cell lines, the 4- to

5-fold reduction in uptake is very similar to drug resistance factors of 5 to 7 fold, and demonstrates that impairment in cisplatin accumulation can account for 70-90% of the total resistance in these models[18]. With progressive increases in resistance, the contribution of reduced drug uptake to overall resistance becomes less; this is likely due to the fact that the difference in uptake between sensitive and resistance cells is limited to a maximum of ~5 fold (Figure 6). It is also noteworthy that, in addition to NSCLC and ovarian cancers, impaired drug accumulation in cisplatin resistance is exhibited in many other tumor types, including head and neck, melanoma, testicular, and breast[18].

The underlying basis for the reduction in drug accumulation in resistant cells is not well understood. However, it is generally recognised that this reduction is not due to an increased rate of cisplatin efflux[53,61], which is consistent with a lack of over-expression of the multidrug resistance (MDR) P-glycoprotein (P-gp) efflux pump in the ovarian OV202/hp cisplatin-resistant tumor model[62]. Similarly, the sensitivity of P-gp over-expressing human leukemic HL60/Dox cells to cisplatin was unchanged by the P-gp inhibitor, cepharanthin[63]. The lack of a role of P-gp in cisplatin resistance is further reinforced by the demonstration that the strongly MDR-phenotypic SKVLB1 cell line and the isogenic MDR-negative parental SKOV3 cell line were equally sensitive to cisplatin[64]. On the other hand, a clinical study in advanced ovarian cancer using a cisplatin-based treatment regimen has demonstrated that P-gp over-expression is associated with a poor chemotherapeutic response[65]. The lung resistance-related protein (LRP) can also regulate transport of several drugs, and patients with advanced ovarian cancers having increased levels of LRP had a greatly reduced response rate[66]. It is clear that further studies are needed to clarify and/or amplify the roles of P-gp and LRP in cisplatin resistance.

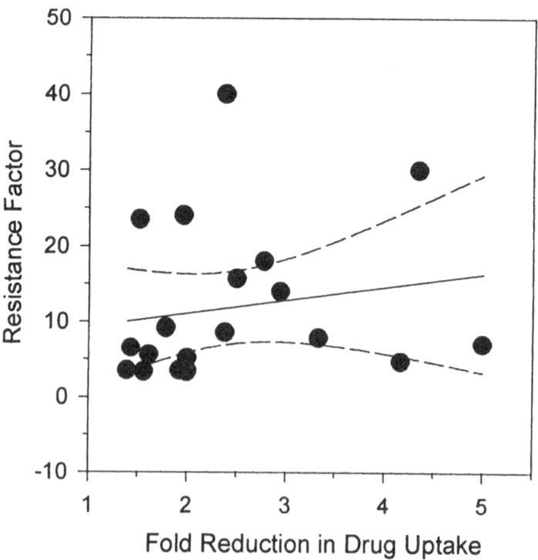

Figure 6. Correlation between resistance factor and fold reduction in cisplatin uptake. The solid line is a linear regression fit, with broken lines indicating the 95% confidence interval. Each point represents data from an individual study in a distinct pair of sensitive/resistant isogenic tumor models. [Data from Kelland[18]].

A reduced rate of cellular uptake appears to be the most likely cause of low cisplatin accumulation, but the mechanism remains obscure. Since reduced uptake can be demonstrated over a wide range of extracellular cisplatin concentrations[67], it is probable that resistance occurs as a result of changes in the non-saturable uptake process of passive drug diffusion. There is limited evidence, however, that an energy dependent active transport involving Na^+K^+-ATPase or a gated ion channel has a role in cisplatin uptake[61,8], and, therefore, an alteration in this system in cisplatin resistance cannot be ruled out. Several membrane proteins have also been identified in cisplatin-resistant tumor cells[18], but further studies are needed to define if any of them have a role in cisplatin uptake and/or resistance. Similarly, the role of the ABC transport proteins MRP1 and MRP2 (cMOAT) also needs to be resolved as both an increase[69] and a decrease[70] in their expression has been reported in conjunction with cisplatin resistance.

Accumulation of platinum analogs designed to circumvent cisplatin resistance is reported to be either reduced[67,71–73] or unchanged[73,74] in cisplatin-resistant cell lines. Thus, cisplatin resistance caused by a defect in uptake can be circumvented in part through structural modifications in the drug molecule, particularly if such modifications lead to an increase in lipophilicity of the antitumor agent.

3.1.2 Glutathione and thiol-related proteins

When cisplatin enters the cell, the much lower chloride concentration (~4 mM) in the cytoplasm facilitates aquation reactions, which results in irreversible interactions between the reactive cisplatin species and a number of cytoplasmic constituents, including the abundant intracellular proteins. Following aquation, cisplatin can also react with the nucleophilic GSH (Figure 7) and the cysteine-rich metallothionein. Levels of these thiol-containing molecules can increase following cisplatin exposure and affect resistance by reducing the availability of "free" cytotoxic drug levels in the cell.

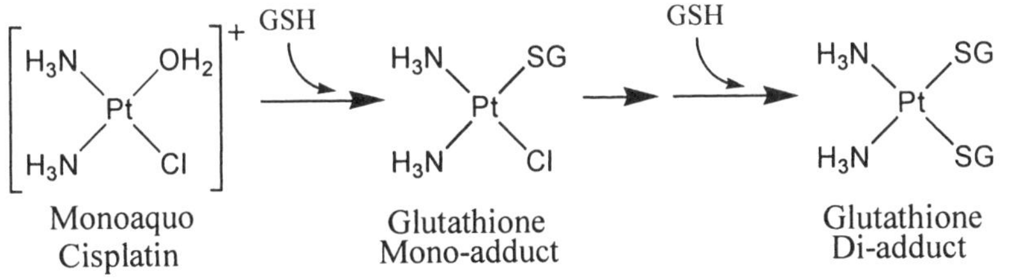

$[Pt(NH_3)_2(OH_2)Cl]^+$ —GSH→ $Pt(NH_3)_2(SG)Cl$ → —GSH→ $Pt(NH_3)_2(SG)_2$

Monoaquo Cisplatin — Glutathione Mono-adduct — Glutathione Di-adduct

Figure 7. Reactions of monoaquated cisplatin with nucleophilic glutathione (GSH) to form inactive conjugation products.

An increase in GSH is found in many cisplatin-resistant tumor models[18], and has been supported by studies with isogenic models established from an individual patient following the first and second relapse after cisplatin therapy[51]. In ovarian tumor models selected for a high level of cisplatin resistance (9 to >400 fold), elevated GSH (4 to 50 fold) was a prominent feature[75,76]. The large increases in GSH were associated with increased expression of the γ-glutamylcysteine synthetase (γ-GCS) gene[75,76], the translation product of which is the rate-limiting enzyme in GSH biosynthesis. Thus, changes in GSH occurred as a result of a transcriptional/translational event in response to cisplatin exposure. Moreover, when resistant cells were grown in absence of cisplatin, resistance diminished and this was accompanied by a concomitant decrease in GSH[76], which suggests that GSH levels and resistance are closely connected. Indeed, Hamaguchi *et al.*[76] have reported a good correlation between GSH levels and IC_{50} of cisplatin in a panel of highly resistant isogenic ovarian tumor models. A similar correlation has also been reported in a panel of unrelated ovarian tumor cell lines[77]. In contrast, studies with a panel of 15 human ovarian tumor xenografts[78] and a mixed collection of 23 human colon, gastric, lung and breast tumor xenografts[79] indicated no correlation between tumor GSH levels and sensitivity to cisplatin. This suggests that increased GSH as a mechanism of resistance may be more important *in vitro* than *in vivo*, but this remains to be clarified. As alluded to earlier, increase in GSH is not a universal occurrence in resistant cells[60].

How an increase in levels of GSH can affect cisplatin resistance remains unclear. It is, however, acknowledged that GSH interacts non-enzymatically with aquated cisplatin and inactivates the antitumor agent, and this can provide a plausible explanation for the relationship between an increase in GSH and resistance. A recent report from Goto *et al.*[80] indicates that conjugation between cisplatin and GSH can also occur enzymatically by GSH-S-transferase π (GSTπ), which is a member of a family of enzymes involved in xenobiotic detoxification reactions (see, for example, Chapter 4 in this volume by Ds. D. Hamilton and colleagues). Irrespective of how the GSH-cisplatin conjugate is formed, there is much inconsistency in the reported data since sensitivity to cisplatin is enhanced only minimally (<2 fold) in cell lines depleted of GSH by over 75% following exposure to L-buthionine-SR-sulfoximine (BSO), a specific inhibitor of γ-GCS[77,81-83]. Moreover, GSH depletion does not appear to lead to any selective sensitisation of cisplatin-resistant cells over the parental isogenic sensitive line[83,84]. This suggests that increased GSH may contribute to cisplatin resistance through an additional mechanism, such as that implicated in DNA repair[18]. Another putative mechanism may relate to the ability of GSH to inhibit apoptosis following drug treatment, possibly by buffering an endogenously-induced oxidative stress[85,86]. In this regard, it is known that cells expressing the anti-apoptotic Bcl-2 protein have correspondingly higher intracellular GSH levels[87,88], which may contribute to the antioxidant functions of Bcl-2 to inhibit apoptosis[89,90].

As indicated earlier, GSTπ is reported to catalyse the conjugation between cisplatin with GSH[80]. This is consistent with the observation that a low level of GSTπ correlated with an 82% overall survival rate with cisplatin in head and neck cancers, whereas a high level of the enzyme was associated with only a 46% survival rate[91]. These data are supported by *in vitro* findings, which indicate that GST activity is increased up to 5 fold following the development of cisplatin resistance in lung, breast and head and neck tumor models[60]. Nevertheless, a direct role of GST in cisplatin resistance has not been defined. Indeed, some studies have reported no correlation between GST and relative sensitivities of human tumor xenografts to cisplatin[78,79].

Metallothioneins (MT) are rich in the thiol-containing amino acid cysteine, and can detoxify heavy metals, such as cadmium, and can also react with aquated cisplatin to inactivate the antitumor agent in much the same way as GSH. It is not surprising, therefore, that over-expression of MT has been associated with cisplatin resistance in both murine and human tumor models[92]. A 2- to 5-fold elevation in cellular MT content was noted in the majority of resistant models investigated. Similar data have also been reported from investigations in human small cell lung tumor models[93]. Other studies have failed to observe changes in MT levels in resistant cell lines[94,95] or between human ovarian tumor biopsies taken before and after cisplatin-based therapy[96]. These variations in the reported data again emphasize that increases in MT are also not an absolute requirement for cells to attain the resistant phenotype. Conversely, substantial elevations in MT may correlate with cisplatin resistance *in vivo*, but not *in vitro*[97]. This supports the notion that in some cases resistance mechanisms may only be expressed in an *in vivo* setting[56].

3.1.3 DNA damage repair and tolerance

Since DNA adducts of cisplatin are the principal lesions inducing cell death, it is not surprising that enhanced repair of adducts will diminish persistence and lead to resistance. Enhanced repair has been demonstrated in cisplatin-resistant murine L1210 leukemia cells[98] and in a number of human cell lines, including those of ovarian, testicular and cervical origin[57,99–101]. As with other mechanisms, repair is not universally present in all cisplatin-resistant cell lines. It was not observed, for instance, in resistant human cell lines derived from the ovary or the colon[72]. When increased repair is indeed present, the contribution of this mechanism to overall resistance is thought to be of the order of 1.5 to 2.0 fold only[102]. Enhanced repair as a mechanism of resistance also applies to cisplatin analogs, such as dichloro-diethylenediamine-platinum(II)[103] and diaminocyclohexane-sulfato-platinum(II)[104]. This information, in conjunction with the knowledge that cisplatin-resistant L1210/DDP cells lack cross-resistance to the diaminocyclohexane analog, has led investigators to suggest that modulation of repair is not a mechanism of circumvention of cisplatin resistance with the diaminocyclohexane analog[104]. There is, however, an indication of differential repair of specific adducts induced by a platinating agent, and studies with diaminocyclohexane- and diethylenediamine-platinum analogs demonstrate that repair was in the order GpXpG > G (monfunctional adduct) > ApG > GpG[105]. Since GpG adducts of cisplatin are not readily repaired, they have been implicated as the most cytotoxic lesion[106]. Conversely, the inactivity of transplatin is attributed to a substantially greater rate of repair of its adducts[107]. There appears to be a limit to the extent that repair capacity can be increased in resistance. This is supported by the finding that in cisplatin-resistant L1210 cells, enhanced repair of the GpG adduct in cells that were 20-fold resistant was similar to that in cells with 100-fold resistance[103].

The major route of platinum adduct removal is by the process of NER, which is defective in diseases such as xeroderma pigmentosum (XP) and Cockayne's syndrome, and this defect normally leads to drug hypersensitivity[102]. NER has broad specificity, and no differences have been observed in the excision of adducts induced by cisplatin and the analogs JM216 and oxaliplatin[25]. Although the NER complex consists of at least 17 different proteins[108], many of the studies implicate only a few proteins in causing an increase in the excision repair activity in resistant tumor cells[109]. From transfection studies using UV repair-deficient CHO cells, it is clear that over-expression of the excision repair cross-complementing (ERCC) gene ERCC1, but not ERCC3 (XPB), results in cisplatin resistance[110]. A 2-fold increase in ERCC1 mRNA levels has also been noted in ovarian tumor samples from platinum-refractory patients[111]. The only other consistent change that has been reported in resistance is over-expression in the repair-related XPA gene[111].

It is useful to discuss also the role of MMR in the context of resistance. Despite the fact that MMR is not directly involved in repair of cisplatin adducts, it has an important function in recognising DNA adducts and activating apoptosis[112]. The MMR complex consists of a number of proteins, including hMSH2 and hMLH1, with hMSH2 being directly involved in specifically recognising GpG adducts of cisplatin[113,114]. Therefore, loss of expression or mutations of the MMR genes leads to a defect in efficient recognition of DNA adducts, and resistance ensues[115–117]. It is useful to note that the extent of resistance attributable to MMR defect is significant, and accounts for a 2- to 5-fold increase in resistance. Of greater interest is the specificity of MMR for cisplatin adducts, as adducts of certain analogs, such as oxaliplatin and JM216, are not recognized by the MMR complex[116]. This suggests that other recognition proteins may play a role in the activity of these analogs against cisplatin-resistant tumor cells.

Ideally, repair of DNA should occur prior to DNA replication to avoid mutations being introduced into the genome. However, resistance can arise if cells enhance their capacity to replicate DNA past the adduct, and then initiate post-replication repair[102]. This can increase the ability of cells to tolerate high levels of DNA adducts induced by cisplatin. Interestingly, replicative bypass is increased 3 to 6 fold by defects in hMLH1 or hMSH6, which links MMR to the bypass mechanism[117]. Consistent with this is the finding that oxaliplatin adducts, which are not recognised by MMR, are not subject to increased bypass by a defect in MMR[117]. This relationship between increased replicative bypass and MMR is, however, challenged by the finding that in cisplatin-resistant ovarian 2008/C13* cells, MMR status is normal yet the cells demonstrate a 5-fold increase in replicative bypass of cisplatin adducts compared to isogenic sensitive 2008 tumor cells[118]. Irrespective of whether the mechanism of DNA damage tolerance is linked to MMR, reports indicate that tolerance to cisplatin adducts appears to be of substantial importance in cisplatin resistance[57,59]. Indeed, damage tolerance provided a significantly better correlation with the extent of resistance than did drug accumulation, DNA adduct repair or GSH content[59].

3.2 Molecular Mechanisms of Resistance

It is well understood that once DNA adducts are formed and detected by recognition proteins, signal transduction pathways are activated to induce cell cycle arrest or apoptosis. These pathways are not well defined, but a few essential genes have been identified, such as the p53 tumor suppressor and bax genes, that can facilitate the apoptotic process. However, the apoptotic effects of cisplatin can be impeded by such factors as alteration in the gene or functional status of p53, elevation of Mdm2 protein levels, and increased expression of specific members of the bcl2 family. A simplified scheme incorporating some of the known molecular factors leading to resistance is shown in Figure 8. Note that molecular mechanisms include mutation in DNA damage recognition proteins, which was discussed earlier.

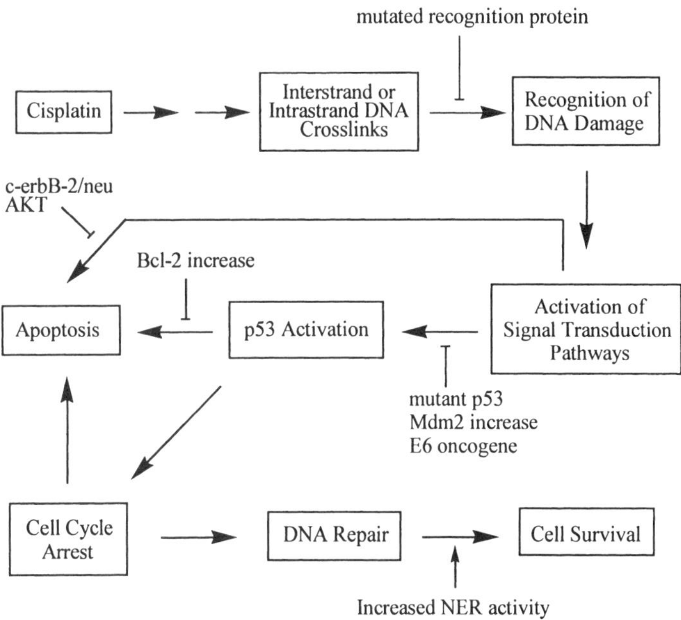

Figure 8. Cisplatin-induced molecular events causing cell death (apoptosis) or cell survival and modulation of the sequence of events by molecular mechanisms of resistance.

3.2.1 Tumor suppressor p53

Expression of the wild-type p53 gene is critical to cell cycle control and apoptosis. Loss of p53 function through mutation or other means is associated with cisplatin resistance, presumably through an absence of a p53-mediated apoptotic signal[28,34,119]. This resistance to the platinating agent has been demonstrated clinically in a variety of tumor types, including those originating from the ovary and head and neck[91,120–122]. However, in other clinical studies, cisplatin sensitivity or resistance did not correlate with tumor p53 status[123,124]. Similar conflicting data have been reported from *in vitro* studies, which demonstrate that the sensitivity of tumor cells harboring wild-type p53 can be both decreased[125] or increased[40] by abolishing p53 function. Furthermore, it is noteworthy that the p53-null SKOV-3 cell line can still undergo apoptosis when exposed to cisplatin[126]. A significant recent finding is the association of wild-type p53 with highly resistant ovarian tumor cell lines[48]. Based on results derived from immunoblots, this resistance has been attributed to a lack of cisplatin-mediated induction of wild-type p53, which would be required to activate the apoptotic pathway[48,57]. Thus, it is likely that other intracellular factors in resistant tumors must play significant roles in regulating the dependency on p53 for therapeutic outcomes following antitumor drug treatment.

In cells harbouring wild-type p53, the apoptotic function of this protein is regulated by a number of factors. Intracellularly, p53 is normally maintained at very low levels or in an inactive state by its binding to the Mdm2 protein[127]. When DNA is damaged, the binding between Mdm2 and p53 is disrupted and results in p53 induction, which is attributable to a greater stability of free p53[127–129]. Furthermore, DNA damage induces phosphorylation and acetylation on specific sites of p53 that may promote its dissociation from Mdm2 and activate apoptosis[127,130]. In this regard, it is pertinent to mention that HMG1 has a role in p53 phosphorylation[30] which appears to point to an additional function for this DNA damage recognition protein in the cytotoxic process. From these considerations, the potential for increased Mdm2 levels and defects in specific kinases to affect cisplatin resistance is clearly apparent. However, these potentials have not been thoroughly investigated. Although resistance to cisplatin has been demonstrated in an *in vitro* study employing transfection with an mdm2 vector[131], a clinical study indicates that over-expression of mdm2 did not affect clinical response of ovarian cancers to cisplatin-based chemotherapy[132]. In addition to Mdm2, activity of wild-type p53 can also be attenuated by the human papillomavirus (HPV), which has been detected clinically in cancer of the cervix. In this case, the protein product of the E6 oncogene in HPV 16 binds to p53 and disrupts transactivation functions[133]. Although inactivation by E6 can confer platinum drug resistance, this is not always the case[40,48].

In the context of p53, it is appropriate to address its role on the issue of DNA damage tolerance. From the many reports published on the subject, it is clear that lack of p53 function will lead to a loss of an apoptotic signal[28,34]. Thus, it is reasonable to suggest that greater DNA damage will be required to affect cell death. From studies with ovarian cancer cell lines, it appears likely that a lack of wild-type p53 function is resposnsible for the increase in DNA damage tolerance as a mechanism of cisplatin resistance[134].

3.2.2 Bcl-2 family

Members of the Bcl-2 family are localised in the mitochondria and can have either pro-apoptotic (Bax, Bak, Bid, Bim) or anti-apoptotic (Bcl-2, Bcl-XL, Bcl-W) functions[135,136]. The members form either homodimers (e.g., Bcl-2/Bcl-2) or heterodimers (e.g., Bcl-2/Bax), and this is dependent on the levels of each component that are present. Only an excess level of homodimers can inhibit (e.g., Bcl-2/Bcl-2) or induce (e.g., Bax/Bax) apoptosis. Although the effect of cisplatin in modulating the interaction among the Bcl-2 family members is largely unknown, there are limited data that need to be discussed. Bax, for instance, can be transactivated by wild-type p53, and an increase in the Bax to Bcl-2 ratio by cisplatin-induced p53 has been reported to activate the apoptotic process[137]. On the other hand, experimental over-expression of bcl-2 was shown to result in the expected appearance of resistance to cisplatin, which was further compounded by the over-expression of mutant p53[125,138,139]. Paradoxically, however, increased tumor expression of bcl-2 in ovarian cancer patients receiving cisplatin was associated with improved survival, and not reduced survival as might have been anticipated from pre-clinical data[125]. This clinical finding has recently been supported by pre-clinical data[140].

Our present understanding indicates that pro-apoptotic homodimers of the Bcl-2 family affect apoptosis by first stimulating the mitochondria to release cytochrome c, which in turn activates a series of proteases, beginning with the cysteine protease caspase-9[136,141]. Using specific inhibitors of caspases, Kondo *et al.*[131] have indeed demonstrated involvement of caspase-1 (or ICE) in cisplatin-induced apoptosis. Conversely, the increased levels of the anti-apoptotic Bcl-X_L has been associated with inactivation of caspase-3 in a cisplatin-resistant ovarian tumor model due to a diminished ability to activate the apoptotic cell death program[142].

3.2.3 Other molecular factors

Although very little data is available, additional factors that lead to resistance need to be briefly mentioned here. They include activation of the anti-apoptotic PI-3 kinase-AKT/PKB pathway by p21-Ras oncoprotein signalling or by loss of the tumor suppressor pTEN[136]. The anti-apoptotic signal arises as a result of AKT-mediated phosphorylation of caspase-9, which is thereby inactivated[143]. However, the impact of these molecular events on cisplatin resistance is not known. On the other hand, amplification and/or over-expression of c-erbB-2/neu leads to experimental and clinical resistance to cisplatin[144–147], but in this case the mechanism is unclear.

CONCLUSION

Based on the information reviewed in this chapter, it is evident that resistance to cisplatin is multifactorial, which diminishes the clinical utility of this agent. The existence of multiple factors contributing to resistance within a given tumor raises a major dilemma in the design of novel therapeutics or clinical protocols that have the potential to circumvent some, if not all, of the major cellular impediments to increase response rates in refractory disease. Although this may appear to be an insurmountable hurdle with the many mechanisms of resistance that have been identified, it is comforting to know that our understanding of signal transduction processes continues unimpeded, which may eventually allow identification of novel genes or redundant pathways that could serve as targets for designer therapeutics. It should also be borne in mind that even in the absence of such knowledge, some progress can still be made, as exemplified by the clinical activity of oxaliplatin against refractory cancers[9].

ACKNOWLEDGMENT

Supported by NIH Grants CA77332 and CA82361. My sincere thanks to Donna L. Williams and Kay Biescar for assistance in preparing this manuscript.

REFERENCES

1. Tanimura H, Weinstein J, Ortuzar W, *et al.* Identification of non-cross resistant platinum compounds among agents submitted to the National Cancer Institute's (NCI's) anticancer drug screen using the DISCOVERY computer program (Meeting abstract). Proc Amer Assoc Cancer Res, 36:A1816, 1995.
2. Prestayko AW, D'Aoust JC, Issell BF, Crooke ST. Cisplatin (cis-diamminedichloroplatinum II). Cancer Treat Rev, 6:17-39, 1979.
3. Roberts JJ, Pera MF, Jr. DNA as a target for anticancer coordination compounds. *In*: Platinum, Gold, and Other Metal Chemotherapeutic Agents: Chemistry and Biochemistry, SJ Lippard (ed.), American Chemical Society, Washington, DC, 3-25, 1983.
4. Ozols RF. Ovarian cancer: new clinical approaches. Cancer Treat Rev, 18 Suppl A:77-83, 1991.
5. Giaccone G. Clinical perspectives on platinum resistance. Drugs, 59 Suppl 4:9-17, 2000.
6. Kelland LR, Sharp SY, O'Neill CF, *et al.* Mini-review: discovery and development of platinum complexes designed to circumvent cisplatin resistance. J Inorg Biochem, 77:111-115, 1999.
7. Gore M, Fryatt I, Wiltshaw E, *et al.* Cisplatin/carboplatin cross-resistance in ovarian cancer. Br J Cancer, 60:767-769, 1989.
8. Eisenhauer E, Swerton K, Sturgeon J, *et al.* Carboplatin therapy for recurrent ovarian carcinoma: National Cancer Institute of Canada experience and a review of the literature. *In*: P Bunn, R Canetta, R Ozols, M Rozencweig (eds.), Carboplatin: Current Perspectives and Future Directions. W.B. Saunders Company, Philadelphia, PA, 133-140, 1990.
9. Faivre S, Kalla S, Cvitkovic E, *et al.* Oxaliplatin and paclitaxel combination in patients with platinum- pretreated ovarian carcinoma: an investigator-originated compassionate-use experience. Ann Oncol, 10:1125-1128, 1999.
10. Shi L, Nishioka WK, Th'ng J, *et al.* Premature p34cdc2 activation required for apoptosis [see comments]. Science, 263:1143-1145, 1994.
11. Shapiro GI, Harper JW. Anticancer drug targets: cell cycle and checkpoint control. J Clin Invest, 104:1645-1653, 1999.
12. O'Connor PM, Fan S. DNA damage checkpoints: implications for cancer therapy. Progr Cell Cycle Res, 2:165-173, 1996.
13. el Khateeb M, Appleton TG, Gahan LR, *et al.* Reactions of cisplatin hydrolytes with methionine, cysteine, and plasma ultrafiltrate studied by a combination of HPLC and NMR techniques. J Inorg Biochem, 77:13-21, 1999.
14. Kelland LR. Preclinical perspectives on platinum resistance. Drugs, 59 Suppl 4:1-8, 2000.
15. Eastman A. The formation, isolation and characterization of DNA adducts produced by anticancer platinum complexes. Pharmacol Ther, 34:155-166, 1987.
16. Roberts JJ, Friedlos F. Quantitative estimation of cisplatin-induced DNA interstrand cross-links and their repair in mammalian cells: relationship to toxicity. Pharmacol Ther, 34:215-246, 1987.

17. Pinto AL, Lippard SJ. Binding of the antitumor drug cis-diamminedichloroplatinum(II) (cisplatin) to DNA. Biochim Biophys Acta, 780:167-180, 1985.
18. Kelland LR. New platinum antitumor complexes. Crit Rev Oncol Hematol, 15:191-219, 1993.
19. Perez C, Leng M, Malinge JM. Rearrangement of interstrand cross-links into intrastrand cross-links in cis-diamminedichloroplatinum(II)-modified DNA. Nucleic Acids Res, 25:896-903, 1997.
20. Malinge JM, Giraud-Panis MJ, Leng M. Interstrand cross-links of cisplatin induce striking distortions in DNA. J Inorg Biochem, 77:23-29, 1999.
21. Jennerwein MM, Eastman A, Khokhar A. Characterization of adducts produced in DNA by isomeric 1,2-diaminocyclohexaneplatinum(II) complexes. Chem Biol Interact, 70:39-49, 1989.
22. Eastman A. Glutathione-mediated activation of anticancer platinum(IV) complexes. Biochem Pharmacol, 36:4177-4178, 1987.
23. Bellon SF, Coleman JH, Lippard SJ. DNA unwinding produced by site-specific intrastrand cross-links of the antitumor drug cis-diamminedichloroplatinum(II). Biochem, 30:8026-8035, 1991.
24. Turchi JJ, Henkels KM, Hermanson IL, Patrick SM. Interactions of mammalian proteins with cisplatin-damaged DNA. J Inorg Biochem, 77:83-87, 1999.
25. Chaney SG, Vaisman A. Specificity of platinum-DNA adduct repair. J Inorg Biochem, 77:71-81, 1999.
26. Donahue BA, Augot M, Bellon SF, *et al.* Characterization of a DNA damage-recognition protein from mammalian cells that binds specifically to intrastrand d(GpG) and d(ApG) DNA adducts of the anticancer drug cisplatin. Biochem, 29:5872-5880, 1990.
27. He Q, Liang CH, Lippard SJ. Steroid hormones induce HMG1 overexpression and sensitize breast cancer cells to cisplatin and carboplatin. Proc Natl Acad Sci USA, 97:5768-5772, 2000.
28. Kastan MB, Onyekwere O, Sidransky D, *et al.* Participation of p53 protein in the cellular response to DNA damage. Cancer Res, 51:6304-6311, 1991.
29. Hainaut P. The tumor suppressor protein p53: a receptor to genotoxic stress that controls cell growth and survival. Curr Opin Oncol, 7:76-82, 1995.
30. Jayaraman L, Moorthy NC, Murthy KG, *et al.* High mobility group protein-1 (HMG-1) is a unique activator of p53. Genes Dev, 12:462-472, 1998.
31. Sionov RV, Haupt Y. The cellular response to p53: the decision between life and death. Oncogene, 18:6145-6157, 1999.
32. Hollstein M, Sidransky D, Vogelstein B, Harris CC. p53 mutations in human cancers. Science, 253:49-53, 1991.
33. Oltvai ZN, Korsmeyer SJ. Checkpoints of dueling dimers foil death wishes. Cell, 79:189-192, 1994.
34. Hartwell LH, Kastan MB. Cell cycle control and cancer. Science, 266:1821-1828, 1994.
35. Thorlacius S, Borresen AL, Eyfjord JE. Somatic p53 mutations in human breast carcinomas in an Icelandic population: a prognostic factor. Cancer Res, 53:1637-1641, 1993.
36. Michieli P, Chedid M, Lin D, *et al.* Induction of WAF1/CIP1 by a p53-independent pathway. Cancer Res, 54:3391-3395, 1994.
37. Zhang W, Grasso L, McClain CD, *et al.* p53-independent induction of WAF1/CIP1 in human leukemia cells is correlated with growth arrest accompanying monocyte/macrophage differentiation. Cancer Res, 55:668-674, 1995.
38. Haapajarvi T, Pitkanen K, Laiho M. Human melanoma cell line UV responses show independency of p53 function. Cell Growth Differ, 10:163-171, 1999.
39. Segal-Bendirdjian E, Mannone L, Jacquemin-Sablon A. Alteration in p53 pathway and defect in apoptosis contribute independently to cisplatin-resistance. Cell Death Differ, 5:390-400, 1998.
40. Fan S, Smith ML, Rivet DJ, *et al.* Disruption of p53 function sensitizes breast cancer MCF-7 cells to cisplatin and pentoxifylline. Cancer Res, 55:1649-1654, 1995.
41. Hawkins DS, Demers GW, Galloway DA. Inactivation of p53 enhances sensitivity to multiple chemotherapeutic agents. Cancer Res, 56:892-898, 1996.
42. Ozols RF, Corden BJ, Jacob J, *et al.* High-dose cisplatin in hypertonic saline. Ann Intern Med, 100:19-24, 1984.

43. Ozols RF, Hamilton TC, Reed E, *et al.* High dose cisplatin and drug resistance: Clinical and laboratory correlations. *In*: Platinum and Other Metal Coordination Compounds in Cancer Chemotherapy, M Nicolini (ed.), Martinus Nijhoff, Boston, MA, 197-206, 1988.
44. Schilder RJ, Ozols RF. New therapies for ovarian cancer. Cancer Invest, 10:307-315, 1992.
45. Andrews PA, Howell SB. Cellular pharmacology of cisplatin: perspectives on mechanisms of acquired resistance. Cancer Cells, 2:35-43, 1990.
46. Kelley SL, Rozencweig M. Resistance to platinum compounds: mechanisms and beyond. Eur J Cancer Clin Oncol, 25:1135-1140, 1989.
47. Jodrell DI, Egorin MJ, Canetta RM, *et al.* Relationships between carboplatin exposure and tumor response and toxicity in patients with ovarian cancer. J Clin Oncol, 10:520-528, 1992.
48. Hagopian GS, Mills GB, Khokhar AR, *et al.* Expression of p53 in cisplatin-resistant ovarian cancer cell lines: modulation with the novel platinum analog (1R,2R-diaminocyclohexane)(trans-diacetato)(dichloro)-platinum(IV). Clin Cancer Res, 5:655-663, 1999.
49. Hills CA, Kelland LR, Abel G, *et al.* Biological properties of ten human ovarian carcinoma cell lines: calibration in vitro against four platinum complexes. Br J Cancer, 59:527-534, 1989.
50. Kelland LR, Barnard CF, Evans IG, *et al.* Synthesis and in vitro and in vivo antitumor activity of a series of trans platinum antitumor complexes. J Med Chem, 38:3016-3024, 1995.
51. Wolf CR, Hayward IP, Lawrie SS, *et al.* Cellular heterogeneity and drug resistance in two ovarian adenocarcinoma cell lines derived from a single patient. Int J Cancer, 39:695-702, 1987.
52. Kelland LR, Mistry P, Abel G, *et al.* Mechanism-related circumvention of acquired cis-diamminedichloroplatinum(II) resistance using two pairs of human ovarian carcinoma cell lines by ammine/amine platinum(IV) dicarboxylates. Cancer Res, 52:3857-3864, 1992.
53. Teicher BA, Holden SA, Kelley MJ, *et al.* Characterization of a human squamous carcinoma cell line resistant to cis-diamminedichloroplatinum(II). Cancer Res, 47:388-393, 1987.
54. Richon VM, Schulte N, Eastman A. Multiple mechanisms of resistance to cis-diamminedichloroplatinum(II) in murine leukemia L1210 cells. Cancer Res, 47:2056-2061, 1987.
55. Eastman A, Schulte N, Sheibani N, Sorenson CM. Mechanisms of resistance to platinum drugs. *In*: Nicolini M (ed.), Platinum and Other Metal Coordination Compounds in Cancer Chemotherapy, Martinus Nijhoff, Boston, MA, 178-196, 1988.
56. Teicher BA, Herman TS, Holden SA, *et al.* Tumor resistance to alkylating agents conferred by mechanisms operative only in vivo. Science, 247:1457-1461, 1990.
57. Siddik ZH, Mims B, Lozano G, Thai G. Independent pathways of p53 induction by cisplatin and X-rays in a cisplatin-resistant ovarian tumor cell line. Cancer Res, 58:698-703, 1998.
58. Fraval HN, Roberts JJ. Excision repair of cis-diamminedichloroplatinum(II)-induced damage to DNA of Chinese hamster cells. Cancer Res, 39:1793-1797, 1979.
59. Johnson SW, Laub PB, Beesley JS, *et al.* Increased platinum-DNA damage tolerance is associated with cisplatin resistance and cross-resistance to various chemotherapeutic agents in unrelated human ovarian cancer cell lines. Cancer Res, 57:850-856, 1997.
60. Teicher BA, Holden SA, Herman TS, *et al.* Characteristics of five human tumor cell lines and sublines resistant to cis-diamminedichloroplatinum(II). Int J Cancer, 47:252-260, 1991.
61. Andrews PA, Velury S, Mann SC, Howell SB. cis-Diamminedichloroplatinum(II) accumulation in sensitive and resistant human ovarian carcinoma cells. Cancer Res, 48:68-73, 1988.
62. Bible KC, Boerner SA, Kirkland K, *et al.* Characterization of an ovarian carcinoma cell line resistant to cisplatin and flavopiridol. Clin Cancer Res, 6:661-670, 2000.
63. Wada H, Saikawa Y, Niida Y, *et al.* Selectively induced high MRP gene expression in multidrug-resistant human HL60 leukemia cells. Exp Hematol, 27:99-109, 1999.

64. Smith CD, Carmeli S, Moore RE, Patterson GM. Scytophycins, novel microfilament-depolymerizing agents which circumvent P-glycoprotein-mediated multidrug resistance. Cancer Res, 53:1343-1347, 1993.
65. Baekelandt MM, Holm R, Nesland JM, *et al.* P-glycoprotein expression is a marker for chemotherapy resistance and prognosis in advanced ovarian cancer. Anticancer Res, 20:1061-1067, 2000.
66. Izquierdo MA, van der Zee AG, Vermorken JB, *et al.* Drug resistance-associated marker Lrp for prediction of response to chemotherapy and prognoses in advanced ovarian carcinoma. J Natl Cancer Inst, 87:1230-1237, 1995.
67. Yoshida M, Khokhar AR, Siddik ZH. Biochemical pharmacology of homologous alicyclic mixed amine platinum(II) complexes in sensitive and resistant tumor cell lines. Cancer Res, 54:3468-3473, 1994.
68. Gately DP, Howell SB. Cellular accumulation of the anticancer agent cisplatin: a review. Br J Cancer, 67:1171-1176, 1993.
69. Kool M, de Haas M, Scheffer GL, *et al.* Analysis of expression of cMOAT (MRP2), MRP3, MRP4, and MRP5, homologues of the multidrug resistance-associated protein gene (MRP1), in human cancer cell lines. Cancer Res, 57:3537-3547, 1997.
70. Shen DW, Goldenberg S, Pastan I, Gottesman MM. Decreased accumulation of [14C]carboplatin in human cisplatin-resistant cells results from reduced energy-dependent uptake. J Cell Physiol, 183:108-116, 2000.
71. Kido Y, Khokhar AR, Siddik ZH. Differential cytotoxicity, uptake and DNA binding of tetraplatin and analogous isomers in sensitive and resistant cancer cell lines. Anticancer Drugs, 4:251-258, 1993.
72. Schmidt W, Chaney SG. Role of carrier ligand in platinum resistance of human carcinoma cell lines. Cancer Res, 53:799-805, 1993.
73. Mellish KJ, Kelland LR, Harrap KR. In vitro platinum drug chemosensitivity of human cervical squamous cell carcinoma cell lines with intrinsic and acquired resistance to cisplatin. Br J Cancer, 68:240-250, 1993.
74. Coluccia M, Nassi A, Boccarelli A, *et al.* In vitro and in vivo antitumour activity and cellular pharmacological properties of new platinum-iminoether complexes with different configuration at the iminoether ligands. J Inorg Biochem, 77:31-35, 2000.
75. Godwin AK, Meister A, O'Dwyer PJ, *et al.* High resistance to cisplatin in human ovarian cancer cell lines is associated with marked increase of glutathione synthesis. Proc Natl Acad Sci USA, 89:3070-3074, 1992.
76. Hamaguchi K, Godwin AK, Yakushiji M, *et al.* Cross-resistance to diverse drugs is associated with primary cisplatin resistance in ovarian cancer cell lines. Cancer Res, 53:5225-5232, 1993.
77. Mistry P, Kelland LR, Abel G, *et al.* The relationships between glutathione, glutathione-S-transferase and cytotoxicity of platinum drugs and melphalan in eight human ovarian carcinoma cell lines. Br J Cancer, 64:215-220, 1991.
78. Kolfschoten GM, Pinedo HM, Scheffer PG, *et al.* Development of a panel of 15 human ovarian cancer xenografts for drug screening and determination of the role of the glutathione detoxification system. Gynecol Oncol, 76:362-368, 2000.
79. D'Incalci M, Bonfanti M, Pifferi A, *et al.* The antitumour activity of alkylating agents is not correlated with the levels of glutathione, glutathione transferase and O6-alkylguanine-DNA-alkyltransferase of human tumour xenografts. Eur J Cancer, 34:1749-1755, 1998.
80. Goto S, Iida T, Cho S, *et al.* Overexpression of glutathione S-transferase pi enhances the adduct formation of cisplatin with glutathione in human cancer cells. Free Radic Res, 31:549-558, 1999.
81. Andrews PA, Murphy MP, Howell SB. Differential potentiation of alkylating and platinating agent cytotoxicity in human ovarian carcinoma cells by glutathione depletion. Cancer Res, 45:6250-6253, 1985.
82. Goddard P, Valenti M, Kelland LR. The role of glutathione (GSH) in determining sensitivity to platinum drugs in vivo in platinum-sensitive and -resistant murine leukaemia and plasmacytoma and human ovarian carcinoma xenografts. Anticancer Res, 14:1065-1070, 1994.

83. Meijer C, Mulder NH, Timmer-Bosscha H, *et al.* Relationship of cellular glutathione to the cytotoxicity and resistance of seven platinum compounds. Cancer Res, 52:6885-6889, 1992.
84. Hamilton TC, Winker MA, Louie KG, *et al.* Augmentation of adriamycin, melphalan, and cisplatin cytotoxicity in drug-resistant and -sensitive human ovarian carcinoma cell lines by buthionine sulfoximine mediated glutathione depletion. Biochem Pharmacol, 34:2583-2586, 1985.
85. Chiba T, Takahashi S, Oguri-Hyakumachi N, *et al.* Increased intracellular glutathione levels protect human T leukemia cells from Fas-mediated apoptosis. FASEB J, 9:A523, 1995.
86. Slater AF, Nobel CS, Maellaro E, *et al.* Nitrone spin traps and a nitroxide antioxidant inhibit a common pathway of thymocyte apoptosis. Biochem J, 306:771-778, 1995.
87. Meyn RE, Mirkovic N, Voehringer DW, Story MD. Bcl-2 inhibits radiation-induced apoptosis by upregulating the antioxidant properties of the cell. Proc Amer Assoc Cancer Res, 37:A159, 1996.
88. Kane DJ, Sarafian TA, Anton R, *et al.* Bcl-2 inhibition of neural death: decreased generation of reactive oxygen species. Science, 262:1274-1277, 1993.
89. Hockenbery DM, Oltvai ZN, Yin XM, *et al.* Bcl-2 functions in an antioxidant pathway to prevent apoptosis. Cell, 75:241-251, 1993.
90. Chiao C, Carothers AM, Grunberger D, *et al.* Apoptosis and altered redox state induced by caffeic acid phenethyl ester (CAPE) in transformed rat fibroblast cells. Cancer Res, 55:3576-3583, 1995.
91. Shiga H, Heath EI, Rasmussen AA, *et al.* Prognostic value of p53, glutathione S-transferase pi, and thymidylate synthase for neoadjuvant cisplatin-based chemotherapy in head and neck cancer. Clin Cancer Res, 5:4097-4104, 1999.
92. Kelley SL, Basu A, Teicher BA, *et al.* Overexpression of metallothionein confers resistance to anticancer drugs. Science, 241:1813-1815, 1988.
93. Kasahara K, Fujiwara Y, Nishio K, *et al.* Metallothionein content correlates with the sensitivity of human small cell lung cancer cell lines to cisplatin. Cancer Res, 51:3237-3242, 1991.
94. Andrews PA, Murphy MP, Howell SB. Metallothionein-mediated cisplatin resistance in human ovarian carcinoma cells. Cancer Chemother Pharmacol, 19:149-154, 1987.
95. Schilder RJ, Hall L, Monks A, *et al.* Metallothionein gene expression and resistance to cisplatin in human ovarian cancer. Int J Cancer, 45:416-422, 1990.
96. Murphy D, McGown AT, Crowther D, *et al.* Metallothionein levels in ovarian tumours before and after chemotherapy. Br J Cancer, 63:711-714, 1991.
97. Toyoda H, Mizushima T, Satoh M, *et al.* HeLa cell transformants overproducing mouse metallothionein show in vivo resistance to cis-platinum in nude mice. Jpn J Cancer Res, 91:91-98, 2000.
98. Sheibani N, Jennerwein MM, Eastman A. DNA repair in cells sensitive and resistant to cis-diamminedichloroplatinum(II): host cell reactivation of damaged plasmid DNA. Biochem, 28:3120-3124, 1989.
99. Lai GM, Ozols RF, Smyth JF, *et al.* Enhanced DNA repair and resistance to cisplatin in human ovarian cancer. Biochem Pharmacol, 37:4597-4600, 1988.
100. Kelland LR, Mistry P, Abel G, *et al.* Establishment and characterization of an in vitro model of acquired resistance to cisplatin in a human testicular nonseminomatous germ cell line. Cancer Res, 52:1710-1716, 1992.
101. Chao CC, Lee YL, Cheng PW, Lin-Chao S. Enhanced host cell reactivation of damaged plasmid DNA in HeLa cells resistant to cis-diamminedichloroplatinum(II). Cancer Res, 51:601-605, 1991.
102. Chaney SG, Sancar A. DNA repair: enzymatic mechanisms and relevance to drug response. J Natl Cancer Inst, 88:1346-1360, 1996.
103. Eastman A, Schulte N. Enhanced DNA repair as a mechanism of resistance to cis-diamminedichloroplatinum(II). Biochem, 27:4730-4734, 1988.
104. Jennerwein MM, Eastman A, Khokhar AR. The role of DNA repair in resistance of L1210 cells to isomeric 1,2-diaminocyclohexaneplatinum complexes and ultraviolet irradiation. Mutat Res, 254:89-96, 1991.

105. Page JD, Husain I, Sancar A, Chaney SG. Effect of the diaminocyclohexane carrier ligand on platinum adduct formation, repair, and lethality. Biochem, 29:1016-1024, 1990.
106. Szymkowski DE, Yarema K, Essigmann JM, *et al.* An intrastrand d(GpG) platinum crosslink in duplex M13 DNA is refractory to repair by human cell extracts. Proc Natl Acad Sci USA, 89:10772-10776, 1992.
107. Heiger-Bernays WJ, Essigmann JM, Lippard SJ. Effect of the antitumor drug cis-diamminedichloroplatinum(II) and related platinum complexes on eukaryotic DNA replication. Biochem, 29:8461-8466, 1990.
108. Sancar A. Mechanisms of DNA excision repair. Science, 266:1954-1956, 1994.
109. Reed E. Platinum-DNA adduct, nucleotide excision repair and platinum based anti-cancer chemotherapy. Cancer Treat Rev, 24:331-344, 1998.
110. Lee KB, Parker RJ, Bohr V, *et al.* Cisplatin sensitivity/resistance in UV repair-deficient Chinese hamster ovary cells of complementation groups 1 and 3. Carcinogenesis, 14:2177-2180, 1993.
111. Dabholkar M, Vionnet J, Bostick-Bruton F, *et al.* Messenger RNA levels of XPAC and ERCC1 in ovarian cancer tissue correlate with response to platinum-based chemotherapy. J Clin Invest, 94:703-708, 1994.
112. Fink D, Aebi S, Howell SB. The role of DNA mismatch repair in drug resistance. Clin Cancer Res, 4:1-6, 1998.
113. Mello JA, Acharya S, Fishel R, Essigmann JM. The mismatch-repair protein hMSH2 binds selectively to DNA adducts of the anticancer drug cisplatin. Chem Biol, 3:579-589, 1996.
114. Duckett DR, Drummond JT, Murchie AI, *et al.* Human MutSalpha recognizes damaged DNA base pairs containing O6-methylguanine, O4-methylthymine, or the cisplatin-d(GpG) adduct. Proc Natl Acad Sci USA, 93:6443-6447, 1996.
115. Brown R, Hirst GL, Gallagher WM, *et al.* hMLH1 expression and cellular responses of ovarian tumour cells to treatment with cytotoxic anticancer agents. Oncogene, 15:45-52, 1997.
116. Fink D, Nebel S, Aebi S, *et al.* The role of DNA mismatch repair in platinum drug resistance. Cancer Res, 56:4881-4886, 1996.
117. Vaisman A, Varchenko M, Umar A, *et al.* The role of hMLH1, hMSH3, and hMSH6 defects in cisplatin and oxaliplatin resistance: correlation with replicative bypass of platinum-DNA adducts. Cancer Res, 58:3579-3585, 1998.
118. Mamenta EL, Poma EE, Kaufmann WK, *et al.* Enhanced replicative bypass of platinum-DNA adducts in cisplatin-resistant human ovarian carcinoma cell lines. Cancer Res, 54:3500-3505, 1994.
119. Pietenpol JA, Tokino T, Thiagalingam S, *et al.* Sequence-specific transcriptional activation is essential for growth suppression by p53. Proc Natl Acad Sci USA, 91:1998-2002, 1994.
120. Righetti SC, Perego P, Corna E, *et al.* Emergence of p53 mutant cisplatin-resistant ovarian carcinoma cells following drug exposure: spontaneously mutant selection. Cell Growth Differ, 10:473-478, 1999.
121. Marx D, Meden H, Ziemek T, *et al.* Expression of the p53 tumour suppressor gene as a prognostic marker in platinum-treated patients with ovarian cancer. Eur J Cancer, 34:845-850, 1998.
122. Cabelguenne A, Blons H, de Waziers I, *et al.* p53 alterations predict tumor response to neoadjuvant chemotherapy in head and neck squamous cell carcinoma: a prospective series. J Clin Oncol, 18:1465-1473, 2000.
123. Burger H, Nooter K, Boersma AW, *et al.* Expression of p53, Bcl-2 and Bax in cisplatin-induced apoptosis in testicular germ cell tumour cell lines. Br J Cancer, 77:1562-1567, 1998.
124. Qureshi KN, Griffiths TR, Robinson MC, *et al.* TP53 accumulation predicts improved survival in patients resistant to systemic cisplatin-based chemotherapy for muscle-invasive bladder cancer. Clin Cancer Res, 5:3500-3507, 1999.
125. Herod JJ, Eliopoulos AG, Warwick J, *et al.* The prognostic significance of Bcl-2 and p53 expression in ovarian carcinoma. Cancer Res, 56:2178-2184, 1996.

126. Ormerod MG, O'Neill C, Robertson D, *et al.* cis-Diamminedichloroplatinum(II)-induced cell death through apoptosis in sensitive and resistant human ovarian carcinoma cell lines. Cancer Chemother Pharmacol, 37:463-471, 1996.
127. Lakin ND, Jackson SP. Regulation of p53 in response to DNA damage. Oncogene, 18:7644-7655, 1999.
128. Fritsche M, Haessler C, Brandner G. Induction of nuclear accumulation of the tumor-suppressor protein p53 by DNA-damaging agents. Oncogene, 8:307-318, 1993.
129. Shieh SY, Ikeda M, Taya Y, Prives C. DNA damage-induced phosphorylation of p53 alleviates inhibition by MDM2. Cell, 91:325-334, 1997.
130. Meek DW. Mechanisms of switching on p53: a role for covalent modification? Oncogene, 18:7666-7675, 1999.
131. Kondo S, Barnett GH, Hara H, *et al.* MDM2 protein confers the resistance of a human glioblastoma cell line to cisplatin-induced apoptosis. Oncogene, 10:2001-2006, 1995.
132. Mano Y, Kikuchi Y, Yamamoto K, *et al.* Bcl-2 as a predictor of chemosensitivity and prognosis in primary epithelial ovarian cancer. Eur J Cancer, 35:1214-1219, 1999.
133. Kessis TD, Slebos RJ, Nelson WG, *et al.* Human papillomavirus 16 E6 expression disrupts the p53-mediated cellular response to DNA damage. Proc Natl Acad Sci USA, 90:3988-3992, 1993.
134. Siddik ZH, Hagopian GS, Thai G, *et al.* Role of p53 in the ability of 1,2-diaminocyclohexane-diacetato-dichloro-Pt(IV) to circumvent cisplatin resistance. J Inorg Biochem, 77:65-70, 1999.
135. Farrow SN, Brown R. New members of the Bcl-2 family and their protein partners. Curr Opin Genet Dev, 6:45-49, 1996.
136. Hanahan D, Weinberg RA. The hallmarks of cancer. Cell, 100:57-70, 2000.
137. Eliopoulos AG, Kerr DJ, Herod J, *et al.* The control of apoptosis and drug resistance in ovarian cancer: influence of p53 and Bcl-2. Oncogene, 11:1217-1228, 1995.
138. Strasser A, Harris AW, Jacks T, Cory S. DNA damage can induce apoptosis in proliferating lymphoid cells via p53-independent mechanisms inhibitable by Bcl-2. Cell, 79:329-339, 1994.
139. Miyake H, Hara I, Yamanaka K, *et al.* Synergistic enhancement of resistance to cisplatin in human bladder cancer cells by overexpression of mutant-type p53 and Bcl-2. J Urol, 162:2176-2181, 1999.
140. Beale PJ, Rogers P, Boxall F, *et al.* BCL-2 family protein expression and platinum drug resistance in ovarian carcinoma. Br J Cancer, 82:436-440, 2000.
141. Henkels KM, Turchi JJ. Cisplatin-induced apoptosis proceeds by caspase-3-dependent and -independent pathways in cisplatin-resistant and -sensitive human ovarian cancer cell lines. Cancer Res, 59:3077-3083, 1999.
142. Gebauer G, Mirakhur B, Nguyen Q, *et al.* Cisplatin-resistance involves the defective processing of MEKK1 in human ovarian adenocarcinoma 2008/C13 cells. Int J Oncol, 16:321-325, 2000.
143. Cardone MH, Roy N, Stennicke HR, *et al.* Regulation of cell death protease caspase-9 by phosphorylation. Science, 282:1318-1321, 1998.
144. Slamon DJ, Godolphin W, Jones LA, *et al.* Studies of the HER-2/neu proto-oncogene in human breast and ovarian cancer. Science, 244:707-712, 1989.
145. Benz CC, Scott GK, Sarup JC, *et al.* Estrogen-dependent, tamoxifen-resistant tumorigenic growth of MCF-7 cells transfected with HER2/neu. Breast Cancer Res Treat, 24:85-95, 1993.
146. Tsai CM, Yu D, Chang KT, *et al.* Enhanced chemoresistance by elevation of p185neu levels in HER-2/neu-transfected human lung cancer cells. J Natl Cancer Inst, 87:682-684, 1995.
147. Yu D, Liu B, Tan M, *et al.* Overexpression of c-erbB-2/neu in breast cancer cells confers increased resistance to Taxol via mdr-1-independent mechanisms. Oncogene, 13:1359-1365, 1996.

Chapter 14

MODIFICATION OF RADIOSENSITIVITY FOLLOWING CHEMOTHERAPY EXPOSURE: POTENTIAL IMPLICATIONS FOR COMBINED-MODALITY THERAPY

Richard A. Britten
Department of Radiation Oncology, Eastern Virginia Medical School, Norfolk, Virginia, USA

1. GENERAL OVERVIEW OF CHEMORADIATION TREATMENT

Treatment protocols for many tumor sites often consist of a combination of poly-chemotherapy with loco-regional radiotherapy. In many instances, these treatments are given in close temporal proximity to each other, either within a few hours (concomitant) or within a few weeks of each other (sequential). In other instances, radiotherapy may be given at some considerable time after completion of chemotherapy to achieve a measure of loco-regional control in tumors that have recurred following front-line chemotherapy. The optimum integration of chemotherapy and radiotherapy in all three situations has yet to be fully established. Careful consideration of the impact of clinically relevant chemoresistance on radiation response in these various scenarios, and appropriate adjustments, may lead to qualitative differences in patient quality of life, and hopefully quantitative improvements in disease free survival.

In this chapter, we will outline the pre-clinical studies that have formed the historical basis for the use of combined modality therapy (CMT) and review the clinical effectiveness of the derivative clinical trials. In many instances, the clinical experience has been less favourable than originally expected. Some of the possible cellular and molecular reasons for these lower response rates will be outlined, with a particular emphasis on some of the emerging concepts relating to cellular survival mechanisms and on the changing use of certain chemotherapy agents.

2. IMPACT OF THE DEVELOPMENT OF CHEMORESISTANCE ON CELLULAR RADIOSENSITIVITY

2.1 General Rationale for Combined Modality Therapy at the Tumor/Cellular Level

The underlying principles for using combined chemotherapy and radiation therapy have been eloquently outlined elsewhere[1,2]. A key advantage of using CMT lies in the spatial and temporal co-operation between the two modalities with regard to both dose-limiting normal tissue toxicity and to the tumor itself. At the cellular level, a major justification for the use of CMT protocols is that radiation and chemotherapy induce different DNA lesions (which are likely to be processed by different repair pathways) or have different cellular sites of action (e.g., microtubules in the case of vinca alkaloids and taxanes). At the simplest level, the assumption is that tumor cells that are *de novo* chemoresistant due to elevated detoxification/metabolizing enzymes are likely to retain sensitivity to radiation. This scenario is particularly pertinent to drugs that are substrates for P-glycoprotein as well as cyclophosphamide, hydroxyurea and 5-fluoruracil (5FU). Similarly, in those instances where tumor cells are chemoresistant due to elevated DNA repair pathways, these cells may still be sensitive to radiation because the lesions that are thought to be primarily responsible for radiation-induced cell death, i.e., DNA double strand breaks, are rarely induced by chemotherapy agents. Thus, in a tumor that is inherently chemoresistant or has undergone clonal drift during chemotherapy (i.e., is enriched for chemoresistant clones), the subsequent treatment of that tumor by radiotherapy should equally eliminate chemo-resistant and –sensitive clones. This hypothesis does not, however, take into consideration the possibility that the development of clinical chemoresistance might impact on radioresponsiveness at the cellular level either directly by modifying cellular radiosensitivity or indirectly by modifying the proliferation of tumor and normal cells.

2.2 Pre-clinical Studies on Independent Cell Killing by Radiation and Chemotherapeutic Agents

The above biological rationale for CMT protocols has been accepted for some time. Surprisingly, however, there have been few studies that have directly compared the inherent sensitivity of human tumor cells to chemotherapeutic agents and radiation. The most abundant data on the relationship between *de novo* cellular chemosensitivity and radiosensitivity is for cisplatin, which is probably a reflection of its widespread use in combination with radiation in the treatment of many solid tumors. Three major studies to date all suggest that *de novo* resistance to cisplatin does not confer any preferential resistance to radiation[3–5]. Importantly, p53 status did not seem to impact upon this relationship, because the same relationship was observed in a variety of human tumor cell lines of differing histologies and p53 status[3,5] and in 19 sub-cloned early-passage cervical cancer cell lines[4], all of which were HPV16 or 18 infected.

From a clinical perspective, even fewer studies have addressed the relative sensitivity of tumors to chemotherapy versus radiotherapy. An initial response to chemotherapy has been shown to predict for a good response to radiotherapy in head and neck tumors[6]. This may have a cellular basis, i.e., cellular chemosensitivity may be associated with cellular radiosensitivity. However, clinical radioresponsiveness has not been conclusively linked to the cellular radiosensitivity of head and neck tumor cells[7–9]. The hypoxic tumor sub-volume, on the other hand, *has* been significantly related to poor clinical radioresponsiveness[10]. There may therefore be a connection between good response to cisplatin and low incidence of hypoxia. Transient hypoxia exposure (24 h) leads to a 2-3 fold increase in cisplatin resistance in glioma cells[11]. Exactly why hypoxia induces this decrease in cisplatin cytotoxicity is not known; however, hypoxia does alter the expression of many genes, including the HAP1 repair endonuclease[12], and presumably other DNA repair enzymes. Moreover, in the clinical setting, tumors with a high hypoxic fraction are more likely to be poorly vascularized and thus will receive less total cisplatin than well-perfused (less hypoxic) tumors. The fact that hypoxic cells are not actively dividing *and* are exposed to lower drug doses is an ideal situation for the development of chemoresistance, which in some instances may adversely affect radiosensitivity. The ERCC1 nucleotide excision repair protein plays a major role in the repair of DNA-adducts induced by bi-functional alkylating agents[13]. In some studies, high *ERCC1* mRNA levels have been reported to correlate with poor clinical response to cisplatin-based chemotherapy[14,15]. Thus, tumors that fail cisplatin treatment are likely to be enriched with high-*ERCC1* expressing clones. An alternative explanation for the poor response of cisplatin-refractory tumors to subsequent radiotherapy may lie in the fact that ERCC1 impacts upon the hypoxic sensitivity of mammalian cells to radiation[16]. There is also some preliminary data to suggest that high *ERCC1* expression is related to a more aggressive (invasive) tumor phenotype[15].

There is little evidence that taxanes induce any cross-resistance to radiotherapy. In fact, *de novo* cellular resistance to the taxane paclitaxel (Taxol®) was reported to be associated with a radiosensitive phenotype[17]. This has been suggested to be due to the opposing impact that the ras/raf/MAPK signaling pathway has on cellular resistance to paclitaxel and radiation. Understanding the involvement of signal transduction pathways in determining chemo- or radio-responsiveness is still in its infancy (see chapter 5 in this volume by Drs. S. Grant and colleagues), but may need to be increasingly considered as signal transduction inhibitors, e.g., farnesyl transferase inhibitors[18], raf-1[19] and c-myc phosphorothioate[20] antisense oligomers, are used increasingly to treat chemo-refractory tumors. Importantly, it may be necessary to evaluate the radiosensitivity of tumor cells that are refractory to these signal transduction inhibitors as they may have up-regulated signaling pathways, and many of the above relationships may be completely altered in such cells.

2.3 Concomitant Chemotherapy and its Impact Upon Subsequent Radiation Response

The administration of concomitant chemotherapy with radiation treatment may be highly advantageous as the tumor can be exposed to more net cytotoxic insults (due to different dose limiting tissues for chemotherapy and radiotherapy). This in itself may prevent the emergence of resistant clones to either modality (assuming that there is no differential effect of radiation on chemo-resistant and -sensitive clones). Moreover, these protocols offer the possibility of synergism (supra-additive cell killing) due to the reported radiosensitizing properties of drugs such as cisplatin[21,22]. Another factor that is often overlooked is that exposure to drugs such as cisplatin can invoke an arrest of cycling cells that can last for up to 3 days[23,24]. Thus, the concomitant administration of cisplatin, or antimetabolite drugs such as hydroxyurea and 5FU, could substantially reduce the level of tumor cell repopulation between radiation fractions.

Although there have been many reports on the radiosensitizing properties of cisplatin in mammalian cells, only a small proportion of these have used human tumor cells[4,25-27]. Most of these studies reported little, if any, radiosensitization by cisplatin in human tumor cells. In one study, cisplatin was shown to differentially sensitize murine cells but not human tumor cells[26]. Clinically achievable cisplatin concentrations (1 μg/ml; a concentration determined in biopsy material) led to radiosensitization in only 21% of cervical cancer cell lines, and actually reduced the clinically relevant radiosensitivity (i.e., surviving fraction at 2 Gy, SF_2) in 57% of the cell lines. Moreover, clinically achievable cisplatin concentrations did not selectively radiosensitize hypoxic human cervical tumor cells[4].

The higher level of local control achieved by cisplatin/radiotherapy regimes over radiotherapy alone[28,29] is likely to be due to the independent cytotoxicity of each modality or to cisplatin-induced reduction in inter-fraction repopulation. It has been suggested[30] that the apparently superior patient survival rate following cisplatin/radiotherapy in cervical cancer[28,29] is due to the large percentage of patients whose radiotherapy lasted for more than 50 days even in the absence of cisplatin. Studies at the Princess Margaret Hospital in Toronto have shown that for every day over 40 days there is a 1% loss of survival (at 5 yr)[31]. When radiotherapy is prolonged beyond 40 days, there will be a considerably higher level of tumor cell repopulation and even accelerated repopulation[32]. The addition of cisplatin would both reduce the total number of clonogens and also the rate of repopulation, provided that the tumor was cisplatin sensitive. Cisplatin-containing CMT can realistically only be improved if it can be ascertained exactly how cisplatin is leading to improved patient survival.

Assessing the relevance of these *in vitro* findings in the clinical setting will depend on the ability to rapidly identify those patients whose tumors are cisplatin resistant. Should similar effects occur in the clinic, then the combination of cisplatin with radiotherapy might not be universally beneficial. Patients whose tumors are cisplatin resistant are unlikely to derive any additional tumor control benefits from the inclusion of cisplatin to their radiotherapy regimen, and could potentially experience *lower* control rates due to cisplatin-induced radioprotection[4]. A number of genetic markers of cisplatin resistance have been identified *in vitro*[14,15] as well as *in vivo*[33], and some form of molecular triage might be necessary for the prescription of cisplatin-based CMT to chemoresistant tumors. Perhaps more importantly, it may be necessary to identify those tumors that may be rendered *less* radioresponsive by prior exposure to cisplatin. In these instances, it may be more desirable to give cisplatin towards the end of radiotherapy to ensure maximum tumor eradication within the radiation field. *In vitro* studies suggest that as many as 52% of tumor cell lines may be less susceptible to radiation following a 3-h cisplatin exposure[4]. This reduction in radiosensitivity could be attributable to several factors. Cisplatin is known to be a potent inducer of several early-response genes[34–36], and it is possible that cisplatin exposure (which precedes irradiation by at least as 3 h) may invoke a radioprotective mechanism. Prolonged exposure to cisplatin commonly reduces the radiosensitivity of human tumor cells[37–49], which could reflect the rapid induction of some of the same mechanisms responsible for collateral radioresistance in cells with acquired cisplatin resistance. There has been at least one gene cloned, XRCC3, that when absent or mutated imparts hypersensitivity to both cisplatin and radiation[50]. Should this gene, or one of similar function, be an early response gene, there could clearly be a rapid reduction in radiosensitivity. A key step in the repair of DNA interstrand cross-links, such as those induced by cisplatin, is the formation of DSBs. This step appears to be a pre-requisite to a recombination phase of repair mediated by RAD52[23,51]. In yeast, these DSBs appear after about 1 h of drug exposure[51]. Thus, when radiation is administered following cisplatin exposure, DSB repair pathways may be up-regulated and thus able to process radiation-induced DSBs more effectively. Cisplatin-DNA adducts (especially DNA interstrand cross-links) inhibit the activity of DNA-PK[52], an important mediator of DSB repair. It is possible that there may be a compensatory up-regulation of DNA-PK activity/expression following the sequestration of DNA-PK to cisplatin adducts. Another DNA repair pathway that might be modified following short cisplatin exposures is an illegitimate recombination pathway that is suppressed following the induction of cisplatin resistance and collateral radioresistance[53]. The activity of this pathway is higher in radiosensitive than radioresistant tumor cells[54].

2.4 Neo-adjuvant Chemotherapy and its Impact Upon Subsequent Radiation Response

As discussed above, the spatial interactions of CMT (i.e., each modality acting at a different physical location within the body), combined with the different limiting normal tissue toxicities of the component modalities, suggest that neo-adjuvant chemotherapy with loco-regional radiotherapy could increase both distant and local tumor control. The use of neo-adjuvant chemotherapy is also believed to be advantageous because the chemotherapy-induced reduction of the tumor volume (clonogens) will reduce the number of tumor cells that are subject to radiobiological hypoxia, and thus improve response to radiotherapy.

Many clinicians prefer to administer chemotherapy prior to commencement of radiation therapy due to concerns about radiation-induced occlusions of tumor micro-vasculature and subsequent lack of penetration of chemotherapy into the tumor. However, there are many instances where neo-adjuvant chemotherapy is administered for non-biological reasons. For example, in health care systems where a centralized patient care system is not in place, chemotherapy may be administered prior to radiotherapy simply because of referral practices. Moreover, radiation is frequently used as a second-line treatment (in a palliative setting) for patients whose tumors have recurred following chemotherapy. It is still unclear if tumors become refractory to chemotherapy due to the emergence (out-growth) of inherently chemoresistant clones, or due to the induction of chemoresistance. However, given that a single short (3 h) exposure of tumor cells to cisplatin can reduce cellular radiosensitivity, the basic assumptions underlying combined modality therapies may not pertain to tumors that have been repeatedly exposed to high chemotherapy doses. If neo-adjuvant chemotherapy and the possible induction of drug resistance has any impact upon subsequent radiation response, it may be necessary to re-evaluate the use of elective neo-adjuvant chemotherapy and/or alter radiation scheduling or dose.

2.5 Chemoresistant Human Tumors Exhibit a Modified Radiation Response

Some clinical trials have suggested that patients treated with induction chemotherapy followed by radiation may have higher local recurrence rates[55–58] and lower survival rates[59] than those historically achieved by radiotherapy alone. In some trials this phenomenon can be explained by patients refusing to complete radiation treatment after experiencing chemotherapy-induced toxicity[59]. In others, the authors suggest that the higher local recurrence rate may be due to a reduced tumor cell radiosensitivity in those patients failing induction chemotherapy. Chemorefractory tumors may indeed have a reduced radioresponsiveness given that the induction of *in vitro* resistance to Adriamycin[37,60–67], vinca alkaloids[65,68], alkylating agents[37,60,69–71], cytosine arabinoside (Ara-C)[72] and cisplatin[37–49] is widely associated with the modulation of clinically relevant radiosensitivity in human tumor cell lines (Table 1). Collateral radioresistance is most frequently reported; however, this is by no means a universal phenomenon, and no change or even an increase in radiosensitivity has also been reported in some studies[44,73–77]. This apparently disparate modification of radiosensitivity following the induction of drug resistance is perhaps not surprising given the diverse mechanisms whereby a tumor cell can become resistant to a single drug. For example, the induction of cisplatin resistance in the 2780 ovarian cancer line is associated with altered drug uptake and detoxification[78,79] and aspects of DNA repair[53,80,81], as well as the uncharacterized DNA-damage tolerance phenomenon[82]. However, both the nature and extent to which radiosensitivity is modified following the induction of cisplatin resistance in 8 human cell lines could be predicted by the equation:

$$SF_2[cDDP] = SF_2[Wt] + (constant - SF_2[Wt])$$

–where $SF_2[Wt]$ denotes the SF_2 of the parental line prior to cisplatin exposure, and $SF_2[cDDP]$ denotes SF_2 of the cisplatin resistant cell line. In that study, a constant of 0.51 was observed[44]. This suggests that cell lines with an SF_2 less than 0.51 will become more resistant after cisplatin exposure, whereas cell lines whose initial radiosensitivity is greater than 0.51 will be rendered more radiosensitive. A similar analysis of the currently available clonogenic survival data (Table 1) indicates that such a relationship persists (P=0.0002) in a wide diversity of human tumor cell lines that have acquired chemoresistance (Figure 1), except that an SF_2 of 0.65 is the consensus transition point for drug-induced radioprotection. In tumor cells that have SF_2 values greater than this level of radiosensitivity, cisplatin resistance has little impact upon radiosensitivity, except in the RT112 cell line. However, it should be noted that cisplatin resistance in this cell line is associated with a monosomic chromosome 19[83], and thus potentially with a lower level of XRCC1 expression, which is associated with an increased radiosensitivity[84].

This relationship may explain the apparently disparate effects of the development of cisplatin resistance on radiosensitivity in different tumor cell lines, but more importantly it may have important ramifications for treatment outcome. There are, however, several reasons why it is dangerous to assume that the above phenomena occur *in vivo*. The frequency and severity of drug exposure and the level of *in vitro* cisplatin resistance are substantially different from the *in vivo* situation. Moreover, it is unclear if these radiomodifying processes occur within a time frame comparable to that over which induction chemotherapy schedules are administered (3-4 months). Furthermore, even in the comparatively controlled *in vitro* situation, with low levels of clonal heterogeneity and uniform drug exposure, varying levels of cisplatin resistance and collateral radioresistance can be induced[47]. However, ***if*** there is a differential modulation of radiosensitivity by cisplatin in radiosensitive versus radioresistant tumors in the clinical setting, patients with tumors that are ordinarily radioresponsive could undergo a significant reduction in radioresponsiveness if they were to receive cisplatin-based chemotherapy prior to irradiation. This hypothesis is indeed substantiated in some xenograft systems, where clinically relevant drug exposures do induce a diminished radioresponsiveness[67,85,86], although other studies suggest that *in vivo* drug treatment does not lead to the induction of radioresistance[87]. Unfortunately, it is not clear whether this is due to the inherent radiosensitivity of the tumor cells used. There is some circumstantial clinical evidence that also supports this hypothesis. Cisplatin given prior to radiotherapy leads to reduced radioresponsiveness in historically radioresponsive tumors, such as ovarian carcinoma[57], Hodgkin's disease[55], squamous cell carcinoma of the head and neck[56], and small cell lung cancer[58]. In such tumors, it may be desirable to administer drugs such as cisplatin towards the end of radiotherapy. In addition to preventing delays in the commencement of radiotherapy, the use of cisplatin treatment in the third week of radiotherapy, for example, may be additionally beneficial in suppressing accelerated repopulation between the radiation fractions. A more aggressive means of circumventing drug-induced radioresistance is the use of "sandwich" CMT, as proposed by Looney[88]. This regimen of alternating weeks of radiotherapy and chemotherapy was reported to be well tolerated and to lead to improved survival.

Table 1. Clinically-relevant radiosensitivity (SF_2) of tumor cells that have acquired chemoresistance.

Tumor type	Cell line	Drug	RI	SF_2[Wt]	SF_2[Res]	Reference
Bladder	RT112	cDDP	3.2	0.70	0.46	44
	"	MMC	ND	0.70	0.58	§
Breast	MCF7	L-PAM	3	0.30	0.44	60, 61
	"	Adr	?	0.30	0.66	60, 61
Breast (rat)	MATB13 762	L-PAM	10	0.44	0.55	61
Cervix adeno-carcinoma	HeLa	cDDP	1.7	0.49	0.56	44
Fibroblasts (hamster)	HA-1	cDDP	2.5	0.70	0.74	73
Gastric	AGS-6	L-PAM	50	0.55	0.6	70
Epidermoid of larynx	Hep2	cDDP	3.9	0.62	0.57	44
Head and neck (SCC)	TE3	cDDP	1.9	0.53	0.57	76
Leukemia (ALL)	CCRF-CEM	VLB	420	0.06	0.21	68
	"	MTX	ND	0.06	0.055	68
	"	Ara-C	852	0.41	0.7	72
	"	Ara-C	65	0.41	0.74	72
	"	Ara-C	4.3	0.41	0.66	72
	"	Ara-C	>1000	0.41	0.54	72
	"	Ara-C	>1000	0.41	0.69	72
	GM3639	VCR	159	0.66	0.31	75
Leukemia (CML)	KBM7	4-HC	20	0.13	0.38	90
Glioma	U373MG	cDDP	2.5	0.49	0.32	47
	"	cDDP	5	0.49	0.72	47
Glioma (rat)	9L	CENU	10	0.45	0.42	62
	"	CENU	21	0.45	0.77	62
	"	CENU	25	0.45	0.56	62
Ovarian	OAW42	L-PAM	3.6	0.26	0.47	71
	"	cDDP	7.6	0.26	0.62	41, 42
	"	cDDP	7.6	0.34	0.46	44
	A2780	L-PAM	10	0.27	0.60	37
	"	cDDP	10	0.27	0.57	37
	"	Adr	100	0.27	0.30	37
	"	cDDP	~7	0.24	0.68	48

Continued

	2780/WT	cDDP	5.3	0.38	0.48	44
	AOvC	cDDP	3.4	0.75	0.80	39
	"	cDDP	3.6	0.75	0.90	39
SCLC	SK3	cDDP	3.2	0.65	0.66	38
	MOA2	cDDP	2.2	0.87	0.90	38
	H322	cDDP	1.55	0.55	0.49	44
	NCI-H69	cDDP	5.3	0.38	0.35	40
	GLC4	Adr	8	0.15	0.31	64
	"	Adr	44	0.15	0.47	64
LCLC	COR-L23	cDDP	1.7	0.32	0.39	40, 44
Lung adeno-carcinoma	MOR	cDDP	1.9	0.40	0.62	40, 44

RI, resistance index; SF_2[Wt], SF_2 of parental cell line; SF_2[Res], SF_2 of drug-resistant variant; §Britten, unpublished data; SCC, squamous cell carcinoma, ALL, acute lymphocytic leukemia; CML, chronic myeloid leukemia; SCLC, small cell lung cancer, LCLC, large cell lung cancer; cDDP, cisplatin; MMC, mitomycin C; L-PAM, melphalan, Adr, Adriamycin, VLB, vinblastine; MTX, methotrexate; VCR, vincristine; 4HC, 4-hydroxyperoxycyclophosphamide; CENU, chloroethylnitrosourea.

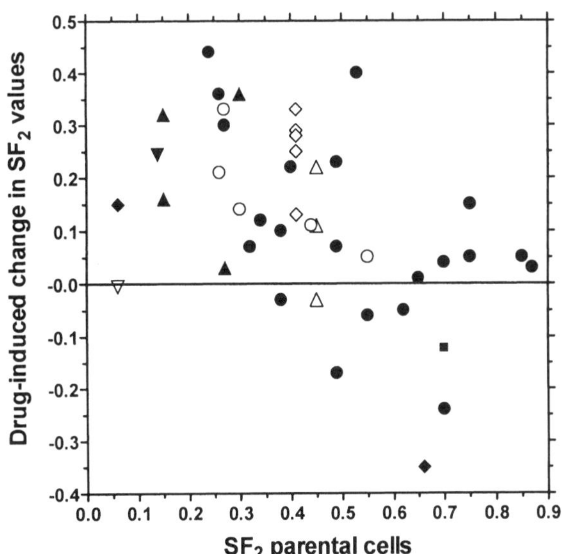

Figure 1. Modification of cellular radiosensitivity (SF_2) following the induction of resistance to cisplatin (●), melphalan (○), mitomycin C (■), Adriamycin (▲), CENU (Δ), 4HC (▼), vinca alkaloids (♦), methotrexate (∇) and Ara-C (◇).

Further improvements in the efficacy of CMT regimens may thus be accrued by careful consideration of how and when bi-functional alkylating agent-based chemotherapy is used in typically radioresponsive tumors. In some instances, this may require changes in chemotherapy scheduling with respect to radiotherapy administration. In other instances, a change in radiation dose might be necessary to obviate any drug-induced radioprotection. An example of the latter scenario is suggested by the work of Andersson and colleagues[89] on acquired cyclophosphamide resistance in CML. These investigators reported that 4HC-resistant CML cells were ~2 fold more resistant to clinically relevant radiation doses than chemotherapy-naïve cells[89]. Extrapolation of these data to the fractionated total body irradiation (TBI) schedules used in the clinic suggested that, when TBI is used as part of the pre-transplant conditioning therapy for allogeneic stem cell transplant for leukemia, there might be as much as a 2.5-log decrease in tumor clonogen eradication resulting from the TBI than would be anticipated in the absence of an effect of chemotherapy on tumor-cell radiosensitivity. It may therefore be necessary/desirable in some patients to administer an extra fraction of radiotherapy to obviate possible chemotherapy-induced collateral radioresistance. In addition, the sequence of delivery of drugs vs. radiotherapy may be important for treatment outcome, as exemplified by studies of Nielsen and colleagues[90] in a mouse model, where a greater level of bone marrow killing was achieved when cyclophosphamide was administered after rather than before the TBI, and this sequence had the additional benefit of being less toxic to the lung.

These concerns are of clinical relevance. Marrow-ablative chemo-radiotherapy followed by allogeneic stem cell transplantation has become a widely accepted treatment strategy for patients with CML; TBI is used as part of the pre-transplant conditioning therapy, aimed at both eliminating the majority of the leukemic cells and at paralyzing the patient's immune system, thus securing subsequent engraftment. The patients most commonly receive chemotherapy prior to TBI to achieve these goals. This approach has led to substantial advances in patient response and survival rates. However, despite these complex clinical manipulations, leukemia recurrence is a frequent event, both in CML and in other types of leukemia. The risk of recurrence is related to the dose of TBI used, and a (fractionated) total dose of 12-14 Gy is sufficient to eliminate the bulk of the leukemic cells in the majority of patients, especially in those who have early disease, such as CML in chronic phase or AML in first complete remission. Unfortunately, the occurrence of acute side effects limit TBI dose escalation above 14.5-15 Gy. For those patients who do not have access to a tissue-compatible donor, an autologous transplant can be considered.

In historically radioresistant tumors, the use of cisplatin/alkylating agent based chemotherapy prior to radiotherapy could be advantageous. The data in Figure 1 suggest that any residual or recurrent tumor following cisplatin treatment is unlikely to be more radioresistant and may even be more responsive to radiotherapy. An obvious concern in any CMT protocol is what impact altering the sequence of chemotherapy and radiotherapy has on the radiosensitivity of either acute or late reacting normal tissues. Given that the average SF_2 of primary human fibroblast cultures is in the range of 0.21 to 0.29[91,92], and assuming that the same relationship depicted in Figure 1 occurs in normal tissues, we could speculate that there may be radioprotection of these tissues. There are few reports of adverse radiotherapy-induced normal tissue complication with cisplatin-based CMT regimens irrespective of scheduling of the two modalities.

3. THE WAY FORWARD: INDIVIDUALIZED MOLECULAR PRESCRIPTION AND SCHEDULING?

The classic empirical approach to integrating CMT will ultimately be used to evaluate the clinical utility of any new innovations. However, it may now be the time to integrate drugs and radiation from a slightly different perspective. One new innovation that may circumvent the emergence of drug resistance and its subsequent impact upon radioresponsiveness is the use of electrochemotherapy. Early clinical studies suggest a higher response to cisplatin when locally applied electric pulses to melanoma tumors are used[93], and in pre-clinical animal studies the addition of electrotherapy improved the efficacy of cisplatin-based CMT[94].

Another new concept is the idea of molecular-based prescription and scheduling of CMT. A number of molecular determinants of cellular sensitivity to both chemotherapeutic agents and radiation have already been identified. The use of DNA microarrays and, in the future, proteomics, are likely to identify even more. Newly-available technologies, such as laser-dissection of histological section coupled with PCR or proteomics, now make it possible to determine if tumor chemorefractiveness is due to acquired chemoresistance or to the selection of inherently chemoresistant clones. Such studies will require sequential sampling of tumor cells during chemotherapy. Peritoneal lavage has been suggested as a safe and relatively non-invasive method of monitoring genetic/biochemical changes for ovarian cancer during chemotherapy[95], but repeat biopsies can be obtained from any tumor that is accessible with minimally-invasive methods such as endoscopes. Once these fundamental questions about the clinical history of chemorefractiveness have been addressed, it may then be possible to rationally integrate radiotherapy and chemotherapy to ensure maximum tumor cell eradication.

Irrespective of the exact nature of clinical chemoresistance, future improvements in the efficacy of combined modality therapy may only be possible if we take into consideration the dynamic nature of tumors undergoing therapy. Most investigations of response determinants are done prior to the commencement of any therapy. At that time there is likely to be a wide diversity of tumor clones present, only a small proportion of which may be important to the final outcome of the treatment. We[96] and others[97–99] have established that there is considerable intra-tumoral heterogeneity of radioresponsiveness in early passage tumor cell lines. A similar situation will almost certainly pertain to chemosensitivity. Using simple mathematical modeling, it was proposed that a clone whose initial abundance was 1% or lower could dominate the radioresponse of the tumor[96]. Thus, *a priori* molecular screening may have only a limited role in triaging patients, for example, in determining whether cisplatin should be used in the initial phases of radiotherapy for cervical cancer (see above). The most exciting use of molecular testing lies in tailoring treatment in the later stages of treatment with radiotherapy. This concept utilizes the likelihood that over the first few weeks of treatment there may be clonal drift, with a preferential enrichment of radioresistant clones (and chemoresistant clones if drugs are administered). Thus, by the 3rd/4th week of radiotherapy (or 3rd/4th cycle of chemotherapy), the clonal spectrum should be very different from the pre-treatment spectrum, and should more closely reflect the clonal composition that may persist at the end of the prescribed treatment. In those instances where repeat biopsies are easily acquired, it may be possible to determine the molecular profile of chemoresistance markers in week 3 of radiotherapy, and decide which, if any, chemotherapy should be used during the later stages of treatment. In addition to deciding whether a particular therapy should be continued to be administered, the principal advantages of this approach are: [1] the ability to switch to alternative chemotherapeutic agents before the tumor has developed full chemoresistance; and [2] to achieve a higher therapeutic ratio. The rationale for the greater therapeutic ratio lies in the fact that chemotherapy-induced normal tissue toxicity should remain constant irrespective of whether chemotherapy is administered early or late during the course of radiotherapy. However, it may be possible to use the changing molecular profile of the tumor during radiotherapy to derive a greater level of tumor cell kill (for the same level of normal tissue toxicity).

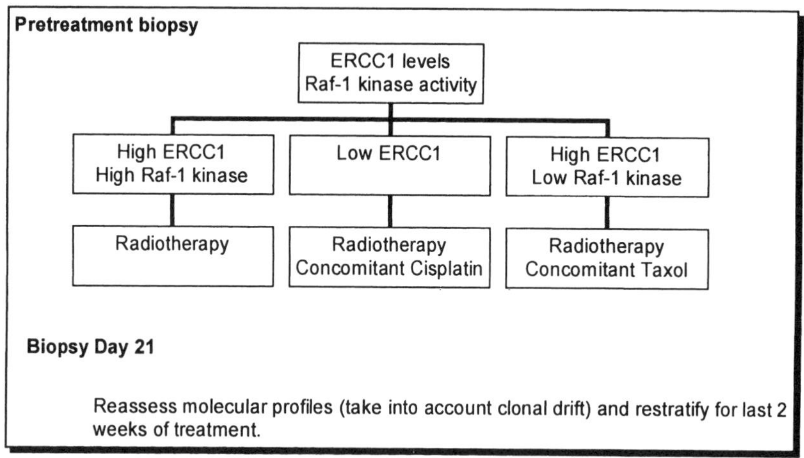

Figure 2. Possible molecular-based treatment decision tree for cancer of the uterine cervix.

Using cervical cancer as an example, it has been shown that Raf-1 is a marker of radiosensitivity[17]. Over the first few weeks of radiotherapy, where there will be a marked elimination of radiosensitive clones, there will theoretically be an increased abundance of low Raf-1 kinase expressing cells. Low Raf-1 kinase activity has been shown to be associated with a high level of paclitaxel cytotoxicity in cervical cancer cells[100]. Given the marked, but opposite, Raf-1 dependencies of radiation and paclitaxel cytotoxicity in cervical cancer, the administration of paclitaxel towards the end of, or after, radiotherapy could lead to a greater level of tumor cell kill than if it were administered earlier in the treatment schedule. The level of normal tissue morbidity outside the radiation field is likely to remain constant. Thus, drugs that have had a limited effectiveness as single agents in a given tumor site, such as paclitaxel in cervical cancer[101], may have an important role in CMT regimens. A potential treatment decision tree for cervical cancer might be along the lines schematically represented in Figure 2.

CONCLUSION

The use of "smart" (molecular directed) treatment planning/prescription may not be too avant garde to consider. Many tumor sites are amenable to repeat biopsy, and scientists have already identified several molecular markers of cellular response to chemotherapy and radiation. The proposed use of gene-chip technologies and proteomics approaches are likely to identify even more in the future. It should then be possible to assess the impact that clinical drug resistance has on radiation response and to employ the appropriate counter-measures to maximize the clinical utility of CMT, and perhaps to more easily ensure that chemotherapy is administered appropriately, i.e., so not to decrease the effectiveness of radiotherapy in tumors where radiotherapy is the treatment of choice.

REFERENCES

1. Tannock IF, Goldenberg GG. Drug resistance and experimental chemotherapy. *In*: The Basic Science of Oncology, 3rd edition, IF Tannock, RP Hill (eds.), McGraw-Hill, New York, NY, 392-419, 1998.
2. Steel GG, Peckham MJ. Exploitable mechanisms in combined radiotherapy-chemotherapy: the concept of additivity. Int J Radiat Oncol Biol Phys, 5:85-91, 1979.
3. Britten RA, Warenius HM. De novo cisplatinum resistance does not influence cellular radiosensitivity. Eur J Cancer, 29A:1315-1320, 1993.
4. Britten RA, Evans AJ, Allalunis-Turner MJ, Pearcey RG. Effect of cisplatin on the clinically relevant radiosensitivity of human cervical carcinoma cell lines. Int J Radiat Oncol Biol Phys, 34:367-374, 1996.
5. Warenius HM, Seabra LA, Maw P. Sensitivity to cis-diamminedichloroplatinum in human cancer cells is related to expression of cyclin D1 but not c-raf-1 protein. Int J Cancer, 67:224-231, 1996.
6. Panis X, Coninx P, Nguyen TD, Legros M. Relation between responses to induction chemotherapy and subsequent radiotherapy in advanced or multicentric squamous cell carcinomas of the head and neck. Int J Radiat Oncol Biol Phys, 18:1315-1318, 1990.
7. Bjork-Eriksson T, West C, Karlsson E, Mercke C. Tumor radiosensitivity (SF2) is a prognostic factor for local control in head and neck cancers. Int J Radiat Oncol Biol Phys, 46:13-19, 2000.
8. Eschwege F, Bourhis J, Girinski T, *et al.* Predictive assays of radiation response in patients with head and neck squamous cell carcinoma: a review of the Institute Gustave Roussy experience. Int J Radiat Oncol Biol Phys, 39:849-853, 1997.

9. Stausbol-Gron B, Overgaard J. Relationship between tumour cell *in vitro* radiosensitivity and clinical outcome after curative radiotherapy for squamous cell carcinoma of the head and neck. Radiother Oncol, 50:47-55, 1999.
10. Stadler P, Becker A, Feldmann HJ, *et al.* Influence of the hypoxic subvolume on the survival of patients with head and neck cancer. Int J Radiat Oncol Biol Phys, 44:749-754, 1999.
11. Liang BC. Effects of hypoxia on drug resistance phenotype and genotype in human glioma cell lines. J Neurooncol, 29:149-155, 1996.
12. Walker LJ, Craig RB, Harris AL, Hickson ID. A role for the human DNA repair enzyme HAP1 in cellular protection against DNA damaging agents and hypoxic stress. Nucleic Acids Res, 22:4884-4889, 1999.
13. Hoy CA, Thompson LH, Mooney CL, Salazar EP. Defective DNA cross-link removal in Chinese hamster cell mutants hypersensitive to bifunctional alkylating agents. Cancer Res, 45:1737-1743, 1985.
14. Dabholkar M, Vionnet J, Bostick-Bruton F, *et al.* Messenger RNA levels of XPAC and ERCC1 in ovarian cancer tissue correlate with response to platinum-based chemotherapy. J Clin Invest, 94:703-708, 1994.
15. Metzger R, Leichman CG, Danenberg KD, *et al.* ERCC1 mRNA levels complement thymidylate synthase mRNA levels in predicting response and survival for gastric cancer patients receiving combination cisplatin and fluorouracil chemotherapy. J Clin Oncol, 16:309-316, 1998.
16. Murray D, Macann A, Hanson J, Rosenberg E. ERCC1/ERCC4 5'-endonuclease activity as a determinant of hypoxic cell radiosensitivity. Int J Radiat Biol, 69:319-327, 1996.
17. Britten RA, Perdue S, Opoku J, Craighead P. Paclitaxel is preferentially cytotoxic to human cervical tumor cells with low Raf-1 kinase activity: implications for paclitaxel-based chemoradiation regimens. Radiother Oncol, 48:329-334, 1998.
18. Adjei AA, Erlichman C, Davis JN, *et al.* A phase I trial of the farnesyl transferase inhibitor SCH66336: evidence for biological and clinical activity. Cancer Res, 60:1871-1877, 2000.
19. Cunningham CC, Holmlund JT, Schiller JH, *et al.* A phase I trial of c-Raf kinase antisense oligonucleotide ISIS 5132 administered as a continuous intravenous infusion in patients with advanced cancer. Clin Cancer Res, 6:1626-1631, 2000.
20. Leonetti C, Biroccio A, Candiloro A, *et al.* Increase of cisplatin sensitivity by c-myc antisense oligodeoxynucleotides in a human metastatic melanoma inherently resistant to cisplatin. Clin Cancer Res, 5:2588-2595, 1999.
21. Dewit L. Combined treatment of radiation and cis-diamminechloroplatinum (II): A review of experimental and clinical data. Int J Radiat Oncol Biol Phys, 13:403-426, 1987.
22. Douple EB, Richmond RC. Platinum complexes as radiosensitizers of hypoxic mammalian cells. Br J Cancer, 37 Suppl III:98-102, 1978.
23. Sorenson CM, Eastman A. Mechanism of cis-diamminedichloroplatinum(II)-induced cytotoxicity: role of G2 arrest and DNA double-strand breaks. Cancer Res, 48:4484-4488, 1988.
24. Bergamo A, Gagliardi R, Scarcia V, *et al. In vitro* cell cycle arrest, *in vivo* action on solid metastasizing tumors, and host toxicity of the antimetastatic drug NAMI-A and cisplatin. Pharmacol Exp Ther, 289:559-564, 1999.
25. Yuhas JM, Tarleton AE, Culo F. Tumor line dependent interactions of irradiation and cis-diamminedichloroplatinum in the multicellular tumor spheroid system. Int J Radiat Oncol Biol Phys, 5:1373-1375, 1979.

26. Leith JT, Eun Sun Lee AB, Vayer AJ Jr, *et al.* Enhancement of the responses of human colon adenocarcinoma cells to X-irradiation and cis-platinum by n-methylformamide (NMF). Int J Radiat Oncol Biol Phys, 11:1971-1976, 1985.
27. Ziegler W, Kopp JM. The effect of combined treatment of HeLa cells with cisplatin and irradiation upon survival and recovery from radiation damage. Radiother Oncol, 8:71-78, 1987.
28. Morris M, Eifel PJ, Lu J, *et al.* Pelvic radiation with concurrent chemotherapy compared with pelvic and para-aortic radiation for high-risk cervical cancer. N Engl J Med, 340:1137-1143, 1999.
29. Rose PG, Bundy BN, Watkins EB, *et al.* Concurrent cisplatin-based radiotherapy and chemotherapy for locally advanced cervical cancer. N Engl J Med, 340:1144-1153, 1999.
30. Pearcey RG, Mohamed IG, Hanson J. Treatment of high-risk cervical cancer. N Engl J Med, 341:695-696, 1999.
31. Fyles A, Keane TJ, Barton M, Simm J. The effect of treatment duration in the local control of cervix cancer. Radiother Oncol, 25:273-279, 1992.
32. Withers HR, Taylor JMG, Maciejewski B. The hazard of accelerated tumor clonogen repopulation during radiotherapy. Acta Oncol, 27:131-146, 1988.
33. Britten RA, Liu D, Tessier A, *et al.* ERCC1 expression as a molecular marker of cisplatin resistance in human cervical tumor cells. Int J Cancer, 89:453-457, 2000.
34. Rubin E, Kharbanda S, Gunji H, *et al.* Cis-diamminedichloroplatinum (II) induces c-*jun* expression in human myeloid leukemia cells: Potential involvement of a protein kinase C-dependent signaling pathway. Cancer Res, 52:878-882, 1992.
35. Eliopoulos AG, Kerr DJ, Maurer HR, *et al.* Induction of the c-myc but not the cH-ras promoter by platinum compounds. Biochem Pharmacol, 50:33-38, 1995.
36. Hayakawa J, Ohmichi M, Kurachi H, *et al.* Inhibition of extracellular signal-regulated protein kinase or c-Jun N-terminal protein kinase cascade, differentially activated by cisplatin, sensitizes human ovarian cancer cell line. J Biol Chem, 274:31648-31654, 1999.
37. Louie KG, Behrens BC, Kinsella TJ, *et al.* Radiation survival parameters of antineoplastic drug-sensitive and -resistant human ovarian cell lines and their modification by buthionine sulfoximine. Cancer Res, 45:2110-2115, 1985.
38. Hida T, Ueda R, Takahashi T, *et al.* Chemosensitivity and radiosensitivity of small cell lung cancer cell lines studied by a newly developed 3-(4,5-dimethylthiazol-2-yl)-2,5-diphenyltetrazolium bromide (MTT) hybrid assay. Cancer Res, 49:4785-4790, 1999.
39. De Pooter CM, Scalliet PG, Elst HJ, *et al.* Resistance patterns between cis-diamminedichloroplatinum(II) and ionizing radiation. Cancer Res, 51:4523-4527, 1991.
40. Twentyman PR, Wright KA, Rhodes T. Radiation response of human lung cancer cells with inherent and acquired resistance to cisplatin. Int J Radiat Oncol Biol Phys, 20:217-220, 1991.
41. Britten RA, Warenius HM, White R, Peacock JH. BSO-induced reduction of glutathione levels increases the cellular radiosensitivity of drug-resistant human tumor cells. Int J Radiat Oncol Biol Phys, 22:769-772, 1992.
42. Britten RA, Peacock JH, Warenius HM. Collateral resistance to photon and neutron irradiation is associated with acquired *cis*-platinum resistance in human ovarian tumour cells. Radiother Oncol, 23:170-175, 1992.
43. Britten RA, Warenius HM, Masters JRW, Peacock JH. The differential induction of collateral resistance to 62.5 MeV ($p \rightarrow Be^{+}$) neutrons and 4 MeV photons by exposure to *cis*-platinum. Int J Radiat Oncol Biol Phys, 26:837-843, 1993.

44. Britten RA, Warenius HM, Carraway AV, Murray D. Differential modulation of radiosensitivity following induction of *cis*-platinum resistance in radio-sensitive and –resistant human tumour cells. Radiat Oncol Invest, 2:25-31, 1994.
45. Poppenborg H, Munstermann G, Knupfer MM, *et al.* C6 cells cross-resistant to cisplatin and radiation. Anticancer Res, 17:2073-2077, 1997.
46. Poppenborg H, Munstermann G, Knupfer MM, *et al.* Cisplatin induces radioprotection in human T98G glioma cells. Anticancer Res, 17:1131-1134, 1997.
47. Raaphorst GP, Wilkins DE, Mao JP, *et al.* Evaluation of cross-resistance between responses to cisplatin, hyperthermia, and radiation in human glioma cells and eight clones selected for cisplatin resistance. Radiat Oncol Invest, 7:153-157, 1999.
48. Raaphorst GP, Maio J, Ng CE, Stewart DJ. Concomitant treatment with mild hyperthermia, cisplatin and low dose-rate irradiation in human ovarian cancer cells sensitive and resistant to cisplatin. Oncol Rep, 5:971-977, 1998.
49. Frit P, Canitrot Y, Muller C, *et al.* Cross-resistance to ionizing radiation in a murine leukemic cell line resistant to cis-dichlorodiammineplatinum(II): role of Ku autoantigen. Mol Pharmacol, 56:141-146, 1999.
50. Tebbs RS, Zhao Y, Tucker JD, *et al.* Correction of chromosomal instability and sensitivity to diverse mutagens by a cloned cDNA of the XRCC3 DNA repair gene. Proc Natl Acad Sci USA, 92:6354-6358, 1995.
51. McHugh PJ, Sones WR, Hartley JA. Repair of intermediate structures produced at DNA interstrand cross-links in Saccharomyces cerevisiae. Mol Cell Biol, 20:3425-3433, 2000.
52. Turchi JJ, Patrick SM, Henkels KM. Mechanism of DNA-dependent protein kinase inhibition by cis-diammine-dichloroplatinum(II)-damaged DNA. Biochem, 36:7586-7593, 1997.
53. Britten RA, Kuny S, Perdue S. Modification of non-conservative double-strand break (DSB) rejoining activity after the induction of cisplatin resistance in human tumour cells. Br J Cancer, 79:843-849, 1999.
54. Britten RA, Liu D, Kuny S, Allalunis-Turner MJ. Differential level of DSB repair fidelity effected by nuclear protein extracts derived from radiosensitive and radioresistant human tumour cells. Br J Cancer, 76:1440-1447, 1997.
55. Johnson RE, Brace KC. Radiation response of Hodgkin's disease recurrent after chemotherapy. Cancer, 19:368-370, 1966.
56. Ensley JF, Jacobs JR, Weaver A, *et al.* Correlation between response to cis-platinum-combination chemotherapy and subsequent radiotherapy in previously untreated patients with advanced squamous cell cancers of the head and neck. Cancer, 54:811-814, 1984.
57. Hoskins WJ, Lichter AS, Wittington R, *et al.* Whole abdominal and pelvic irradiation in patients with minimal and residual disease at second-look surgical reassessment for ovarian carcinoma. Gynecol Oncol, 20:271-280, 1985.
58. Ochs JJ, Tester WJ, Cohen MH, *et al.* "Salvage" radiation therapy for intrathoracic small cell carcinoma of the lung progressing on combination chemotherapy. Cancer Treat Rep, 67:1123-1126, 1988.
59. Tattershall MHN, Ramirez C, Coppleson M. A randomized trial comparing platinum-based chemotherapy followed by radiotherapy vs. radiotherapy alone in patients with locally advanced cervical cancer. Int J Gynecol Cancer, 2:244-251, 1992.
60. Lehnert S, Greene D, Batist G. Radiation response of drug-resistant variants of a human breast cancer cell line. Radiat Res, 118:568-580, 1989.
61. Lehnert S, Greene D, Batist G. Radiation response of drug-resistant variants of a human breast cancer cell line: The effect of glutathione depletion. Radiat Res, 124:208-215, 1990.

62. Saito Y, Nakada Y, Hotta T, *et al.* Glutathione and cellular response of ACNU-resistant rat glioma sublines to drugs and radiation. Int J Cancer, 48:861-865, 1991.
63. Lau DH, Lewis AD, Ehsan MN, Sikic BI. Multifactorial mechanisms associated with broad cross-resistance of ovarian carcinoma cells selected by cyanomorpholino doxorubicin. Cancer Res, 51:181-187, 1991.
64. Meijer C, Mulder NH, Timmer-Bosscha H, *et al.* Role of free radicals in an adriamycin-resistant human small cell lung cancer cell line. Cancer Res, 47:4613-4617, 1987.
65. Pauwels O, Gozy M, Van Houtte P, *et al.* Cross resistance and collateral sensitivity between cytotoxic drugs and radiation in two human bladder cell lines. Radiother Oncol, 39:81-86, 1996.
66. Denecke J, Fiedler K, Hacker-Klom U, *et al.* Multiple drug-resistant C6 glioma cells cross-resistant to irradiation. Anticancer Res, 17:4531-4534, 1997.
67. Budach W, Budach V, Scheulen ME, *et al.* Drug- and radiation-induced resistance in a human neurogenic sarcoma xenografted in nude mice. Cancer Chemother Pharmacol, 31 Suppl 2:S169-173, 1993.
68. Shimm DS, Olson S, Hill AB. Radiation resistance in a multidrug resistant human T-cell leukemia line. Int J Radiat Oncol Biol Phys, 15:931-936, 1988.
69. Lehnert S, Vestergaard J, Batist G, Alaoui-Jamali MA. Radiation resistance in a melphalan-resistant subline of a rat mammary carcinoma. Radiat Res, 139:232-239, 1994.
70. Barranco SC, Townsend CM Jr, Weintraub B, *et al.* Changes in glutathione content and resistance to anticancer agents in human stomach cancer cells induced by treatments with melphalan *in vitro*. Cancer Res, 50:3614-3618, 1990.
71. Britten RA, Warenius HM, White R, *et al.* Melphalan resistant human ovarian tumour cells are cross-resistant to photons, but not to high LET neutrons. Radiother Oncol, 18:357-367, 1990.
72. Martin-Aragon S, Mukherjee SK, Taylor BJ, *et al.* Cytosine arabinoside (ara-C) resistance confers cross-resistance or collateral sensitivity to other classes of anti-leukemic drugs. Anticancer Res, 20:139-150, 2000.
73. Wallner KE, Li GC. Effect of cisplatin resistance on cellular radiation response. Int J Radiat Oncol Biol Phys, 13:587-591, 1987.
74. Poppenborg H, Knupfer MM, Preiss R, *et al.* Cisplatin (CDDP)-induced radiation resistance is not associated with CDDP resistance in 86HG39 and A172 malignant glioma cells. Eur J Cancer, 35:1150-1154, 1999.
75. Cho J, Lee Y, Lutzky J, *et al.* Collateral sensitivity to radiation and cis-platinum in a multidrug-resistant human leukemia cell line. Cancer Chemother Pharmacol, 37:168-172, 1995.
76. Komori K. Cross-resistance to radiation in human squamous cell carcinoma cells with induced cisplatin resistance. Kokubyo Gakkai Zasshi, 65:202-212, 1998.
77. Oshita F, Fujiwara Y, Saijo N. Radiation sensitivities in various anticancer-drug-resistant human lung cancer cell lines and mechanism of radiation cross-resistance in a cisplatin-resistant cell line. J Cancer Res Clin Oncol, 119:28-34, 1992.
78. Batist G, Behrens BC, Makuch R, *et al.* Serial determinations of glutathione levels and glutathione-related enzyme activities in human tumor cells *in vitro*. Biochem Pharmacol, 35:2257-2259, 1986.
79. Scanlon KJ, Kashani-Sabet M. Elevated expression of thymidylate synthase cycle genes in cisplatin-resistant human ovarian carcinoma A2780 cells. Proc Natl Acad Sci USA, 85:650-653, 1988.

80. Parker RJ, Eastman A, Bostick-Bruton F, Reed E. Acquired cisplatin resistance in human ovarian cancer cells is associated with enhanced repair of cisplatin-DNA lesions and reduced drug accumulation. J Clin Invest, 87:772-777, 1991.
81. Masuda H, Tanaka T, Matsuda H, Kusaba I. Increased removal of DNA-bound platinum in a human ovarian cancer cell line resistant to *cis*-diamminedichloroplatinum(II). Cancer Res, 50:1863-1866, 1990.
82. Johnson SW, Perez RP, Godwin AK, *et al.* Role of platinum-DNA adduct formation and removal in cisplatin resistance in human ovarian cancer cell lines. Biochem Pharmacol, 47:689-697, 1994.
83. Walker MC, Povey S, Parrington JM, *et al.* Development and characterization of cisplatin-resistant human testicular and bladder tumour cell lines. Eur J Cancer, 26:742-747, 1990.
84. Thompson LH, Rubin JS, Cleaver JE, *et al.* A screening method for isolating DNA repair-deficient mutants of CHO cells. Somatic Cell Genet, 6:391-405, 1980.
85. Wurschmidt F. Combined modality treatment of the rhabdomyosarcoma R1H of the rat: influence of sequence of cisplatin and fractionated irradiation. Int J Radiat Oncol Biol Phys, 25:73-78, 1993.
86. Jackel M, Tausch-Treml R, Kopf-Maier P. Effect of acquired cisplatin resistance on the response of a xenografted human hypopharynx carcinoma to concurrent radiochemotherapy with cisplatin. Laryngoscope, 104:329-334, 1994.
87. Mattern J, Bak M Jr, Hoever KH, Volm M. Radiosensitivity of drug-resistant human tumour xenografts. Strahlenther Onkol, 165:870-872, 1989.
88. Looney WB. Alternating chemotherapy and radiotherapy. NCI Monogr, 6:85-94, 1988.
89. Andersson BS, Mroue M, Britten RA, *et al.* Mechanisms of cyclophosphamide resistance in a human myeloid leukemia cell line. Acta Oncol, 34:247-251, 1995.
90. Nielsen OS, Safwat A, Overgaard J. The effect of sequence and time interval between cyclophosphamide and total body irradiation on lung and bone marrow damage following bone marrow transplantation in mice. Radiother Oncol, 29:51-59, 1993.
91. Geara FB, Peters LJ, Ang KK, *et al.* Intrinsic radiosensitivity of normal human fibroblasts and lymphocytes after high- and low-dose-rate irradiation. Cancer Res, 52:6348-6352, 1992.
92. Dahlberg WK, Little JB, Fletcher JA, *et al.* Radiosensitivity *in vitro* of human soft tissue sarcoma cell lines and skin fibroblasts derived from the same patients. Int J Radiat Biol, 63:191-198, 1993.
93. Sersa G, Stabuc B, Cemazar M, *et al.* Electrochemotherapy with cisplatin: clinical experience in malignant melanoma patients. Clin Cancer Res, 6:863-867, 2000.
94. Sersa G, Kranjc S, Cemazar M. Improvement of combined modality therapy with cisplatin and radiation using electroporation of tumors. Int J Radiat Oncol Biol Phys, 46:1037-1041, 2000.
95. Fujiwara K, Yamauchi H, Yoshida T, *et al.* Relationship between peritoneal washing cytology through implantable port system (IPS-cytology) and second-look laparotomy in ovarian cancer patients with unmeasurable residual diseases. Gynecol Oncol, 70:231-235, 1998.
96. Britten RA, Evans AJ, Allalunis-Turner MJ, *et al.* Intratumoral heterogeneity as a confounding factor in clonogenic assays for tumour radioresponsiveness. Radiother Oncol, 39:145-153, 1996.
97. Leith JT, Dexter DL, DeWyngaert JK, *et al.* Differential responses to x-irradiation of subpopulations of two heterogeneous human carcinomas *in vitro*. Cancer Res, 42:2556-2561, 1982.

98. Tofilon PJ, Vines CM, Meyn RE, *et al.* Heterogeneity in radiation sensitivity within human primary tumour cell cultures as detected by the SCE assay. Br J Cancer, 59:54-60, 1989.
99. Weichselbaum RR, Beckett MA, Dahlberg W, Dritschilo A. Heterogeneity of radiation response of a parent human epidermoid carcinoma cell line and four clones. Int J Radiat Oncol Biol Phys, 14:907-912, 1988.
100. Rasouli-Nia A, Liu D, Perdue S, Britten RA. High Raf-1 kinase activity protects human tumor cells against paclitaxel-induced cytotoxicity. Clin Cancer Res, 4:1111-1116, 1998.
101. Kudelka AP, Winn R, Edwards CL, *et al.* Activity of paclitaxel in advanced or recurrent squamous cell cancer of the cervix. Clin Cancer Res, 2:1285-1288, 1996.

Chapter 15

CLINICAL PHARMACOLOGY OF MELPHALAN AND ITS IMPLICATIONS FOR CLINICAL RESISTANCE TO ANTICANCER AGENTS

Roy B. Jones
Bone Marrow Transplant Program, University of Colorado Health Science Center, Denver, Colorado, USA

1. INTRODUCTION

Melphalan (L-phenylalanine mustard, Alkeran®) was one of the first bifunctional alkylating agents developed for anticancer use. The initial synthesis was reported by Bergel and Stock[1]. Its design was an outgrowth of studies performed during and following World War II on the mechanisms of mustard gas effects on biological systems. A summary of these early studies by Philips[2] is of historical interest; it also serves as a model description of cancer drug development based upon evaluation of molecules observed to have antitumor effects as a result of empiric observation and congener synthesis.

The chemical structure of melphalan is shown in Figure 1. The bis 2-chlorethylamine functional group is the critical alkylating component of the molecule. For many years melphalan was available for human use only as 2-mg tablets. The approval of an intravenous (i.v.) formulation by the Food and Drug Administration in 1992 has allowed the use of higher doses appropriate for hematopoietic stem cell transplantation. The i.v. formulation is unstable, however, and even admixtures in 0.9% saline decompose at the rate of 1% every 10 minutes. This instability effectively prohibits the study of prolonged infusions of drug and hinders storage of blood fractions containing drug for bulk analysis. A recent report on the use of melphalan formulated in 3% saline[3] and a subsequent clinical trial of melphalan given by 24 h continuous infusion[4] should allow exploration of prolonged infusion schedules. In spite of these difficulties, i.v. melphalan is finding increasing use for high-dose therapy.

Melphalan is a structural analog of the amino acid phenylalanine. The vague structural similarity of the phenyl group to the isopropyl group of leucine permits cellular uptake by the same amino acid carrier. Melphalan is much less water-soluble than leucine, however. At near neutral pH, moderate solubility is limited to small molecular weight alcohols (methanol, ethanol). Melphalan stability can be enhanced by acidification of the solvent. At low concentrations in water or plasma, melphalan is non-enzymatically hydrolyzed to mono- and di-hydroxyethylamine derivatives[5]. These compounds have minimal antitumor activity[6] and can be ignored for purposes of pharmacodynamic analysis.

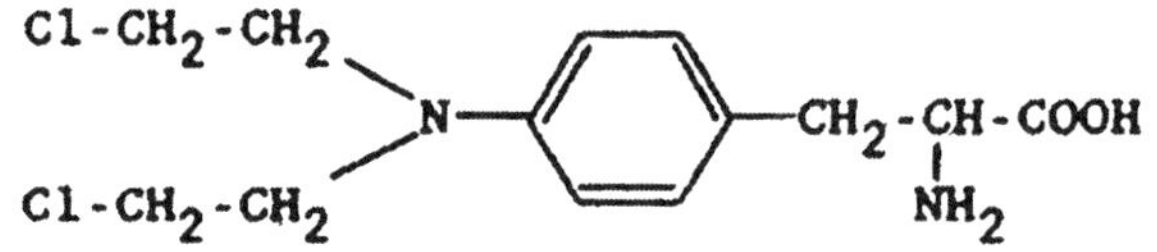

Figure 1. Melphalan.

The extent of protein binding of melphalan is unclear, with reports varying widely from 20%[7] to 90%[8]. Several binding proteins have been identified, including albumin, α-1-acid glycoprotein[8] and metallothionein[9]. The fraction of the binding that is covalent vs. reversible is also a matter of controversy. These topics, and the extent of binding to whole blood cells, require further study.

2. PHARMACOKINETICS AND EXTRACELLULAR PHARMACOLOGY

2.1 Metabolism and Elimination

In plasma, melphalan is non-enzymatically hydrolyzed to mono- and di-hydroxyethylamine derivatives (Figure 2). These derivatives are essentially inactive and are eliminated over several days[10]. A glutathione (GSH) conjugate has been identified[11], consistent with the known role of glutathione-

S-transferase (GST)-mediated melphalan detoxification in tumor cells. Others have reported minimal or no GSH conjugation in isolated, perfused human liver[12]. No metabolites other than those described have been identified, and thus metabolism is felt to play a minor role in melphalan elimination. Both hydrolysis and tissue alkylation are non-rate limited processes and should proceed at a predictable linear rate of elimination independent of drug concentration.

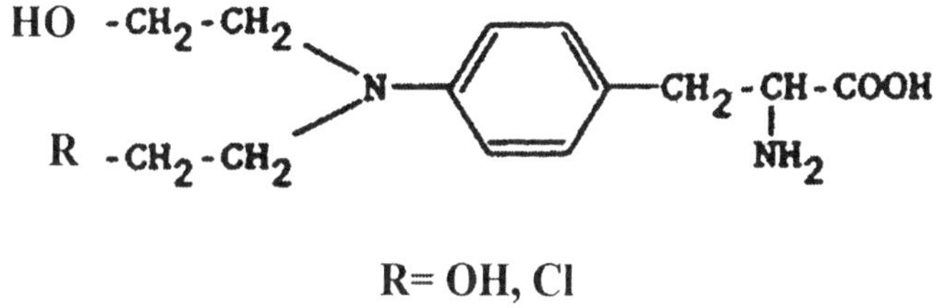

$$HO-CH_2-CH_2 \diagdown N-C_6H_4-CH_2-CH(NH_2)-COOH$$
$$R-CH_2-CH_2 \diagup$$

R= OH, Cl

Figure 2. Mono- and di-hydroxy melphalan.

While 20-35% of orally-administered melphalan has been reported to be excreted in the urine unchanged[7], two other studies report that the pharmacokinetics (PK) of melphalan is minimally changed[13] or not changed at all[14] in patients with moderate-severe renal failure. This suggests that hydrolysis and tissue alkylation are so rapid that urinary excretion of the drug is clinically unimportant. It seems that melphalan can be administered safely and in full dose to patients with severe degrees of renal or hepatic failure.

2.1.1 Oral administration

2.1.1.1 Absorption

The bioavailability of orally administered melphalan varies from 30-100%[15] and gastrointestinal absorption is decreased up to 39% by previously ingested food[16,17]. Taking the drug in the fasted state reduces the variability in absorption[16]. In addition to variability in the extent of absorption, there is considerable variability in the lag time of absorption from minutes to 4 h[18-20]. Leucine or glutamine can inhibit the absorption of oral melphalan by almost 20%, suggesting that this may be an active transport process[8,17,21,22].

Cimetidine, which reduces gastric acidity, can produce a 30% decrease in melphalan absorption[23]. Since it is clear that melphalan is more stable at lower pH, this could be explained by increased instability of melphalan at the higher gastric and upper intestinal pH's produced by cimetidine.

2.1.1.2 Pharmacokinetics

Both the maximal plasma concentration (C_{max}) and area under the plasma concentration vs. time curve (AUC) vary by 2-4 fold between patients following a 10 mg oral dose[20], with C_{max} averaging ~100 ng/ml and the elimination half-life ($T_{½}$-elim) being ~1 h. Choi *et al.*[24] evaluated the use of high-dose oral melphalan as part of a three-drug bone marrow transplant conditioning regimen. The melphalan was administered daily for three days. There was a 6-fold variability in PK parameters between patients and a trend towards lower C_{max} and AUC but stable $T_{½}$-elim for the third dose compared to the first two doses. These observations suggest impaired absorption, perhaps because the third dose was given simultaneously with high doses of cyclophosphamide and thiotepa. These drugs produce gastrointestinal injury, and perhaps transient decrease gastric acid production. Irrespective of mechanism, the high variability in PK parameters observed in this study and subsequently verified by others[25] suggest the desirability of i.v. melphalan when melphalan is used in high-dose therapy.

2.1.2 Intravenous administration

At conventional doses (<30 mg/m^2) a $T_{½}$-elim of 30-60 min and a volume of distribution (Vd) approximating total body water[26] were observed.

The vast majority of i.v. melphalan PK studies have been performed after short infusions (10-60 min) and following high doses (>100 mg/m^2). At these high doses, the AUC and C_{max} tend to increase linearly with dose. The $T_{½}$-elim in most reports has varied from 20-80 min[20,27–31], consistent with lower dose studies as linear PK would predict. These studies variously report a 2-10 fold range of AUC with identical doses, but the majority show a 3-4 fold variation. The etiology of this variation is unclear, but seems unlikely to relate to PK assay methodology.

Because of this AUC variation, Ardiet and colleagues have evaluated the use of a small test dose of melphalan administered prior to either conventional[32] or high-dose[33] melphalan. The therapeutic dose could be adjusted based upon the test dose AUC to produce more uniform drug exposure in either setting. In both cases the method proved feasible and reliable.

Regional administration of melphalan has been studied using both intraperitoneal[34] and isolated limb perfusion[35] methods. In both cases, a 1-2 log differential between regional and systemic melphalan concentrations was noted.

Tranchand *et al.*[36] reported that pretreatment with carboplatin produces wide variability in melphalan PK compared to administration of the same dose of melphalan prior to carboplatin. The cause of this apparent drug-drug interaction is unclear, but in the absence of important metabolism or renal excretion, an interaction at the level of protein binding seems possible. Little additional data has been reported concerning i.v. melphalan drug-drug PK interactions.

3. PHARMACODYNAMICS AND CELLULAR PHARMACOLOGY

Melphalan enters cells primarily through a neutral amino acid active transport pathway which is shared by leucine[37]. *In vitro* studies have demonstrated that high concentrations of leucine can inhibit cellular uptake of melphalan[38], an observation which may have clinical relevance. Melphalan efflux from cells is governed, in part, by the multi-drug resistance (MDR) transport mechanism[39].

At physiologic pH, melphalan spontaneously forms a positively charged aziridinium reactive species which can covalently bind (alkylate) any one of a variety of cellular molecules. These molecules usually contain functional groups with partial negative charge, and particularly contain oxygen, nitrogen, phosphorus, or sulfur atoms with free electron pairs. This would include binding to any structural or functional component of the cell, including the cell membrane and its components[40]. For most alkylating agents, including melphalan, definitive evidence as to what alkylation product (or combination of products) are primarily responsible for toxic or therapeutic effects is lacking.

Because alkylation of a multiplicity of targets is the predominant mode of cytotoxicity, the antitumor effects of melphalan are cell cycle non-specific, a desirable characteristic for drugs used as a single high-dose treatment with hematopoietic stem cell transplantation.

3.1 DNA Alkylation

The major focus of studies of intracellular alkylation products of melphalan has been DNA, primarily because DNA plays a central role in cellular function and replication. The predominant site of alkylation is believed to be the N-7 position of guanine[41,42], but alkylation of adenine (particularly at N-3)[43] and the O-4 position of thymidine are frequently noted.

Both mono-alkylation products and inter- and intrastrand crosslinks can be produced and correlate in certain situations with cytotoxicity and mutagenesis. The mono-alkylation products tend to form rapidly, followed by slower development of crosslinks[44]. In addition, crosslinks between DNA and proteins involved in DNA synthesis and repair have been reported.

3.2 Glutathione (GSH) Binding

GSH is a low molecular weight tripeptide with a free sulfhydryl group present in millimolar concentrations intracellularly. Its major function is believed to be neutralization of reactive, positively-charged toxins (such as alkylating agents). Several groups have described binding of melphalan to GSH[45–47], consistent with this hypothesis. Other observers have noted a lack of GSH binding in normal tissues such as the liver[48] and blood cells[49] under clinical conditions. The latter data cast doubt on the role of GSH in modulating melphalan toxic effects in patients. This question deserves further study and clarification.

4. CLINICAL USE

4.1 Antitumor Activity

Like most alkylating agents, melphalan has a broad spectrum of antitumor activity. Especially when given at high dose, melphalan has demonstrated activity in breast, lung, colon, testis, ovarian, stomach, and renal cancers and in melanoma, sarcoma, myeloma, lymphoma, and leukemia; a variety of pediatric solid tumors have also been noted to respond[50].

The use of oral melphalan has declined in the last 20 years. In contrast, i.v. melphalan use has increased since the early 1990s when it first became available in the U.S. The major application for this drug is its use in high-dose therapy with hematopoietic stem cell support. As a single agent, it has become a standard for the treatment of myeloma[51]. Double doses of melphalan are being used to explore the concept of tandem transplantation[52].

Melphalan is frequently used in combination with other agents for relapsed or high-risk pediatric solid tumors[53]. Preliminary investigations of melphalan alone or in combination therapy for pediatric acute leukemia[54,55] have been conducted.

The BEAM regimen is now a standard approach for relapsed non-Hodgkins lymphomas[56]. Recently, high-dose melphalan as a single agent has been explored in ovarian cancer[57,58]. Ayash *et al.*[59] and Bitran *et al.*[60] have explored the use of high-dose melphalan for metastatic breast cancer, either preceding or following cyclophosphamide/thiotepa-based high-dose chemotherapy, with highly promising preliminary results. Longer follow-up of these latter studies will be of considerable interest.

The increasing use of melphalan coincides with emerging data questioning the desirability of the use of high-dose cyclophosphamide. In many chemotherapy regimens, melphalan serves as a substitute for cyclophosphamide. Among cyclophosphamide's undesirable features is that it is a prodrug, which requires cytochrome (P-450) activation in the liver to attain its antitumor effects. This activation is saturable at higher doses, is subject to modulation by drug-drug interactions at the P-450 level, and is rapidly auto-inducible. All of these factors vary unpredictably between patients and from day to day in multi-day regimens, making reproducible cyclophosphamide delivery virtually impossible[61]. Because melphalan is not metabolized, hydrolyzes at a somewhat predictable rate, and does not require bioactivation, the above-mentioned concerns about cyclophosphamide are not as relevant, and melphalan may become a more attractive substitute for cyclophosphamide in the future.

4.2 Toxicities

At high doses with hematopoietic stem cell support, the most common dose-limiting toxicity of melphalan is oroesophageal mucositis. This toxicity commonly limits single-agent dose escalation to less than 220 mg/m^2. Phillips *et al.*[62] recently reported preliminary data describing pretreatment of patients with amifostine for cytoprotection, followed by a short melphalan infusion. This maneuver has allowed escalation of melphalan to 300 mg/m^2 with only moderate mucositis[62]. Since amifostine does not attenuate antitumor effects in other studies, this approach may allow use of higher doses of melphalan or use of full single-agent dose in multi-drug regimens with greater safety. Further data from this study will be of high interest.

In addition to mucositis, the other gastrointestinal toxicities of nausea, vomiting, and diarrhea are frequently seen but infrequently dose limiting. Hepatic veno-occlusive disease (VOD) is occasionally noted with single agent therapy. When melphalan is added to multi-drug regimens, however, it is likely that it can contribute to higher rates of VOD[63,64]. Further pulmonary toxicity is occasionally noted with melphalan[65], so this, too, must be a concern when melphalan is added to multi-drug regimens containing other known pulmonary toxins.

Other recognized toxicities of alkylating agents, including gonadal dysfunction, alopecia, teratogenesis/mutagenesis, and immunosuppression, will not be discussed further here.

When melphalan is used without hematopoietic stem cell support, myelosuppression is the most common dose-limiting toxicity. Chronic oral dosing with melphalan has been associated with an increased risk of secondary leukemia[66], but others have observed that secondary leukemia after high-dose melphalan may more closely relate to the cumulative amount of chemotherapy given prior to the transplant[67].

5. ANTITUMOR RESISTANCE MECHANISMS

Evaluation of mechanisms by which tumor cells develop resistance to melphalan is complex and requires a preliminary review of the pharmacology of the drug. Theoretically, resistance could develop through perturbation of any of the pharmacologic pathways affecting melphalan absorption, distribution, cell membrane penetration, intracellular distribution, binding, metabolism, or drug elimination. The issue becomes even more complex in view of the multiplicity of cellular targets for melphalan binding. This review will ignore factors that might influence melphalan absorption and emphasize factors that pertain to i.v. melphalan use.

By using Medline, the search terms melphalan and resistance, and the time interval 1980-1999, 41 reports were identified where cellular pharmacologic factors associated with the development of melphalan resistance were reported in sufficient detail to be evaluable for this chapter. A variety of cell lines and experimental conditions were used to develop this database. Multiple reports from the same group of investigators using the same experimental conditions were condensed as "one publication" for purposes of this analysis. Because of space limitations, aggregate data from this review will be presented without systematic references to the individual studies reviewed. The various categories of tumor resistance are described in Table 1.

Table 1. Tumor resistance categories.

Tumor resistance categories
Pharmacokinetic Factors
- Absorption
- Distribution
- Elimination
- Metabolism
Tumor Effects
Cell Membrane Effects
Cellular Factors
- Glutathione/Glutathione S-transferase
- DNA polymerase/Topoisomerase
- DNA repair enzymes
- Apoptosis

5.1 Pharmacokinetic Resistance Factors

I.v. melphalan is fully absorbed and no important metabolites have been noted, as described above. Major changes in renal function do not appear to affect melphalan action. Thus, there are no known bases for PK resistance development in patients. This contrasts sharply with cyclophosphamide, as mentioned above. For a discussion of the clinical pharmacology of cyclophosphamide, see chapter 16 by Drs. McCune and Slattery in this volume.

5.2 Tumor Effects

Penetration of drug into tumors (as opposed to single cells or small cell aggregates) is often limited by tumor vasculature, oxygenation, and pH. Poor tumor vasculature will retard penetration of any drug. Hypoxia and lower pH often occur together and in association with poor perfusion of large tumor masses. Lower pH will decrease the rate of hydrolysis (inactivation) of melphalan and thus favors increased antitumor effect[68,69]. Melphalan is therefore an appropriate drug for use in patients with large, centrally hypoxic tumor masses when the tumor type is known to be sensitive to this drug.

5.3 Cell Membrane Effects

Leucine and glutamine can competitively inhibit the active transport of melphalan into cells (see section 2.1.1.1). Additionally, there is a report of melphalan inducing apoptosis through a membrane effect[70]. Hantel and Ayala[71] reported an association between decreased melphalan transport and resistance, but four other reports failed to detect such an association. The data suggest that membrane transport mutations may be an infrequent cause of melphalan resistance.

The MDR membrane transport mechanism mediated by p170/P-glycoprotein allows a variety of tumor cells to export lipid soluble drugs from the intracellular space (see chapter 3 in this volume by Dr. L. Deng and colleagues). This transport system can export melphalan[72], and thus is clearly a possible resistance mechanism in human tumors. A variety of inhibitors of the MDR pathway are being explored for co-administration with cancer agents, but none has been thoroughly tested with melphalan. Furthermore, it is possible that dose-intensive treatments alone may be able to overcome this resistance mechanism.

5.4 Intracellular Effects

5.4.1 Glutathione/glutathione-S-transferase modulation

GSH depletion, either intrinsic or produced by pretreatment with drugs such as diethyl maleate, was evaluated in 14 reports, 7 of which demonstrated an association between decreases in GSH content and melphalan sensitivity. More commonly, the tumor cell GSH content was experimentally altered as opposed to being intrinsically high or low. Thus, while intrinsic GSH levels may be substantially different from average in a minority of tumor cells, it is clearer that GSH modulation, for example, by other alkylating agents in a combination chemotherapy regimen, may alter melphalan sensitivity. This concept is discussed in more detail below.

Most GST conjugates are formed enzymatically through the action of GST. Of 10 reports noting tumor cells with decreased levels of GST activity, 5 noted increased melphalan sensitivity. This enzyme activity was also artificially altered by pretreatment with ethacrynic acid[73] or sulfasalazine[74]. These pretreatments produced the same effect as melphalan treatment of cells that were intrinsically deficient in GST[75].

In summary, melphalan detoxification by GSH is likely to be an important pathway to deactivate the drug. Thus, artificial reduction in intracellular GSH concentration or GST activity increases the sensitivity of tumor cells to melphalan. The mechanism by which these pretreatments could produce a therapeutic index improvement, however, are less clear. The GSH content and GST activity of tumor cells is often comparable to that of normal tissues.

5.4.2 DNA polymerase and topoisomerase

DNA polymerase and topoisomerase I and II are critical enzymes for DNA synthesis. Five of 8 reports evaluating polymerase activity in melphalan-resistant and -sensitive cell lines found an association between low polymerase activity and melphalan sensitivity. Two of 4 reports noted an association between low topoisomerase activity and melphalan sensitivity. These reports, taken together, document a moderate but not strong association between low DNA synthesis/repair enzyme activity and melphalan sensitivity.

5.4.3 DNA repair enzymes

The association between nucleotide excision repair enzyme activity and melphalan resistance has been studied extensively. Sixteen of 22 reports evaluating low intrinsic nucleotide excision repair activity and melphalan sensitivity found an association. These data suggest that low repair enzyme activity may be relatively common in tumor cell lines and that it frequently is associated with sensitivity to melphalan.

Melphalan is a bifunctional alkylating agent which can form a diethylamine interstrand or intrastrand crosslinks between nucleotides. Methylating agents such as nitrosoureas or DTIC can have their single strand DNA adducts repaired by the suicide repair enzyme O^6-guanine methyltransferase, but no similar enzyme has been identified for bifunctional, mustard-type alkylating agents. 3-methyl adenine adducts can be removed by the enzyme 3-methyladenine DNA glycosylase[76] whose activity has been found to be increased in melphalan-resistant cells in one of two reports.

5.4.4 Apoptosis

Sheikh *et al.*[70] suggested that membrane-associated events produced by UV-irradiation and melphalan can initiate apoptosis and result in tumor cell death. Since apoptosis can explain some but not all tumor cell killing by alkylating agents, understanding these membrane-initiated events in greater detail would be important to further mechanistic understanding of melphalan cytotoxicity[77].

6. TUMOR RESISTANCE AND MULTI-AGENT TREATMENT

Consideration of cytotoxic drug resistance in tumors and drug toxicity to normal tissues emphasizes both the theoretical strengths and weaknesses of alkylating agents used in cancer treatment. Alkylating agents interact with a multiplicity of cellular targets, the damaging of any one of which might produce cell death. Since multiple pathways might be involved in the production of cytotoxicity or apoptosis, it is theoretically likely that the development of high-level, stable, alkylating agent resistance in tumor cells would be difficult. This is the case, even in artificial laboratory systems. *In vitro*, maximal single alkylating agent resistance can often be overcome by dose escalations of less than 10 fold[78]. Furthermore, alkylating agent resistance developed after initial treatment is often unstable *in vivo*, lasting only a few weeks[79], followed by reversion to a more sensitive phenotype. These observations suggest that increasing the dose of melphalan will increase its potential for tumor killing, but also its toxicity to normal tissues.

It is likely that any alkylating agent will to some extent damage any intracellular resistance mechanism described above, as all of these contain electron-rich amino acid or nucleic acid residues that can be alkylated. Thus, the use of several alkylating agents in combination might overcome tumor resistance through two separate pathways:

- independent targeting of different cytotoxic mechanisms favored by the chemistry and pharmacology of each agent; and
- damaging pathways whose activation can produce resistance to a second alkylating agent, thus rendering the cell more sensitive to that agent.

The implication of these hypotheses is that the use of multiple alkylating agents is favored for maximal antitumor effect, and the scheduling of these agents so that one agent might enhance tumor sensitivity to additional agents is critical for treatment success, particularly with melphalan. These hypotheses have been confirmed experimentally[80–82].

The study of melphalan used in combination with non-alkylating agents to reduce tumor resistance has received less study. Since melphalan is capable of damaging many cellular repair processes, as described above, its use prior to or simultaneously with other antineoplastic agents which do not require metabolic activation might be expected to increase their antitumor effect.

Unfortunately, the study of normal tissues to evaluate the effect of single or multiple alkylating agent treatment on cytotoxicity (and tissue-based toxicity) is inadequate. Thus, while it seems clear that increasing dose and number of alkylating agents will increase tumor killing, it is normal tissue toxicity which forms a practical barrier to these treatments. Defining methods to enhance the therapeutic index (ratio of antitumor effect to normal tissue toxicity) is critical for improvement of these treatment strategies. The use of amifostine (a normal tissue cytoprotectant) with melphalan is a promising example of this approach[62].

7. MELPHALAN AND FUTURE HIGH-DOSE CANCER THERAPY STRATEGIES

The increasing use of melphalan in regimens of high-dose chemotherapy with hematopoietic stem cell support reflects a change in the spectrum of patients being treated. For example, there are increasing numbers of myeloma patients receiving this therapy. It may also reflect an increasing recognition of the pharmacologic desirability of high-dose melphalan. The drug has a broad spectrum of activity for hematopoietic cancers and solid tumors. It activates spontaneously and is not subject to metabolic deactivation. The rate of inactivation by hydrolysis is predictable, except for situations that markedly change the pH or chloride ion concentration, and these are usually non-physiologic events.

Recent data derived from the use of cyclophosphamide dose escalation for breast cancer[83,84] and the other undesirable PK effects described above will likely result in increasing substitution of melphalan for cyclophosphamide in high-dose regimens in the future. A major limitation to the use of melphalan in multi-drug regimens is its dose-limiting mucosal toxicity, particularly when used with other agents that produce mucositis. Amifostine may ameliorate this toxicity[62], and perhaps the VOD toxicity it produces in combination[85]. This should further enlarge melphalan's spectrum of use.

The use of melphalan in combination with busulfan and cyclophosphamide has been explored[86]. Furthermore, when melphalan and cyclophosphamide were used together with cisplatin, a serious increase in renal toxicity was recorded[87]. The combination of melphalan with busulfan, either with[88] or without[89] thiotepa, has been used for hematologic neoplasms and breast cancer. Total body irradiation and melphalan, either with[90] or without[91] etoposide, have also been evaluated in the treatment of hematologic neoplasms.

CONCLUSION

The pharmacologic properties of i.v. melphalan make it a promising alkylating agent to evaluate more fully in the future. This is particularly true since the only rate limited step involved in melphalan action, its energy-dependent cellular uptake, seems to be functional even in most resistant tumor cell lines. The optimal use of this drug will be facilitated by a thorough consideration of the pharmacologic principles that underlie its action.

REFERENCES

1. Bergel F, Stock JA. Cyto-active amino acid and peptide derivatives: part I: substituted phenylalanines. J Chem Soc, 76:2409-2412, 1954.
2. Philips FS. Recent contributions to the pharmacology of bis (2-haloethyl) amines and sulfides. Pharmacol Rev, 2:281-323, 1950.
3. Pinguet F, Martel P, Rouanet P, *et al.* Effect of sodium chloride concentration and temperature on melphalan stability during storage and use. Amer J Hosp Pharm, 51:2701-2704, 1994.
4. Pinguet F, Culine S, Bressolle F, *et al.* A phase I and pharmacokinetic study of melphalan using a 24 hr continuous infusion in patients with advanced malignancies. Clin Cancer Res, 6:57-63, 2000.
5. Chang SY, Alberts DS, Farquhar D, *et al.* Hydrolysis and protein binding of melphalan. J Pharmaceut Sci, 67:682-684, 1978.
6. Colvin M, Chabner BA. Alkylating agents. *In*: Cancer Chemotherapy, Principles and Practice, BA Chabner, J Collins (eds.), JB Lippincott, Philadelphia, PA, 276-313, 1990.
7. Reece PA, Hill HS, Green RM, *et al.* Renal clearance and protein binding of melphalan in patients with cancer. Cancer Chemother Pharmacol, 22:348-352, 1988.
8. Gera S, Musch E, Osterheld HKO, *et al.* Relevance of the hydrolysis and protein binding

of melphalan to the treatment of multiple myeloma. Cancer Chemother Pharmacol, 22:348-352. 1999.

9. Yu X, Wu Z, Fenselau C. Covalent sequestration of melphalan by metallothionein and selective alkylation of cysteines. Biochem, 34:3377-3385, 1995.
10. Ahmed AE, Hsu T-F. Quantitative analysis of melphalan and its major hydrolysate in patients and animals by reversed-phase high-performance liquid chromatography. J Chromatogr, 222:453-460, 1981.
11. Dulik DM, Fenselau C. Conversion of melphalan to 4-(glutathionyl)phenylalanine. Drug Metab Dispos, 15:195-199, 1987.
12. Vahrmeijer AL, Snel CAW, Steenvoorden DPT, *et al.* Lack of glutathione conjugation of melphalan in the isolated in situ liver perfusion in humans. Cancer Res, 56:4709-4714, 1996.
13. Kergueris MF, Milpied N, Moreau P, *et al.* Pharmacokinetics of high-dose melphalan in adults: influence of renal function. Anticancer Res, 14:2379-2382, 1994.
14. Tricot G, Alberts DS, Johnson C, *et al.* Safety of autotransplants with high-dose melphalan in renal failure: a pharmacokinetic and toxicity study. Clin Cancer Res, 2:947-952, 1996.
15. Alberts DS, Chang SY, Chen HSG, *et al.* Systemic availability of oral melphalan. Cancer Treat Rev, 6:51-55, 1979.
16. Bosanquet AG, Gilby ED. Comparison of fed and fasted states on the absorption of melphalan in multiple myeloma. Cancer Chemother Pharmacol, 12:183-186, 1984.
17. Reece PA, Kotasek D, Morris RG, *et al.* The effect of food on oral melphalan absorption. Cancer Chemother Pharmacol, 16:194-197, 1986.
18. Woodhouse KW, Hamilton P, Lennard A, *et al.* The pharmacokinetics of melphalan in patients with multiple myeloma: an intravenous/oral study using a conventional dose regimen. Eur J Clin Pharmacol, 24:283-285, 1983.
19. Pallante SL, Fenselau G, Mennel RG, *et al.* Quantitation by gas chromatography-chemical ionization-mass spectrometry of phenylalanine mustard in plasma of patients. Cancer Res, 40:2268-2272, 1980.
20. Taha ARK, Ahmad RA, Gray H, *et al.* Plasma melphalan and prednisolone concentrations during oral therapy for multiple myeloma. Cancer Chemother Pharmacol, 9:57-60, 2000.
21. Adair CG, Elnay JC. The effect of dietary amino acids on the gastrointestinal absorption of melphalan and chlorambucil. Cancer Chemother Pharmacol, 19:343-346, 1987.
22. Reece PA, Dale BM, Morris RG, *et al.* Effect of L-leucine on oral melphalan kinetics in patients. Cancer Chemother Pharmacol, 20:256-258, 1987.
23. Sviland L, Robinson A, Procter SJ, *et al.* Interaction of cimetidine with oral melphalan. A pharmacokinetic study. Cancer Chemother Pharmacol, 20:173-175, 1987.
24. Choi KE, Ratain MJ, Williams SF, *et al.* Plasma pharmacokinetics of high-dose oral melphalan in patients treated with trialkylator chemotherapy and autologous bone marrow reinfusion. Cancer Res, 49:1318-1321, 1989.
25. Boros L, Peng YM, Alberts DS, *et al.* Pharmacokinetics of very high-dose oral melphalan in cancer patients. Amer J Clin Oncol, 13:19-22, 1990.
26. Alberts DS, Chang SY, Chen H-SG, *et al.* Kinetics of intravenous melphalan. Clin Pharmacol Ther, 26:73-80, 1979.
27. Gouyette A, Hartmann O, Pico J-L. Pharmacokinetics of high-dose melphalan in children and adults. Cancer Chemother Pharmacol, 16:184-189, 1986.

28. Ardiet C, Tranchand B, Biron P, *et al.* Pharmacokinetics of high-dose intravenous melphalan in children and adults with forced diuresis. Cancer Chemother Pharmacol, 16:300-305, 1986.
29. Peters W, Stuart A, Klotman M, *et al.* High dose combination cyclophosphamide, cisplatin, and melphalan with ABMS: a clinical and pharmacologic study. Cancer Chemother Pharmacol, 23:377-383, 1989.
30. Moreau P, Kergueris MF, Milpied N, *et al.* A pilot study of 220 mgm^2 melphalan followed by autologous stem cell transplantation in patients with advanced haematological malignancies: pharmacokinetics and toxicity. Br J Haematol, 95:527-530, 1996.
31. Pinguet F, Martel P, Fabbro M, *et al.* Pharmacokinetics of high-dose intravenous melphalan in patients undergoing peripheral blood hematopoietic progenitor-cell transplantation. Anticancer Res, 17:605-612, 1997.
32. Ploin DY, Tranchand B, Guastalla JP, *et al.* Pharmacokinetically guided dosing for intravenous melphalan: a pilot study in patients with advanced ovarian adenocarcinoma. Eur J Cancer, 28A:1311-1315, 1992.
33. Tranchand B, Ploin DY, Minuit M-P, *et al.* High-dose melphalan dosage adjustment: possibility of using a test dose. Cancer Chemother Pharmacol, 23:95-100, 1989.
34. Howell SB, Pfeifle CE, Olshen RA. Intraperitoneal chemotherapy with melphalan. Ann Int Med, 101:14-18, 1984.
35. Rauschecker HF, Foth F, Michaelis HC, *et al.* Kinetics of melphalan leakage during hyperthermic isolation perfusion in melanoma of the limb. Cancer Chemother Pharmacol, 27:379-384, 2000.
36. Tranchand B, Ardiet C, Bouffet E, *et al.* Effect of carboplatin on the pharmacokinetics of melphalan administered intravenously. Bull Cancer (Paris), 81:43-46, 1994.
37. Begleiter A, Lam H-YP, Grover J, *et al.* Evidence for active transport of melphalan by two amino acid carriers in L5178Y lymphoblasts in vitro. Cancer Res, 39:353-359, 1979.
38. Vistica DT, Toal JN, Rabinowitz M. Amino-acid conferred protection against melphalan: characteristics of melphalan transport and correlation of uptake with cytotoxicity in cultured L1210 leukemia cells. Biochem Pharmacol, 27:2865-2870, 1978.
39. Goldenberg GJ, Froese EK. Antagonism of the cytocidal activity and uptake of melphalan by tamoxifen in human breast cancer cells in vitro. Biochem Pharmacol, 34:763-770, 1985.
40. Skipper HE, Aabo K, Bennett LL, Langham WH. Overall tracer studies with 14C-labeled nitrogen mustard in normal and leukemic mice. Cancer, 4:1025-1027, 1951.
41. Brookes P, Lawley PD. Molecular mechanisms of cytotoxic action of difunctional alkylating agents and resistance to its action. Nature, 206:480-483, 1965.
42. Hoes I, Lemiere F, Van Dongen W, *et al.* Analysis of melphalan adducts of 2'-deoxynucleotides in calf thymus DNA hydrolysates by capillary high-performance liquid chromatography-electrospray tandem mass spectrometry. J Chromatogr B Biomed Sci Appl, 736:43-59, 1999.
43. Povirk LF, Shuker DE. DNA damage and mutagenesis induced by nitrogen mustards. Mutat Res, 318:205-226, 1994.
44. Ross WE, Ewig RAG, Kohn KW. Differences between melphalan and nitrogen mustard in the formation and removal of DNA crosslinks. Cancer Res, 38:1052-1056, 1978.
45. Dulik DM, Fenselau C, Hilton J. Characterization of melphalan-glutathione adducts whose formation is catalyzed by glutathione transferases. Biochem Pharmacol, 35:3405-3409,

1986.
46. Dulik DM, Fenselau C. Conversion of melphalan to 4-(glutathionyl)phenylalanine. A novel mechanism for conjugation by glutathione S-transferases. Drug Metab Dispos, 15:195-199, 1987.
47. Hall AG, Matheson E, Hickson ID, *et al.* Purification of an alpha class glutathione S-transferase from melphalan-resistant Chinese hamster ovary cells and demonstration of its ability to catalyze melphalan-glutathione adduct formation. Cancer Res, 54:3369-3372, 1994.
48. Vahrmeijer AL, Snel CAW, Steenvoorden DPT, *et al.* Lack of glutathione conjugation of melphalan in the isolated in situ liver perfusion in humans. Cancer Res, 56:4709-4714, 1996.
49. Hogarth L, English M, Price L, *et al.* The effect of treatment with high dose melphalan, cisplatin or carboplatin on levels of glutathione in plasma, erythrocytes, mononuclear cells and urine. Cancer Chemother Pharmacol, 37:479-485, 1996.
50. Sarosy G, Leyland-Jones B, Soochan P, Cheson BD. The systemic administration of intravenous melphalan. J Clin Oncol, 6:1768-1782, 1988.
51. Barlogie B, Jagannath S. Autotransplants in myeloma. Bone Marrow Transplant, 10 Suppl 1:37-44, 1992.
52. Vesole DH, Barlogie B, Jagannath S, *et al.* High-dose therapy for refractory multiple myeloma: improved prognosis with better supportive care and double transplants. Blood, 84:950-956, 1994.
53. Pritchard J, McElwain TJ, Graham-Pole J. High-dose melphalan with autologous marrow for treatment of advanced neuroblastoma. Br J Cancer, 45:86-94, 1982.
54. Maraninchi D, Pico JL, Hartmann O, *et al.* High-dose melphalan with or without marrow transplantation: a study of dose-effect in patients with refractory and/or relapsed acute leukemias. Cancer Treat Rep, 70:445-448, 1986.
55. Michel G, Maraninchi D, Demiocq F, *et al.* Repeated courses of high-dose melphalan and unpurged autologous bone marrow transplantation in children with acute-nonlymphoblastic leukemia in first complete remission. Bone Marrow Transpl, 3:105-111, 1988.
56. Mills W, Chopra R, McMillan A *et al.* BEAM chemotherapy and autologous bone marrow transplantation for patients with relapsed or refractory non-Hodgkin's lymphoma. J Clin Oncol, 13:588-595, 1995.
57. Mulder PO, Willemse B, Aalders JG, *et al.* High-dose chemotherapy with autologous bone marrow transplantation in patients with refractory ovarian cancer. Eur J Cancer Clin Oncol, 25, 645-649. 1989.
58. Stoppa A, Maraninchi D, Viens P, *et al.* High doses of melphalan and autologous marrow rescue in advanced common epithelial ovarian carcinomas: A retrospective analysis in 35 patients. *In*: Autologous Bone Marrow Transplantation: Proceedings of the Fourth International Symposium, K Dicke, G Spitzer, A Zander (eds.), 509-515, 1989.
59. Ayash U, Elias A, Wheeler C, *et al.* Double dose-intensive chemotherapy with autologous marrow and peripheral progenitor cell support for metastatic breast cancer: a feasibility study. J Clin Oncol, 12:37-44, 1994.
60. Bitran JD, Samuels B, Klein L, *et al.* Tandem high-dose chemotherapy supported by hematopoietic progenitor cells yields prolonged survival in stage IV breast cancer. Bone Marrow Transplant, 17:157-162, 1996.

61. Nieto Y, Xu X, Cagnoni PJ, *et al.* Non-predictable pharmacokinetic behavior of cyclophosphamide when combined with high doses of cisplatin and BCNU. Clin Cancer Res, 5:747-751, 1999.
62. Phillips GL, Hale GA, Howard DS, *et al.* Amifostine (AMJ) cytoprotection (CP) of escalating doses of melphalan (MEL) and autologous hematopoietic stem cell transplantation (AHSCT): a phase I-II study. Proc Amer Soc Clin Oncol, 19:49a, 2000.
63. Fermand JP, Chevert S, Ravard P, *et al.* High-dose chemoradiotherapy and autologous blood stem cell transplantation in multiple myeloma: results of a phase II trial involving 63 patients. Blood, 82:2005-2009, 1993.
64. Ayash L, Elias A, Reich E, *et al.* Double dose-intensive chemotherapy with autologous marrow and peripheral blood progenitor cell (PBPC) support for metastatic breast cancer (Meeting abstract). Breast Cancer Treat Res, 27:183-183, 1993.
65. Codling BW, Chakera TM. Pulmonary fibrosis following therapy with melphalan for multiple myeloma. J Clin Pathol, 25:668-673, 1972.
66. Hartmann O, Oberlin O, Lemerle J, *et al.* Acute leukemia in two patients with high-dose melphalan and autologous marrow transplantation for malignant solid tumors. J Clin Oncol, 2:1424-1425, 1984.
67. Govindarajan R, Jagannath S, Flick JT, *et al.* Preceding standard therapy is the likely cause of MDS after autotransplants for multiple myeloma. Br J Hemat, 95:349-356, 1996.
68. Teicher BA, Holden SA, al Achi A, Herman TS. Classification of antineoplastic treatments by their differential toxicity toward putative oxygenated and hypoxic tumor subpopulations in vivo in the FSaIIC murine fibrosarcoma. Cancer Res, 50:3339-3344, 1990.
69. Skarsgard LD, Skwarchuk MW, Vinczan A, *et al.* The cytotoxicity of melphalan and its relationship to pH, hypoxia and drug uptake. Anticancer Res, 15:219-223, 1995.
70. Sheikh MS, Antinore MJ, Huang Y, Fornace AJ Jr. Ultraviolet-irradiation-induced apoptosis is mediated via ligand independent activation of tumor necrosis factor receptor 1. Oncogene, 17:2555-2563, 1998.
71. Hantel A, Ayala S. Mechanisms contributing to melphalan (M) resistance (Mr) in human colon cancer cell lines (Hcccl). Proc Amer Assoc Cancer Res, 32:A2127, 1991.
72. Uanivee B, Averiul DA. Melphalan resistance and photoaffinity labelling of P-glycoprotein in multidrug-resistant Chinese hamster ovary cells: reversal of resistance by cyclosporin A and hyperthermia. Biochem Pharmacol, 58:291-302, 1999.
73. Hansson J, Berhane K, Castro VM, *et al.* Sensitization of human melanoma cells to the cytotoxic effect of melphalan by the glutathione transferase inhibitor ethacrynic acid. Cancer Res, 51:94-98, 1991.
74. Gupta V, Jani JP, Jacobs S, *et al.* Activity of melphalan in combination with the glutathione transferase inhibitor sulfasalazine. Cancer Chemother Pharmacol, 36:13-19, 1995.
75. Jungnelius U, Hao XY, Skog S, *et al.* Cell cycle dependent sensitivity of human melanoma cells to melphalan is correlated with the activity and cellular concentration of glutathione transferases. Carcinogenesis, 15:99-103, 1994.
76. Geleziunas R, McQuillan A, Malapetsa A, *et al.* Increased DNA synthesis and repair-enzyme expression in lymphocytes from patients with chronic lymphocytic leukemia resistant to nitrogen mustards. J Natl Cancer Inst, 83:557-564, 1991.
77. Brown JM, Wouters BG. Apoptosis, p53, and tumor cell sensitivity to anticancer agents.

Cancer Res, 59:1391-1399, 1999.
78. Batist G, Torres-Garcia S, Demuys JM, *et al.* Enhanced DNA cross-link removal: the apparent mechanism of resistance in a clinically relevant melphalan-resistant human breast cancer cell line. Mol Pharmacol, 36:224-230, 1989.
79. Teicher BA, Ara G, Keyes SR, *et al.* Acute in vivo resistance in high-dose therapy. Clin Cancer Res, 4:483-491, 1998.
80. Holden SA, Teicher BA, Ayash U, *et al.* A preclinical model for sequential high-dose chemotherapy. Cancer Chemother Pharmacol, 36:61-64, 1995.
81. Bubley GJ, Ogata GK, Dupuis NP, Teicher BA. Detection of sequence-specific antitumor alkylating agent DNA damage from cells treated in culture and from a patient. Cancer Res, 54:6325-6329, 1994.
82. Frei E III, Ara G, Teicher B, *et al.* Double high-dose chemotherapy with stem cell rescue (HD-SCR) in patients with breast cancer - effect of sequence. Cancer Chemother Pharmacol, 45:239-246, 2000.
83. Fisher B, Anderson S, Wickerham DL, *et al.* Increased intensification and total dose of cyclophosphamide in a doxorubicin-cyclophosphamide regimen for the treatment of primary breast cancer: findings from National Surgical Adjuvant Breast and Bowel Project B-22. J Clin Oncol, 15:1858-1869, 1997.
84. Fisher B, Anderson S, DeCillis A, *et al.* Further evaluation of intensified and increased total dose of cyclophosphamide for the treatment of primary breast cancer: findings from National Surgical Adjuvant Breast and Bowel Project B-25. J Clin Oncol, 17:3374-3388, 1999.
85. Zuazu I, Brunet S, Fernandez MT, Domingo-Albos A. Hepatic veno-occlusive disease in a patient undergoing bone marrow autotransplant after busulfan and melphalan conditioning (letter). Med Clin (Barc), 94:119, 1990.
86. Phillips GU, Shepherd JD, Barnett MJ, *et al.* Busulfan, cyclophosphamide, and melphalan conditioning for autologous bone marrow transplantation in hematologic malignancy. J Clin Oncol, 9:1880-1888, 1991.
87. Peters W, Stuart A, Klotman M, *et al.* High dose combination cyclophosphamide, cisplatin, and melphalan with ABMS: a clinical and pharmacologic study. Cancer Chemother Pharmacol, 23:377-383, 1989.
88. Martino R, Badell I, Brunet S, *et al.* High-dose busulfan and melphalan before bone marrow transplantation for acute nonlymphoblastic leukemia. Bone Marrow Transplant, 16:209-212, 1995.
89. Bensinger WI, Schiffman KS, Holmberg U, *et al.* High-dose busulfan, melphalan, thiotepa and peripheral blood stem cell infusion for the treatment of metastatic breast cancer. Bone Marrow Transplant, 19:1183-1189, 1997.
90. Gandola U, Lombardi F, Siena S, *et al.* Total body irradiation and high-dose melphalan with bone marrow transplantation at Istituto Nazionale Tumori, Milan, Italy. Radiother Oncol, 18 Suppl 1:105-109, 1990.
91. Keating A, Crump M. High dose etoposide, melphalan, total body irradiation and ABMT for acute myeloid leukemia in first remission. Leukemia, 6 Suppl 4:90-91, 1992.

Chapter 16

PHARMACOLOGICAL CONSIDERATIONS OF PRIMARY ALKYLATORS

Jeannine S. McCune[1,2] and John T. Slattery[1,3]
[1]*Department of Clinical Research, Fred Hutchinson Cancer Research Center, Seattle, Washington, USA*
[2]*Department of Pharmacy, University of Washington, Seattle, Washington, USA*
[3]*Department of Pharmaceutics, University of Washington, Seattle, Washington, USA*

1. INTRODUCTION

The alkylating agents, in combination with other antineoplastic agents or radiation, are frequently used in preparative regimens for conventional hematopoietic stem cell transplantation (HSCT). The alkylating agents are well suited for preparative regimens for HSCT because of their activity against a number of tumor types; a relative lack of cross-resistance among these agents; and because myelosuppression is frequently the dose-limiting toxicity at standard doses.[1] Data from pre-clinical models indicate that the degree of tumor-cell kill is directly proportional to the dose of an alkylating agent, suggesting that the 2-20 fold dose-escalation achieved through the use of HSCT may improve response rates.[2,3] However, there are substantial toxicities associated with the preparative regimens that include alkylating agents.

The doses of alkylating agents are usually individualized based on the patient's weight or body surface area (BSA) to try to reduce the interpatient variability in drug effect. The interpatient variability in the pharmacokinetics of the alkylating agents results in a large range (up to 10 fold) of the area-under-the-concentration-time curve (AUC) when alkylating agents are dosed on the basis of weight or BSA.[4–7] In addition, a number of alkylating agents (i.e., cyclophosphamide, ifosfamide and thiotepa) have metabolites that contribute to response and toxicity. The variability in the AUC of the metabolites can be greater than that of the parent compound.[5,8–12] The considerable between-patient differences in the AUC of the alkylating agents and their metabolites may impact on the efficacy and toxicity of a preparative regimen when relationships between outcome and the AUC of the alkylating agents and/or their metabolites exist.

The wide range in the AUC of the alkylating agents may be reduced through the use of adaptive dosing methods. Therapeutic drug monitoring (TDM) and the use of pretreatment characteristics (e.g., genotype, serum creatinine) known to affect the AUC of an alkylating agent are two such methods.[13] An example of adaptive dosing is the use of glomerular filtration rate obtained prior to treatment to estimate carboplatin clearance in patients receiving standard dose carboplatin.[14] TDM is conducted by determining the AUC after administration of an alkylating agent and subsequent doses are adjusted to bring the AUC within the desired range. TDM is best implemented if: [1] considerable variability is present in the AUC of the alkylating agent after administration of a dose based on BSA or weight; [2] the concentration of the alkylating agent and its metabolites can be measured in plasma with sensitive, precise and reproducible assays; and [3] relationships are defined between outcome (e.g., relapse rates, rejection rates and toxicity) and the AUC of the alkylating agent or its metabolites. The use of TDM has been hindered by the doubt that its benefit justifies the effort or cost. However, TDM of antineoplastic agents to achieve a target AUC can be used as a mechanism to overcome resistance in patients with cancer. For example, the use of TDM of the antimetabolite methotrexate improved response rates in children with B-cell acute lymphoblastic leukemia (66 ± 7% in the standard BSA dosing arm vs. 76 ± 6% in those undergoing TDM, P=0.02).[15]

The substantial toxicity rate of preparative regimens for HSCT makes the use of adaptive dosing attractive to potentially diminish toxicity without increasing the risk of relapse and rejection. The interpatient variability in the pharmacokinetics of the alkylating agents and the pharmacodynamic relationships are just now being realized. This chapter will address: [1] the inter-patient variability in the AUC of alkylating agents and their relevant metabolites after administration of a dose based on weight or BSA to patients undergoing HSCT; and [2] the concentration-effect relationships of alkylating agents and their metabolites in alkylator-based preparative regimens and the potential for adaptive dosing to improve outcome.

2. BUSULFAN

2.1 Pharmacokinetic Characteristics of Busulfan

High-dose busulfan (1 mg/kg p.o. every 6 h x 16 doses) is one of the most frequently used components of preparative regimens for HSCT. Busulfan is predominantly metabolized, with less than 2% of an oral busulfan dose eliminated unchanged in the urine of humans.[16] The only known pathway for busulfan elimination involves glutathione (GSH) conjugation to form γ-glutamyl-β-(S-tetrahydrothiophenium ion) alanyl-glycine (THT^+). Glutathione S-transferase (GST) catalyzes THT^+ formation, with GSTA1-1 being the most active human form of GST catalyzing this reaction examined to date.[17,18]

There is substantial interpatient variability in the apparent oral clearance (CL/F) and thus the AUC at a given dose (mg/kg) of oral busulfan, with younger children (age <4 years) having a higher CL/F. The mean CL/F of busulfan varies ~3 fold (2.64 to 6.60 ml/min/kg) in small studies of patients over 4 years of age.[19,20] The coefficient of variation (standard deviation/mean) of CL/F adjusted for actual body weight (ml/min/kg) was 21% in 279 adult patients, the largest patient population analyzed for busulfan pharmacokinetics.[21] The clearance of Busulfex® exhibits similar variability, with a coefficient of variation of 25% in 59 patients.[22]

Weight, disease and age are factors that may influence the clearance of oral busulfan. The absolute CL/F (not adjusted for body weight) of busulfan is elevated in obese patients (body mass index (BMI) >27 kg/m^2) in comparison to normal weight patients (BMI of 18 to 27 kg/m^2).[21] Expressing busulfan CL/F relative to adjusted ideal body weight (AIBW, defined as ideal body weight plus 25% of the difference between actual and ideal body weight) or BSA eliminates the differences in busulfan CL/F among these groups. However, the interpatient variability in busulfan CL/F when expressed relative to AIBW or BSA is still sizable, with a coefficient of variation of 21% among all patients.[21] A few studies have suggested that busulfan CL/F varies based on the underlying disease, although definitive conclusions are hindered by the absence of a mechanistic rationale for these differences and the low number of patients in these studies (<75 patients per disease).[21,23,24]

Busulfan CL/F is enhanced in young children (≤4 years old) compared to adults and older children (>10 years old). The difference in busulfan CL/F between adults and young children could be due to poor absorption or enhanced elimination of busulfan in young children. The absorption rate constant is similar between young children and adults.[25,26] Other data suggest an enhanced ability of children less than 4 years of age to metabolize busulfan.[27,28] Young children (≤4 years old) have an elevated ratio of the AUC of the THT^+ to the AUC of busulfan in comparison to adolescents and adults (0.0631 ± 0.0237 vs. 0.0421 ± 0.0120, children vs. adolescents and adults, P=0.0098).[27] The 50% increase in this ratio is consistent with the difference in the mean CL/F between these two populations. Busulfan conjugation is 77% higher in epithelial cells obtained from the small intestine of younger children (1-3 years) relative to that in older children (9-17 years). Since the conjugation of busulfan with GSH to THT^+ is mediated by GSTA1-1, these data suggest that GSTA1-1 expression is elevated in the enterocytes of young children.

2.2 Pharmacodynamics of Busulfan

Busulfan AUC or average steady-state plasma concentration (C_{SS}) have been related to relapse, rejection and toxicity in a variety of patient populations patients receiving the busulfan/cyclophosphamide (BU/CY) preparative regimen for HSCT. In this discussion we will present all AUC and because C_{SS} results as relationships between busulfan C_{SS} and outcome because AUC data are easily converted to C_{SS} (C_{SS}=AUC divided by the time between doses) and C_{SS} is frequently used to express busulfan exposure after high-dose busulfan. Busulfan C_{SS} has been related to outcome only in patients receiving BU/CY. In the BU/CY regimen, oral busulfan is typically administered at 6-h intervals over 4 days (total of 16 doses), followed by various cyclophosphamide doses (total of 120 to >200 mg/kg), administered by i.v. bolus over 2 to 4 days. Close attention should be given in the interpretation of these reports because of the potential changes in the concentration-effect relationships between busulfan C_{SS} and outcome with each patient population and with each preparative regimen. Patients of varying ages, diseases (myeloid, lymphoid, and solid tumors, and nonmalignant disorders), stem cell donor (autologous or allogeneic) and cyclophosphamide doses are often combined in the reports. It should be recognized that when busulfan is combined with agents other than or in addition to cyclophosphamide (e.g., total body irradiation (TBI), melphalan, or thiotepa), relationships between busulfan C_{SS} and outcome are expected to differ from those observed for the BU/CY regimen. This has been observed in adults receiving the BU/CY/TBI regimen[29] and in children receiving busulfan with either thiotepa, melphalan, cyclophosphamide/melphalan or cyclophosphamide/thiotepa.[30]

2.2.1 Busulfan exposure and disease relapse in the BU/CY preparative regimens for HSCT

The relationship between busulfan exposure and disease relapse has been addressed in few studies with enough patients having a single disease treated with a fixed BU/CY preparative regimen.[4,31,32] The first observation that higher busulfan exposure results in lower relapse rates was in 45 adult patients receiving BU/CY prior to HLA-matched grafts.[4] All patients received busulfan 1 mg/kg p.o. every 6 h (total of 16 mg/kg) followed by cyclophosphamide 60 mg/kg i.v. every 24 h (total of 120 mg/kg). The majority (39 of 45) of these patients had chronic myelogenous leukemia (CML) in chronic phase, with the remaining patients having CML in accelerated phase. The variability of C_{SS} after administration of a 1 mg/kg dose of busulfan was substantial, with an ~3-fold range (642 to 1,749 ng/ml), and a median C_{SS} of 917 ng/ml. The cumulative incidence of relapse was 38% in patients with busulfan C_{SS} below the median and 0% in those with a busulfan C_{SS} above the median (*P*=0.0003). Busulfan C_{SS} was the only statistically significant determinant of relapse in univariate or multivariate analysis that included other potential determinants such as age, interval from diagnosis to transplant, donor gender, and cytomegalovirus status of the patient and donor. The 3-year survival estimates were 0.82 and 0.64 for patients with a busulfan C_{SS} above and below the median of 917 ng/ml, respectively (P=0.33). The power to detect this difference in survival rate was 24%, demonstrating the need for studies evaluating the concentration-effect relationship between busulfan C_{SS} and outcome in larger patient populations.[4]

Studies in other patient populations have not suggested a relationship between busulfan exposure and relapse. No relationship was found between busulfan C_{SS} and mixed chimerism in 64 children and young adults with β-thalassemia receiving genotypically HLA-matched grafts.[31] Two different doses of the BU/CY regimen were administered: busulfan 14 mg/kg and cyclophosphamide 200 mg/kg (n=36) or busulfan 14 or 16 mg/kg and cyclophosphamide 120 mg/kg (n=28). In addition, busulfan C_{SS} did not predict the occurrence of relapse in patients with acute myelogenous leukemia receiving the BU/CY regimen (total busulfan dose of 16 to 20 mg/kg, administered every 6 or 12 h; cyclophosphamide 120 mg/kg, 200 mg/kg or 6,000 mg/m^2) followed by autologous (n=27) or allogeneic (n=25) grafts.[32] However, the low number of patients receiving one type of graft may have precluded defining a relationship between busulfan C_{SS} and relapse.[32]

2.2.2 Busulfan exposure and engraftment in the BU/CY preparative regimens

The relation between busulfan C_{SS} and engraftment has been examined in various studies of HSCT patients receiving BU/CY.[31,33,34] Low doses of busulfan are associated with graft rejection in children receiving the BU/CY regimen.[35,36] Slattery *et al.*[33] found that having a busulfan C_{SS} >600 ng/ml resulted in lower rejection rates in adult and pediatric patients receiving allogeneic grafts. Eight of 15 patients with a busulfan C_{SS} <600 ng/ml rejected in comparison to 1/23 with the higher exposure (P=0.0028).[33] A similar relationship between busulfan exposure and rejection was found in a retrospective analysis of 38 children receiving allogeneic grafts from various sources.[37] A busulfan C_{SS} <600 ng/ml was related to autologous recovery or mixed chimerism. Eight of the 23 children with a busulfan C_{SS} <600 ng/ml rejected their graft, compared with 0 of 8 children with a busulfan C_{SS} >600 ng/ml (P=0.018).[37] Subsequently, these investigators implemented TDM and adjusted busulfan doses to maintain a busulfan C_{SS} of 600-900 ng/ml in 24 children to try to improve outcome.[34] The first administered dose of busulfan in the BU/CY preparative regimen was adjusted based on the CL/F obtained from pharmacokinetic sampling after administration of a test dose (0.5 mg/kg) of busulfan 4 days prior to initiation of high-dose busulfan. The use of a test dose resulted in 54% of the patients having a target C_{SS} of 600-900 ng/ml with the first dose of high-dose busulfan. In the remaining patients, the busulfan C_{SS} obtained from the first busulfan dose of the preparative regimen was used for subsequent dose adjustments. The dose necessary to achieve a busulfan C_{SS} of 600-900 ng/ml ranged from 10.9 to 29 mg/kg. Performing busulfan TDM in this manner resulted in an improvement in the rate of successful engraftment from 74% to 96%.[34]

A relationship between busulfan C_{SS} and graft rejection was not observed in children with β-thalassemia receiving genotypically HLA-matched grafts. Six of the 64 patients had an C_{SS} <200 ng/ml; however, the low frequency of rejection (7.5%) suggests that these children received grafts better matched in minor histocompatibility antigens than those from the other studies.[31,33,34]

2.2.3 Busulfan exposure and toxicity in the BU/CY preparative regimen for HSCT

Several investigators have reported a relationship between elevated busulfan exposure and veno-occlusive disease of the liver (VOD) in patients receiving BU/CY.[33,38–42] These data indicated that hepatic VOD is more common in patients receiving BU/CY with a busulfan C_{SS} >900-1025 ng/ml.[33,39,40]

Various investigators have reported that busulfan C_{SS} does not influence toxicity in patients receiving BU/CY, potentially due to inherent differences in the likelihood of busulfan toxicity between populations.[43] The relationship between busulfan C_{SS} and toxicity may be disease-specific. In 45 CML adult patients receiving BU/CY (cyclophosphamide 120 mg/kg), only one patient developed severe regimen-related toxicity even though the median C_{SS} was 917 ng/ml.[4] In a study in which patients received the BU/CY regimen (cyclophosphamide 120 mg/kg in 18 patients; 200 mg/kg in 2 patients), busulfan C_{SS} did not influence the occurrence of VOD in a group of 19 adults and 1 adolescent of various diagnoses (11 with CML).[44] Thirteen of the 20 patients had a busulfan C_{SS} >1025 ng/ml (the number of patients with a C_{SS} >900 ng/ml was not defined); however, only three patients in the study had VOD. The low number of patients having VOD in these studies makes it unlikely that a specific cause could be identified.

Identification of contributing factors in the occurrence of hepatic VOD is necessary in children since up to 25% develop VOD after receiving BU/CY, with severe VOD occurring in 3%.[34,45] The studies demonstrating a relationship between busulfan exposure and VOD have included few young children. Seventy and 100%, respectively, of the patients in the Slattery *et al.*[33] and the Dix *et al.*[40] studies, were adults and adolescents, while the age range of patients included in the Grochow study[39] was not specified (it is assumed that they were adults). Three reports involving children suggest that the relationship between busulfan C_{SS} and hepatic VOD differ between children and adults receiving the BU/CY regimen.[31,37,46] The majority of children in the pediatric reports (56%[31] to 100%[37,46]) received cyclophosphamide at 200 mg/kg in comparison to the 120 mg/kg dose administered to the adults in whom a relationship between busulfan C_{SS} and VOD has been observed.[33,40] In two of the three pediatric studies in which a busulfan exposure-toxicity relationship was not found, busulfan C_{SS} exceeded the toxicity threshold defined in adults (900 ng/ml) in only 2-3% of the patients studied.[31,37] A relationship between VOD and busulfan C_{SS} was not found in 23 children (aged 2.5 to 13 years) with β-thalassemia who received busulfan dosed on the basis of body weight (16 mg/kg) or BSA (600 mg/m^2) in addition to 200 mg/kg of cyclophosphamide.[46] However, only 3 cases of VOD occurred and the number of children with a busulfan C_{SS} >900 ng/ml was not specified. In contrast, Vassal *et al.*[45] reported an increased incidence of VOD in children receiving BU/CY (cyclophosphamide doses not specified, melphalan was also used in some children) as busulfan exposure is increased to achieve C_{SS} equal to that of adults receiving 16 mg/kg.

2.3 Conclusions on Adaptive Dosing of Busulfan

The majority of studies have demonstrated a relationship between busulfan C_{SS} and outcome in patients receiving the BU/CY preparative regimen. Many centers use TDM because of the variability in the clearance of both oral and i.v. busulfan and its narrow therapeutic index. Adjusting the dose of busulfan to achieve a target C_{SS} appears to minimize the toxicities of the BU/CY regimen, particularly VOD, while improving engraftment and relapse rates.

3. CYCLOPHOSPHAMIDE

3.1 Pharmacokinetics of Cyclophosphamide

The oxazaphosphorine cyclophosphamide is frequently used in preparative regimens for HSCT in combination with other alkylating agents, such as busulfan, cisplatin, carmustine, or thiotepa. Less than 20% of cyclophosphamide is protein bound and its volume of distribution ranges from 0.54-1.1 L/kg.[47] The mean elimination half-life of cyclophosphamide varies from 4.8-6.8 h.[5,9,48] Cyclophosphamide predominately undergoes hepatic elimination, with 10-30% of an i.v. dose excreted unchanged in the urine.[5,49–51] The majority (91-96%) of cyclophosphamide undergoing hepatic elimination is metabolized to hydroxycyclophosphamide (HCY) by multiple isozymes of cytochrome P450 (CYP) (see Figure 1)[52]. This translates into 64-86% of an i.v. cyclophosphamide dose when renal elimination is considered. A minor fraction (4-9%) of cyclophosphamide is metabolized by the liver to deschloroethylcyclophosphamide, translating into 2.8 to 8.1% of an i.v. dose when renal elimination is considered. HCY tautomerizes to aldophosphamide, and the concentrations of these two metabolites have not been quantified independently.[53] HCY/aldophosphamide have five subsequent metabolic fates: metabolism to 4-ketocyclophosphamide by CYP; metabolism to carboxyethylphosphoramide mustard (CEPM) by aldehyde dehydrogenase 1A1 (ALDH-1A1); formation of 4-glutathioylcyclophosphamide; formation of hydroxypropylphosphoramide mustard; and formation of the cytotoxic metabolite phosphoramide mustard (PM).[52,54] The urotoxic metabolite acrolein results from the conversion of HCY/aldophosphamide to PM.[47,52]

Figure 1. Metabolic schema of cyclophosphamide and its metabolites.

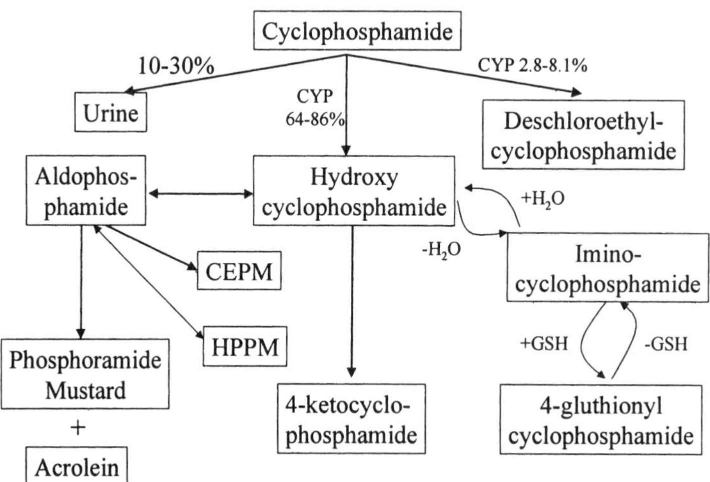

CEPM: O-carboxyethyl-phosphoramide mustard
CYP: Cytochrome P-450
HPPM: Hydroxypropylphosphoramide mustard
GSH: Glutathione

Pharmacokinetic data on the metabolites of cyclophosphamide should be interpreted with special attention to the analytical method used.[53,55] In early studies, total alkylating activity was measured using a reaction of the metabolites with 4-(4-nitrobenzyl) pyridine. This assay is non-specific and underestimates the serum concentration of HCY and PM.[9] Quantification of HCY concentrations is difficult because it is extremely unstable in biologic fluids, with a half-life in plasma *in vitro* of less than 3 minutes, although analysis is possible after conversion into stable derivatives.[55] Some analytical methods have relied on trapping HCY in plasma with either semicarbazide or sodium cyanide before analysis, which can form derivatives that are unstable, have long work-ups prior to trapping and/or require the syntheses and use of a deuterium-labeled, chemically unstable internal standard. Other derivatization techniques have been developed for acrolein, formed by the chemical decomposition of HCY, which yield the sum of the concentrations of HCY and acrolein. However, these procedures are limited by the reaction of acrolein with nucleophiles. Since 1995, more clinically applicable methods involving the derivatization with pentafluorophenyl hydroxylamine or *p*-nitrophenylhydrazine (pNPH) have been available.[55,56] These methods are accurate, sensitive and specific and provide the tools to reliably advance the pharmacokinetic and pharmacodynamic data on the metabolites of cyclophosphamide.

Cyclophosphamide dosed on the basis of body weight (mg/kg) or BSA (mg/m^2) results in a wide AUC range of the parent drug, and an even greater variability in the AUC of its metabolites.[5,8] The coefficient of variation of cyclophosphamide clearance was 39% in 355 adults, the largest population studied to date, receiving the first day of the CPB regimen (cyclophosphamide 1,875 $mg/m^2/d$ i.v. bolus day –6 to –4; cisplatin 55 $mg/m^2/day$ continuous i.v. infusion (CI) day –6 to –3; carmustine (BCNU) 600 mg/m^2 i.v. on day –3).[57] The improved analytical methods have been used to generate pharmacokinetic data on the metabolites of cyclophosphamide in patients receiving HSCT (1000 to 2400 mg/m^2 i.v. for 1 to 3 days).[5,55,56,58] The AUC of cyclophosphamide can not be used to predict that of HCY since the AUC of cyclophosphamide and HCY do not correlate ($r^2=0.16$, $P=0.455$).[55] There is a greater amount of interpatient variability in the AUC of the metabolites than that seen with cyclophosphamide. Cyclophosphamide AUC ranges ~3 fold after a dose based on body weight or BSA;[1,5] the AUC of HCY ranges ~6 fold (29.2-179 μM-h), with a 20-68% coefficient of variation.[5,9,55] There is a 6-fold variation in the AUC of CEPM (51.9-332 μM-h) with a coefficient of variation of 40%.[5] The coefficient of variation of the active cytotoxic PM has been reported to be as high as 77% with the AUC ranging from 230-2390 μM-h.[5,9]

A confounding factor in evaluating clearance of cyclophosphamide and its metabolites is the well-known effect of cyclophosphamide or its metabolites upon their own clearance. The increased clearance of cyclophosphamide after administration of higher doses (2,000-2,400 mg/m^2/day) for 2 to 4 days has been well recognized for a number of years.[59,60] The AUC of cyclophosphamide decreases by 24.8% from day 1 to day 2 after i.v. administration of cyclophosphamide (60 mg/kg/day).[5] This increase in the clearance of cyclophosphamide could be caused by an increase in the formation clearance of deschloroethylcyclophosphamide, the renal elimination of unchanged cyclophosphamide, or the formation clearance of HCY. Since the former two processes do not appreciably change over this short time span, the most likely explanation for the change in the AUC of cyclophosphamide is an increased formation of HCY. The formation clearance of HCY can not be calculated precisely *in vivo* because of its subsequent metabolism to several other metabolites. However, an increase in the formation of HCY is likely due to the induction of cytochrome P450 enzymes by cyclophosphamide, which has been demonstrated in human hepatocyte culture.[61] In addition, the AUC of HCY increased 54.7% from day 1 to day 2 of cyclophosphamide administration. This increase is attributable to an increase in the fraction of cyclophosphamide converted to HCY, a decrease in the elimination clearance of HCY, or both. The formation of CEPM via ALDH1A1 has been suggested to be the major pathway of HCY elimination. Acrolein inhibits ALDH1A1 activity, as evidenced *in vitro* and *in vivo* by an average decrease in ALDH1A1 activity by 24% over 2 days of high-dose cyclophosphamide.[5,62,63] Therefore, both an increased formation and decreased elimination of HCY appear to be contributing to the increase in its AUC.

Other components of the preparative regimen may also influence the disposition of cyclophosphamide.[55] The AUC of cyclophosphamide is lower and the ratio of HCY to cyclophosphamide is higher in patients receiving BU/CY than those receiving CY/TBI.[55] This suggests that busulfan or phenytoin increases the formation or decreases the elimination of HCY. In addition, cyclophosphamide is commonly administered as part of the CPB or CTCb (cyclophosphamide 1,500 mg/m^2/day, thiotepa 125 mg/m^2/day, carboplatin 200 mg/m^2/day CI for 4 days) preparative regimens, typically in breast cancer patients. The effects of the platinating agents, thiotepa and carmustine on cyclophosphamide disposition are unknown. However, drug-drug interactions are anticipated since thiotepa is an inhibitor of cytochrome P450 activity in human liver microsomes and therefore the clearance of cyclophosphamide or the formation of its metabolites may be altered.[58]

3.2 Pharmacodynamics of Cyclophosphamide

3.2.1 Cyclophosphamide exposure and response

Only a few reports in diverse patient populations receiving various preparative chemotherapy regimens have evaluated the relationship between the AUC of cyclophosphamide or its metabolites and survival or relapse rates.[48,57,64,65] The first report was in 19 women with metastatic breast cancer who were receiving the CTCb regimen. The ten women who had a higher cyclophosphamide AUC (>5000 μM-h) had a shorter duration of response (median of 5.25 months) than those with lower cyclophosphamide AUC (median duration of response not reached) after a median follow-up of 22 months.

The relationship between response and cyclophosphamide AUC has also been evaluated in patients receiving the CPB regimen.[57,64] Petros *et al.*[64] reported data from 85 breast cancer patients with over 10 positive axillary lymph nodes who received the CPB preparative regimen. The median follow-up was 6 years. Patients with a lower cyclophosphamide AUC had a longer overall survival (P=0.031), but not disease-free survival (P=0.094) based on Kaplan-Meier analysis. However, the AUC of cyclophosphamide was not related to relapse in a heterogeneous population of 355 patients receiving the same preparative regimen.[57] After a minimum follow-up of 1 year, a subgroup analysis was performed based on the patient's primary malignancy. No difference was found in the AUC between patients who had and had not relapsed in those with stage II-III breast cancer (n=115, P=0.36), stage IV breast cancer (n=163, P=0.45), non-Hodgkin's lymphoma (n=44, P=0.15), and Hodgkin's disease (n=13, P=0.84).

The relationship between cyclophosphamide and HCY exposure with survival was evaluated in 41 women with advanced breast cancer receiving a preparative regimen of cyclophosphamide 4,000 mg/m^2/day CI for 4 days; thiotepa 200 mg/m^2/day CI for 4 days, novobiocin (an antibiotic that augments alkylating agent cytotoxicity in experimental models) 4 g/day p.o. for 7 days.[65] The median follow-up was 64.9 months. Progression-free survival was not related to the AUC of cyclophosphamide (P=0.74) or HCY (P-value not reported). In addition, overall survival was not related to the AUC of cyclophosphamide (P=0.12) or HCY (P-value not reported).

3.2.2 Cyclophosphamide exposure and toxicity in patients receiving the CPB or CTCb preparative regimen

A relationship between cardiotoxicity and the AUC of cyclophosphamide has been defined in two reports.[48,64] Cardiac dysfunction was associated with a lower AUC in those patients receiving cyclophosphamide as part of the CTCb regimen. The median cyclophosphamide AUC for the 6 patients who developed congestive heart failure was significantly lower (2888 μM-h) than that of the 13 patients who did not develop congestive heart failure (6121 μM-h, P<0.005).[48] These data were confirmed by Petros *et al.*[64] who reported that a lower cyclophosphamide AUC was found in the 7 of 85 (8%) women who experienced cardiac toxicity after receiving a different (CPB) preparative regimen (P=0.011). However, data from the largest cohort of patients suggests that a relationship between cardiotoxicity and cyclophosphamide AUC does not exist in breast cancer patients receiving the CPB regimen.[66] The AUC of cyclophosphamide did not differ in those who did (n=12) or did not (n=357) experience cardiac toxicity. Potential reasons for the difference between the findings of Ayash *et al.*[48] and Petros *et al.*[64] vs. those of Nieto *et al.*[66] are the small number of patients in the earlier reports or the differences in the definition of cardiac toxicity. In addition, Neito *et al.*[66] reported in a separate publication that toxic death was not related to the sum of the AUCs of cyclophosphamide from days 1-3 in 355 patients receiving CPB (P=0.18).[57] Pulmonary toxicity in patients receiving this regimen was also not related to cyclophosphamide AUC.[7]

3.2.3 Cyclophosphamide exposure and toxicity in patients receiving the cyclophosphamide/total body irradiation (CY/TBI) preparative regimen

Cyclophosphamide is common to many preparative regimens with a high incidence of fatal VOD and may contribute to the hepatotoxicity of the CY/TBI and BU/CY preparative regimens. Data from co-cultures of hepatocytes and endothelial cells indicate that acrolein is a hepatotoxin.[67] McDonald *et al.*[68] recently reported a relationship between the AUC of CEPM, an acid metabolite of HCY, and hepatic VOD in 105 adult CML patients. These patients received a graft from an unrelated donor following the cyclophosphamide (60 mg/kg/day x 2 days) and TBI (12-13.2 Gy) preparative regimen.[8] Forty-two percent of the patients experienced VOD, defined by the McDonald criteria[68], with 17% experiencing moderate to severe VOD. The patients with moderate to severe VOD had a 48% higher CEPM AUC than those without VOD (mean 599 vs. 405 μM-h, P=0.01). The AUC for the other metabolites analyzed (PM, alcophosphamide, ketocyclophosphamide, and deschlorethylcyclophosphamide) were higher in the patients who experienced moderate to severe VOD, with the exception of HCY. Thus, the metabolites of cyclophosphamide must be considered to be at least a participant in VOD observed in CY/TBI regimen, and further work is needed.

3.3 Conclusions on Adaptive Dosing of Cyclophosphamide

Data on the relationship between cyclophosphamide AUC and response have been conflicting. Also, the relationship between cyclophosphamide and its metabolites and cardiac toxicity is unclear in the CPB and CTCb preparative regimens because of conflicting results. Preliminary evidence suggests that the concentration of the metabolite CEPM correlates to the occurrence of VOD in patients receiving the CY/TBI preparative regimen. Although these pharmacodynamic relationships exist, a confounding factor with adaptive dosing of cyclophosphamide is the induction of cytochrome P450 enzymes by cyclophosphamide and the inhibition of ALDH1A1 by acrolein. Further work is needed to identify determinants in the intra-patient variability of the clearance of cyclophosphamide to facilitate adaptive dosing of cyclophosphamide.

4. IFOSFAMIDE

Like cyclophosphamide, ifosfamide is an oxazaphosphorine. The only chemical difference between it and cyclophosphamide is a shift of one chloroethyl group from the exocyclic nitrogen to the oxazaphosphorine nitrogen. Their overall metabolism is similar; however, a higher fraction of ifosfamide is converted to the dechloroethylated metabolites. The differences in the toxicity profiles of ifosfamide and cyclophosphamide have been attributed to these metabolic differences.[69] Chloroacetaldehyde is formed as a by-product of dechloroethylation and is structurally related to acetaldehyde, a metabolite of ethanol, and the sedative chloral hydrate.[69] Chloroacetaldehyde, or one of the dechloroethylated metabolites of ifosfamide, may account for the neurotoxicity that occurs after ifosfamide administration.[69–71] The nephrotoxic effects of ifosfamide have also been attributed to chloroacetaldehyde.[71]

To date, one study has evaluated the effect of ifosfamide concentration on outcome in patients undergoing a HSCT.[6] The relationship between the renal function and ifosfamide concentration was evaluated in 9 patients receiving ifosfamide (4000 mg/m^2/day), carboplatin (400 mg/m^2/day) and etoposide (400 mg/m^2/day) as a CI for 4 days. The clearance of ifosfamide varied 2.7 fold, with a coefficient of variation of 27% in this small patient population. One patient developed anuric renal failure. Based on the observation that this patient had a lower clearance of ifosfamide, these authors suggested that an ifosfamide concentration >153 μM at 16-22 h after the start of the ifosfamide infusion may be predictive for renal dysfunction. However, this work needs to be confirmed in a larger patient population. In addition, the effect of ifosfamide's metabolites on nephrotoxicity should also be examined since the nephrotoxic effects of standard-dose ifosfamide have been attributed to chloroacetaldehyde and the AUC of the metabolites vary more than that of the parent drug.[10,71]

5. CARMUSTINE

Carmustine (BCNU) is primarily used in the CPB preparative regimen, where it is administered at a dose of 600 mg/m^2 as a 2-h infusion after 3 days of cisplatin and cyclophosphamide. Dosing carmustine based on BSA (mg/m^2) results in a 12-fold range and a coefficient of variation of 79% in its AUC.[7,72] Carmustine decomposes spontaneously under physiological conditions to yield a chloroethyl carbonium ion and 2-chloroethyl isocyanate.[73] Although other metabolic pathways (e.g., GSH conjugation) have been found in rodents, the importance of these pathways in human are unknown. Animal data suggests that the variability in carmustine clearance is greater after administration of cyclophosphamide and cisplatin, as occurs in the CPB regimen.[74]

An elevated carmustine AUC (>600 μg-min/ml) has been associated with a higher incidence of acute pulmonary toxicity in 38 patients receiving CPB. Twelve of the 14 (86%) patients with a carmustine AUC >600 μg-min/ml developed acute pulmonary toxicity, while only 33% (8 of 24) with an AUC below this value developed toxicity.[7] However, these data have not been confirmed in trials with larger patient populations (n=52 or 85 patients) receiving the same preparative regimen.[64,75] Since pharmacodynamic relationships have not been firmly defined in this setting, the role of adaptive dosing of carmustine is unclear and TDM would be difficult with the current administration schedule in the CPB regimen. Alteration of the administration schedule of carmustine may change the concentration-effect relationship between carmustine AUC and pulmonary toxicity, based on data indicating that the rate of fatalities from interstitial pneumonitis decreases from 11.8% to 5.56% when carmustine (600 mg/m^2) is administered as a one-time dose or over 4 days.[76]

6. THIOTEPA

Administration of thiotepa dosed on the basis of BSA or weight results in a coefficient of variation of 27 to 58% in its AUC.[11,77–80] The metabolic profile of thiotepa and the contribution of the metabolites to the effect of thiotepa are not completely understood.[81–83] The metabolite TEPA is formed in the liver after oxidative desulfuration. Recent studies have identified two new metabolites, monochloroTEPA and thiotepa-mercapturate; however, other unidentified compounds with alkylating activity are present.[84]

The relationship between thiotepa AUC and response has been studied in a variety of patient populations receiving different preparative regimens. A relationship was not found between the pharmacokinetic parameters of thiotepa and response in 16 patients with various solid tumors receiving thiotepa alone (total dose of 135 to 1215 mg/m^2), followed by an autologous HSCT.[79] In contrast, thiotepa AUC was associated with response (P=0.04) in

20 patients with various malignancies receiving cyclophosphamide and thiotepa as a preparative regimen.[83] These results highlight how the concentration-effect relationships change based on the preparative regimen.

A number of trials have shown a relationship between varying toxicities and thiotepa exposure.[11,80,83] Those patients receiving cyclophosphamide and thiotepa who had a thiotepa AUC >55 μM-h were more likely to experience life-threatening or lethal toxicity (4/6) than those with an AUC <20 μM-h (0/8, $P<0.01$).[83] Hussein *et al.*[80] evaluated the pharmacokinetics of thiotepa in 37 patients receiving cyclophosphamide, cisplatin and escalating doses of thiotepa (300-900 mg/m^2) as part of a Phase I/II study. There was a stronger correlation between mucositis and the AUC of thiotepa (r^2=0.41, P=0.0018) than between mucositis and the dose (r^2=0.19, P=0.129). The incidence of life-threatening or lethal toxicity and thiotepa exposure was not addressed.[80] The relationship between toxicity and the exposure of thiotepa and its metabolite TEPA was examined in 15 allogeneic and autologous HSCT patients receiving thiotepa with busulfan and cyclophosphamide.[11] The occurrence of grade 2-4 regimen related toxicity of the mucosa, liver and central nervous system was not related to thiotepa or TEPA exposure. However, TEPA peak concentrations >1.75 μg/ml and a combined thiotepa and TEPA AUC >30 mg-h/L were associated with grades 2-4 maximum regimen related toxicity (5/6 vs. 0/9, P=0.01 for both comparisons).[11]

The considerable interpatient variability in the clearance of thiotepa may make it a candidate for adaptive dosing, but the concentration-effect relationships that have been found between thiotepa exposure and response or toxicity have been conflicting. The presence of unidentified metabolites with alkylating activity may confound concentration-effect relationships. Further work is needed to identify these metabolites to better define pharmacodynamic relationships for thiotepa and its metabolites since thiotepa is being used increasingly in preparative regimens for HSCT.[85,86]

7. CARBOPLATIN AND CISPLATIN

Carboplatin at doses of 400 mg/m^2 or an AUC of 10 to 20 mg-min/ml is part of various preparative regimens for HSCT (i.e., thiotepa and cyclophosphamide (CTC), paclitaxel with or without cyclophosphamide, or etoposide).[87–89] Carboplatin is typically dosed on the basis of a targeted AUC rather than BSA because of the reduced interpatient variability in carboplatin exposure with AUC-dosing.[14,87] The dose of carboplatin is calculated as the product of the target AUC and the estimated clearance of carboplatin based on the patient's renal function.[14,90] Fifty to seventy percent of carboplatin is renally eliminated.[14,90,91] Various methods are used to estimate carboplatin clearance based on renal function, age and weight. These estimation methods were validated in patients receiving standard dose carboplatin.[14,90,91] Several studies have demonstrated that the Calvert equation, which is commonly used to dose carboplatin outside of the HSCT setting, does not accurately determine carboplatin clearance in HSCT patients receiving high-dose carboplatin (AUC 10-32mg-min/ml).[88,89,92,93] Potential causes for this divergence are: inaccuracies of estimating glomerular filtration rate with measured or calculated creatinine clearance[88,92,93]; the lack of correlation between glomerular filtration rate, estimated with creatinine clearance, and carboplatin clearance in HSCT patients (r^2=0.0004 to 0.33)[88,93]; a large non-renal component of carboplatin clearance with higher-doses[88]; and potential saturation of the renal reabsorption of carboplatin, resulting in higher renal elimination.[89]

Limited sampling schedules have been developed to estimate carboplatin AUC with few blood samples and to conduct adaptive dosing of carboplatin in the HSCT setting.[94] Limited sampling approaches decrease cost relative to more extensive pharmacokinetic sampling, but must be prospectively validated to ensure that the AUC is accurately determined. Validation of limited sampling schedules should be performed in patients receiving the specific preparative regimen of interest. The limited sampling schedule developed for patients receiving carboplatin alone failed when used in those receiving a preparative regimen consisting of CTC.[95] Bayesian models may also have a role in estimating AUC in patients receiving carboplatin as part of a preparative regimen. A Bayesian model with two carboplatin concentration-time points was more precise and less biased than the use of the Calvert equation in 44 patients receiving carboplatin in combination with paclitaxel and cyclophosphamide (7 patients did not receive cyclophosphamide).[88]

There is a paucity of data regarding the pharmacodynamic relationships of carboplatin in patients undergoing HSCT. A cumulative carboplatin AUC >30 mg-min/ml was predictive of ototoxicity in 31 patients receiving carboplatin (400 mg/m^2/day), cyclophosphamide (1500 mg/m^2/day) and thiotepa (120 mg/m^2/day) for 4 consecutive days followed by autologous HSCT.[87] However, carboplatin AUC did not relate to various other non-hematologic toxicities.[87] Hematologic toxicity (neutropenia and thrombocytopenia) was not predicted by carboplatin AUC in these patients, nor in those receiving a preparative regimen of paclitaxel, carboplatin and cyclophosphamide.[88] Wright *et al.*[6] evaluated the relationship between the renal function and the AUC of ultrafilterable platinum (which correlates with intact carboplatin concentrations[96]) in 9 patients receiving ifosfamide (4000 mg/m^2/day), carboplatin (400 mg/m^2/day) and etoposide (400 mg/m^2/day) as a CI for 4 days. Based on the one patient who developed anuric renal failure, these authors suggested that an ultrafilterable platinum >14 μM at 16-22 h after the start of the carboplatin infusion may be predictive for renal dysfunction.

The use of cisplatin in HSCT has been traditionally limited to the CPB regimen, although it has recently been used as part of non-myeloablative stem cell transplantation regimens.[97] There is a 2 to 4 fold range in the AUC of cisplatin after administration of a 55 mg/m^2 dose in the CPB regimen.[1,64] To date, cisplatin exposure has not been associated with cardiotoxicity nor nephrotoxicity in patients receiving the CPB regimen.[64,66]

CONCLUSION

The role of adaptive dosing of the alkylating agents to decrease resistance should be studied further based on the considerable interpatient variability in the clearance of these drugs and the concentration-effect relationships that have been identified. The identification of these pharmacodynamic relationships between busulfan in patients receiving the BU/CY regimen can improve engraftment, relapse and toxicity rates. However, close attention to the preparative regimen is warranted because the concentration-effect relationships may change, as evidenced by data from the BU/CY preparative regimen. Adaptive dosing of cyclophosphamide may also reduce toxicity rates in patients receiving CY/TBI. Further work is needed to more precisely define the concentration-effect relationships of ifosfamide and the platinum analogs in patients undergoing HSCT. Presently, there appears to be little utility of adaptive dosing for carmustine because of the lack of pharmacodynamic relationships and the current 2-h administration schedule which does not allow for dose adjustments. In addition, the presence of unidentified alkylating metabolites of thiotepa makes identification of concentration-effect relationships difficult.

Concentration monitoring may also decrease resistance by identifying pharmacodynamic or pharmacokinetic interactions and lead to the more efficiently design of new preparative regimens. The development of new regimens including alkylators, such as those with radiolabeled antibodies or those used prior to non-myeloablative stem cell transplantation regimens, may lead to decreased relapse, rejection and toxicity rates in patients undergoing HSCT.[97,98]

REFERENCES

1. Jones RB, Matthes S, Dufton C, *et al.* Pharmacokinetic/pharmacodynamic interactions of intensive cyclophosphamide, cisplatin and BCNU in patients with breast cancer. Breast Cancer Res Treat, 26(Suppl):S11-17, 1993.
2. Schabel FM Jr, Griswold DP Jr, Corbett TH, Laster WR Jr. Increasing the therapeutic response rates to anticancer drugs by applying the basic principles of pharmacology. Cancer, 54(6 Suppl):1160-1167, 1984.

3. Eder JP, Elias A, Shea TC, *et al.* A phase I-II study of cyclophosphamide, thiotepa, and carboplatin with autologous bone marrow transplantation in solid tumor patients. J Clin Oncol, 8:1239-1245, 1990.
4. Slattery JT, Clift RA, Buckner CD, *et al.* Marrow transplantation for chronic myeloid leukemia: the influence of plasma busulfan levels on the outcome of transplantation. Blood, 89:3055-3060, 1997.
5. Ren S, Kalhorn TF, McDonald GB, *et al.* Pharmacokinetics of cyclophosphamide and its metabolites in bone marrow transplantation patients. Clin Pharmacol Ther, 64:289-301, 1998.
6. Wright JE, Elias A, Tretyakov O, *et al.* High-dose ifosfamide, carboplatin, and etoposide pharmacokinetics: correlation of plasma drug levels with renal toxicity. Cancer Chemother Pharmacol, 36:345-351, 1995.
7. Jones RB, Matthes S, Shpall EJ, *et al.* Acute lung injury following treatment with high-dose cyclophosphamide, cisplatin, and carmustine: pharmacodynamic evaluation of carmustine. J Natl Cancer Inst, 85:640-647, 1993.
8. McDonald GB, Ren S, Bouvier ME, *et al.* Venoocclusive disease of the liver and cyclophosphamide pharmacokinetics: A prospective study in marrow transplant patients. Hepatol, 17:314A, 1999.
9. Chan KK, Hong PS, Tutsch K, Trump DL. Clinical pharmacokinetics of cyclophosphamide and metabolites with and without SR-2508. Cancer Res, 54:6421-6429, 1994.
10. Boddy AV, Proctor M, Simmonds D, *et al.* Pharmacokinetics, metabolism and clinical effect of ifosfamide in breast cancer patients. Eur J Cancer, 1:69-76, 1995.
11. Przepiorka D, Madden T, Ippoliti C, *et al.* Dosing of thioTEPA for myeloablative therapy. Cancer Chemother Pharmacol, 37:155-160, 1995.
12. O'Dwyer PJ, LaCreta F, Engstrom PF, *et al.* Phase I/pharmacokinetic reevaluation of thioTEPA. Cancer Res, 51:3171-3176, 1991.
13. Newell DR. Can pharmacokinetic and pharmacodynamic studies improve cancer chemotherapy? Ann Oncol, 5(Suppl 4):9-14; discussion 15, 1994.
14. Calvert AH, Newell DR, Gumbrell LA, *et al.* Carboplatin dosage: prospective evaluation of a simple formula based on renal function [see comments]. J Clin Oncol, 7:1748-1756, 1989.
15. Evans WE, Relling MV, Rodman JH, *et al.* Conventional compared with individualized chemotherapy for childhood acute lymphoblastic leukemia. N Engl J Med, 338:499-505, 1998.
16. Ehrsson H, Hassan M, Ehrnebo M, Beran M. Busulfan Kinetics. Clin Pharmacol Ther, 34:86-89, 1983.
17. Gibbs JP, Czerwinski M, Slattery JT. Busulfan-glutathione conjugation catalyzed by human liver cytosolic glutathione S-transferases. Cancer Res, 56:3678-3681, 1996.
18. Czerwinski M, Gibbs JP, Slattery JT. Busulfan conjugation by glutathione S-transferases alpha, mu, and pi. Drug Metab Dispos, 24:1015-1019, 1996.
19. Hassan M, Oberg G, Bekassy AN, *et al.* Pharmacokinetics of high-dose busulphan in relation to age and chronopharmacology. Cancer Chemother Pharmacol, 28:130-134, 1991.
20. Regazzi MB, Locatelli F, Buggia I, *et al.* Disposition of high-dose busulfan in pediatric patients undergoing bone marrow transplantation. Clin Pharmacol Ther, 54:45-52, 1993.
21. Gibbs JP, Gooley T, Corneau B, *et al.* The impact of obesity and disease on busulfan oral

clearance in adults. Blood, 93:4436-4440, 1999.

22. Busulfex Product Information. 1999.
23. Vassal G, Fischer A, Challine D, *et al.* Busulfan disposition below the age of three: alteration in children with lysosomal storage disease. Blood, 82:1030-1034, 1993.
24. Hassan M, Fasth A, Gerritsen B, *et al.* Busulphan kinetics and limited sampling model in children with leukemia and inherited disorders. Bone Marrow Transplant, 18:843-850, 1996.
25. Shaw PJ, Scharping CE, Brian RJ, Earl JW. Busulfan pharmacokinetics using a single daily high-dose regimen in children with acute leukemia. Blood, 84:2357-2362, 1994.
26. Grochow LB, Krivit W, Whitley CB, Blazar B. Busulfan disposition in children. Blood, 75:1723-1727, 1990.
27. Gibbs JP, Murray G, Risler L, *et al.* Age-dependent tetrahydrothiophenium ion formation in young children and adults receiving high-dose busulfan. Cancer Res, 57:5509-5516, 1997.
28. Gibbs JP, Liacouras CA, Baldassano RN, Slattery JT. Up-regulation of glutathione S-transferase activity in enterocytes of young children. Drug Metab Dispos, 27:1466-1469, 1999.
29. Demirer T, Buckner CD, Appelbaum FR, *et al.* Busulfan, cyclophosphamide and fractionated total body irradiation for autologous or syngeneic marrow transplantation for acute and chronic myelogenous leukemia: phase I dose escalation of busulfan based on targeted plasma levels. Bone Marrow Transplant, 17:491-495, 1996.
30. Vassal G, Koscielny S, Challine D, *et al.* Busulfan disposition and hepatic veno-occlusive disease in children undergoing bone marrow transplantation. Cancer Chemother Pharmacol, 37:247-253, 1996.
31. Pawlowska AB, Blazar BR, Angelucci E, *et al.* Relationship of plasma pharmacokinetics of high-dose oral busulfan to the outcome of allogeneic bone marrow transplantation in children with thalassemia. Bone Marrow Transplant, 20:915-920, 1997.
32. Baker KS, Bostrom B, DeFor T, *et al.* Busulfan pharmacokinetics do not predict relapse in acute myelogenous leukemia. Bone Marrow Transplant, 26:607-614, 2000.
33. Slattery JT, Sanders JE, Buckner CD, *et al.* Graft-rejection and toxicity following bone marrow transplantation in relation to busulfan pharmacokinetics [published erratum appears in Bone Marrow Transplant 1996 18:829]. Bone Marrow Transplant, 16:31-42, 1995.
34. Bolinger AM, Zangwill AB, Slattery JT, *et al.* Target dose adjustment of busulfan using pharmacokinetic parameters in pediatric patients undergoing bone marrow transplantation for malignancy or genetic disease. Blood, 94:145a, 1999.
35. Hobbs JR, Hugh-Jones K, Shaw PJ, *et al.* Engraftment rates related to busulphan and cyclophosphamide dosages for displacement bone marrow transplants in fifty children. Bone Marrow Transplant, 1:201-208, 1986.
36. Yeager AM, Wagner JE Jr, Graham ML, *et al.* Optimization of busulfan dosage in children undergoing bone marrow transplantation: a pharmacokinetic study of dose escalation. Blood, 80:2425-2428, 1992.
37. Bolinger AM, Zangwill AB, Slattery JT, *et al.* An evaluation of engraftment, toxicity and busulfan concentration in children receiving bone marrow transplantation for leukemia or genetic disease. Bone Marrow Transplant, 25:925-930, 2000.

38. Grochow LB, Jones RJ, Brundrett RB, *et al.* Pharmacokinetics of busulfan: correlation with veno-occlusive disease in patients undergoing bone marrow transplantation. Cancer Chemother Pharmacol, 25:55-61, 1989.
39. Grochow LB. Busulfan disposition: the role of therapeutic monitoring in bone marrow transplantation induction regimens. Semin Oncol, 20(4 Suppl 4):18-25, 1993.
40. Dix SP, Wingard JR, Mullins RE, *et al.* Association of busulfan area under the curve with veno-occlusive disease following BMT. Bone Marrow Transplant, 17:225-230, 1996.
41. Hassan M, Oberg G, Ljungman P, *et al.* Correlation between hepatic veno-occlusive disease (VOD) and busulphan levels using limited sampling model for dose estimation. Blood, San Diego, CA: 251a, 1997.
42. Kashyap A, Synold T, Parker P, *et al.* First dose area under the curve (AUC) of oral busulfan predicts risk of developing veno-occlusive diseases (VOD) in adult allogeneic bone marrow transplant (BMT) patients. Proc Amer Soc Clin Oncol, 16:215a, 1997.
43. Ringden O, Remberger M, Ruutu T, *et al.* Increased risk of chronic graft-versus-host disease, obstructive bronchiolitis, and alopecia with busulfan versus total body irradiation: long-term results of a randomized trial in allogeneic marrow recipients with leukemia. Nordic Bone Marrow Transplantation Group [see comments]. Blood, 93:2196-2201, 1999.
44. Schuler U, Schroer S, Kuhnle A, *et al.* Busulfan pharmacokinetics in bone marrow transplant patients: is drug monitoring warranted? Bone Marrow Transplant, 14:759-765, 1994.
45. Vassal G, Hartmann O, Benhamou E. Busulfan and veno-occlusive disease of the liver [letter]. Ann Intern Med, 112:881, 1990.
46. Poonkuzhali B, Srivastava A, Quernin MH, *et al.* Pharmacokinetics of oral busulphan in children with beta thalassaemia major undergoing allogeneic bone marrow transplantation. Bone Marrow Transplant, 24:5-11, 1999.
47. Moore MJ. Clinical pharmacokinetics of cyclophosphamide. Clin Pharmacokinet, 20:194-208, 1991.
48. Ayash LJ, Wright JE, Tretyakov O, *et al.* Cyclophosphamide pharmacokinetics: correlation with cardiac toxicity and tumor response. J Clin Oncol, 10:995-1000, 1992.
49. Mouridsen HT, Faber O, Skovsted L. The metabolism of cyclophosphamide. Dose dependency and the effect of long-term treatment with cyclophosphamide. Cancer, 37:665-670, 1976.
50. Chen TL, Passos-Coelho JL, Noe DA, *et al.* Nonlinear pharmacokinetics of cyclophosphamide in patients with metastatic breast cancer receiving high-dose chemotherapy followed by autologous bone marrow transplantation [published erratum appears in Cancer Res, 55:1600, 1995]. Cancer Res, 55:810-816, 1995.
51. Bagley CM Jr, Bostick FW, DeVita VT Jr. Clinical pharmacology of cyclophosphamide. Cancer Res, 33:226-233, 1973.
52. Ren S, Yang JS, Kalhorn TF, Slattery JT. Oxidation of cyclophosphamide to 4-hydroxycyclophosphamide and deschloroethylcyclophosphamide in human liver microsomes. Cancer Res, 57:4229-4235, 1997.
53. Kaijser GP, Beijnen JH. Oxazaphosphorines: Cyclophosphamide and Ifosfamide. *In*: A Clinician's Guide to Chemotherapy Pharmacokinetics and Pharmacodynamics, LB Grochow, MM Ames (eds.), Williams and Wilkins, Baltimore, MD, 229-258, 1998.
54. Dockham PA, Lee MO, Sladek NE. Identification of human liver aldehyde dehydrogenases that catalyze the oxidation of aldophosphamide and retinaldehyde.

Biochem Pharmacol, 43:2453-2469, 1992.

55. Slattery JT, Kalhorn TF, McDonald GB, *et al.* Conditioning regimen-dependent disposition of cyclophosphamide and hydroxycyclophosphamide in human marrow transplantation patients. J Clin Oncol, 14:1484-1494, 1996.
56. Anderson LW, Ludeman SM, Colvin OM, *et al.* Quantitation of 4-hydroxycyclophosphamide/aldophosphamide in whole blood. J Chromatogr B Biomed Appl, 667:247-257, 1995.
57. Nieto Y, Xu X, Cagnoni PJ, *et al.* Nonpredictable pharmacokinetic behavior of high-dose cyclophosphamide in combination with cisplatin and 1,3-bis(2-chloroethyl)-1-nitrosourea [see comments]. Clin Cancer Res, 5:747-751, 1999.
58. Anderson LW, Chen TL, Colvin OM, *et al.* Cyclophosphamide and 4-hydroxycyclophosphamide/aldophosphamide kinetics in patients receiving high-dose cyclophosphamide chemotherapy. Clin Cancer Res, 2:1481-1487, 1996.
59. Graham MI, Shaw IC, Souhami RL, *et al.* Decreased plasma half-life of cyclophosphamide during repeated high- dose administration. Cancer Chemother Pharmacol, 10:192-193, 1983.
60. Moore MJ, Hardy RW, Thiessen JJ, *et al.* Rapid development of enhanced clearance after high-dose cyclophosphamide. Clin Pharmacol Ther, 44:622-628, 1988.
61. Chang TK, Weber GF, Crespi CL, Waxman DJ. Differential activation of cyclophosphamide and ifosphamide by cytochromes P-450 2B and 3A in human liver microsomes. Cancer Res, 53:5629-5637, 1993.
62. Ren S, Kalhorn TF, Slattery JT. Inhibition of human aldehyde dehydrogenase 1 by the 4-hydroxycyclophosphamide degradation product acrolein. Drug Metab Dispos, 27:133-137, 1999.
63. Bunting KD, Townsend AJ. Dependence of aldehyde dehydrogenase-mediated oxazaphosphorine resistance on soluble thiols: importance of thiol interactions with the secondary metabolite acrolein. Biochem Pharmacol, 56:31-39, 1998.
64. Petros WP, Broadwater G, Berry D, *et al.* Association of high-dose cyclophosphamide, cisplatin, and carmustine pharmacokinetics with survival, toxicity and dosing weight in patients with primary breast cancer. Clin Cancer Res, 8:698-705, 2002.
65. Hahm HA, Armstrong DK, Chen TL, *et al.* Novobiocin in combination with high-dose chemotherapy for the treatment of advanced breast cancer: a phase 2 study. Biol Blood Marrow Transplant, 6:335-343, 2000.
66. Nieto Y, Cagnoni PJ, Bearman SI, *et al.* Cardiac toxicity following high-dose cyclophosphamide, cisplatin, and BCNU (STAMP-I) for breast cancer. Biol Blood Marrow Transplant, 6:198-203, 2000.
67. DeLeve LD. Cellular target of cyclophosphamide toxicity in the murine liver: role of glutathione and site of metabolic activation. Hepatol, 24:830-837, 1996.
68. McDonald GB, Hinds MS, Fisher LD, *et al.* Veno-occlusive disease of the liver and multiorgan failure after bone marrow transplantation: a cohort study of 355 patients. Ann Intern Med, 118:255-267, 1993.
69. Wagner T. Ifosfamide clinical pharmacokinetics. Clin Pharmacokinet, 26:439-456, 1994.
70. Goren MP, Wright RK, Pratt CB, Pell FE. Dechloroethylation of ifosfamide and neurotoxicity [letter]. Lancet, 2:1219-1220, 1986.
71. Skinner R, Sharkey IM, Pearson AD, Craft AW. Ifosfamide, mesna, and nephrotoxicity in

children. J Clin Oncol, 11:173-190, 1993.

72. Henner WD, Peters WP, Eder JP, *et al.* Pharmacokinetics and immediate effects of high-dose carmustine in man. Cancer Treat Rep, 70:877-880, 1986.
73. Jones RB, Matthes S, Dufton C, *et al.* Nitrosureas. *In*: A Clinician's Guide to Chemotherapy Pharmacokinetics and Pharmacodynamics, LB Grochow, MM Ames (eds.), Williams and Wilkins, Baltimore, MD, 331-344, 1998.
74. Jones RB, Matthes S, Kemme D, *et al.* Cyclophosphamide, cisplatin, and carmustine: pharmacokinetics of carmustine following multiple alkylating-agent interactions. Cancer Chemother Pharmacol, 35:59-63, 1994.
75. Bearman SI, Overmoyer BA, Bolwell BJ, *et al.* High-dose chemotherapy with autologous peripheral blood progenitor cell support for primary breast cancer in patients with 4-9 involved axillary lymph nodes. Bone Marrow Transplant, 20:931-937, 1997.
76. Phillips GL, Fay JW, Herzig GP, *et al.* Intensive 1,3-bis(2-chloroethyl)-1-nitrosourea (BCNU), NSC #4366650 and cryopreserved autologous marrow transplantation for refractory cancer. A phase I-II study. Cancer, 52:1792-1802, 1983.
77. Henner WD, Shea TC, Furlong EA, *et al.* Pharmacokinetics of continuous-infusion high-dose thiotepa. Cancer Treat Rep, 71:1043-1047, 1987.
78. Ackland SP, Choi KE, Ratain MJ, *et al.* Human plasma pharmacokinetics of thiotepa following administration of high-dose thiotepa and cyclophosphamide. J Clin Oncol, 6:1192-1196, 1988.
79. Lazarus HM, Reed MD, Spitzer TR, *et al.* High-dose i.v. thiotepa and cryopreserved autologous bone marrow transplantation for therapy of refractory cancer. Cancer Treat Rep, 71:689-695, 1987.
80. Hussein AM, Petros WP, Ross M, *et al.* A phase I/II study of high-dose cyclophosphamide, cisplatin, and thioTEPA followed by autologous bone marrow and granulocyte colony-stimulating factor-primed peripheral-blood progenitor cells in patients with advanced malignancies. Cancer Chemother Pharmacol, 37:561-568, 1996.
81. Cohen BE, Egorin MJ, Kohlhepp EA, *et al.* Human plasma pharmacokinetics and urinary excretion of thiotepa and its metabolites. Cancer Treat Rep, 70:859-864, 1986.
82. Hagen B, Neverdal G, Walstad RA, Nilsen OG. Long-term pharmacokinetics of thio-TEPA, TEPA and total alkylating activity following i.v. bolus administration of thio-TEPA in ovarian cancer patients. Cancer Chemother Pharmacol, 25:257-262, 1990.
83. Eder JP, Antman K, Elias A, *et al.* Cyclophosphamide and thiotepa with autologous bone marrow transplantation in patients with solid tumors. J Natl Cancer Inst, 80:1221-1226, 1988.
84. van Maanen MJ, Tijhof IM, Damen JM, *et al.* A search for new metabolites of N,N',N"-triethylenethiophosphoramide. Cancer Res, 59:4720-4724, 1999.
85. Appelbaum FR. Is there a best transplant conditioning regimen for acute myeloid leukemia? Leukemia, 14:497-501, 2000.
86. Zecca M, Pession A, Messina C, *et al.* Total body irradiation, thiotepa, and cyclophosphamide as a conditioning regimen for children with acute lymphoblastic leukemia in first or second remission undergoing bone marrow transplantation with HLA-identical siblings. J Clin Oncol, 17:1838-1846, 1999.
87. van Warmerdam LJ, Rodenhuis S, van der Wall E, *et al.* Pharmacokinetics and pharmacodynamics of carboplatin administered in a high-dose combination regimen with thiotepa, cyclophosphamide and peripheral stem cell support. Br J Cancer, 73:979-984, 1996.

88. Johansen MJ, Madden T, Mehra RC, *et al.* Phase I pharmacokinetic study of multicycle high-dose carboplatin followed by peripheral-blood stem-cell infusion in patients with cancer. J Clin Oncol, 15:1481-1491, 1997.
89. Motzer RJ, Mazumdar M, Sheinfeld J, *et al.* Sequential dose-intensive paclitaxel, ifosfamide, carboplatin, and etoposide salvage therapy for germ cell tumor patients. J Clin Oncol, 18:1173-1180, 2000.
90. Chatelut E, Canal P, Brunner V, *et al.* Prediction of carboplatin clearance from standard morphological and biological patient characteristics [see comments]. J Natl Cancer Inst, 87:573-580, 1995.
91. Egorin MJ, Van Echo DA, Olman EA, *et al.* Prospective validation of a pharmacologically based dosing scheme for the cis-diamminedichloroplatinum(II) analogue diamminecyclobutanedicarboxylatoplatinum. Cancer Res, 45:6502-6506, 1985.
92. Shea T, Graham M, Bernard S, *et al.* A clinical and pharmacokinetic study of high-dose carboplatin, paclitaxel, granulocyte colony-stimulating factor, and peripheral blood stem cells in patients with unresectable or metastatic cancer. Semin Oncol, 22(5 Suppl 12):80-85, 1995.
93. Schilder RJ, Johnson S, Gallo J, *et al.* Phase I trial of multiple cycles of high-dose chemotherapy supported by autologous peripheral-blood stem cells. J Clin Oncol, 17:2198-2207, 1999.
94. van Warmerdam LJ, Rodenhuis S, van Tellingen O, *et al.* Validation of a limited sampling model for carboplatin in a high-dose chemotherapy combination. Cancer Chemother Pharmacol, 35:179-181, 1994.
95. Panday VR, van Warmerdam LJ, Huizing MT, *et al.* A single 24-hour plasma sample does not predict the carboplatin AUC from carboplatin-paclitaxel combinations or from a high-dose carboplatin-thiotepa-cyclophosphamide regimen. Cancer Chemother Pharmacol, 43:435-438, 1999.
96. Gaver RC, Deeb G. High-performance liquid chromatographic procedures for the analysis of carboplatin in human plasma and urine. Cancer Chemother Pharmacol, 16:201-206, 1986.
97. Khouri IF, Giralt S, Saliba R, *et al.* "Mini"-allogeneic stem cell transplantation for relapse/refractory lymphomas with aggressive histologies. Proc Amer Soc Clin Oncol, New Orleans, LA, 47a, 2000.
98. Matthews DC, Appelbaum FR, Eary JF, *et al.* Phase I study of (131)I-anti-CD45 antibody plus cyclophosphamide and total body irradiation for advanced acute leukemia and myelodysplastic syndrome. Blood, 94:1237-1247, 1999.

Chapter 17

GENOMIC APPROACHES TO CLINICAL DRUG RESISTANCE

Sambasivarao Damaraju[1], Michael Sawyer[2] and Brent Zanke[1,2]
Polyomx Program (www.polyomx.org) and Departments of [1]Experimental Oncology and [2]Medicine, Cross Cancer Institute, Edmonton, Alberta, Canada

1. INTRODUCTION

Detailed genomic studies related to drug resistance mechanisms are now possible because of the available information on the human genome. The rapid advances in methodologies, such as microarray analysis for gene expression profiling, and the even larger choice of methods now developed for scoring genetic variations among populations, will have a profound impact on the way we understand health and disease. The drug resistance phenotype in human tumors is a serious setback that limits the usage of chemotherapeutic agents for treating cancers. Drug resistance in tumors may arise due to one of several mechanisms, including altered metabolism, rapid efflux, or decreased uptake. Until recently, our understanding of secondary cellular regulators/factors that contribute to drug resistance was limited due to the lack of appropriate analytical tools. Microarray and genetic polymorphism studies led to the identification and characterization of several metabolic pathways intimately linked to drug resistance. We summarize some of the recent advances in the areas of microarray and genetic polymorphisms and their relevance to health and disease in general and to drug resistance mechanisms in particular. Lastly, we introduce the basic premise underlying the emerging area of metabonomics and how it is relevant to drug resistance.

2. GENE EXPRESSION PROFILING

2.1 Moving Toward Customized Anticancer Drug Therapy and Rational Drug Design

Foulds[1] and Knudson[2] were the first to propose that the evolution of a cancer cell phenotype, such as its growth properties and its susceptibility to anticancer agents, is a Darwinian process resulting from multiple stepwise changes in gene expression. During the past decade, molecular biology has given molecular meaning to these postulates, identifying several classes of genes involved in tumor formation and drug sensitivity—oncogenes, tumor suppressor genes, apoptosis-associated genes, membrane transporters, DNA repair enzymes and drug target enzymes[3]. Since tumor gene and protein bioprofiles are intermediary between genomic mutation and cell behavior, they provide a convenient and accurate malignancy metric that can be exploited for prognosis, selection of therapy, and the discovery of therapeutic targets. Early efforts identified single genes within functional classes, laboriously attempting to sketch the distorted biology of cancer[1,4–6]. The identification of some of these genetic changes formed the foundation for the molecular classification of tumors, the study of tumor markers, and even early attempts to predict tumor drug sensitivity[7,8]. The complexity of cancer genetic changes quickly frustrated attempts to relate complex phenotypes to simple changes. Complete pictures are now coming into focus as the identification of single gene products is relenting to an unprecedented explosion of high throughput and genome-wide biological information about tumors.

2.2 DNA Microarray Gene Expression Profiling

With the completion of the human genome project, the finite reality of gene expression has been appreciated. By the best estimates, no more than 30,000 different gene transcripts exist in humans[9]. These transcripts have been isolated through transcript sequencing and are catalogued, with commercial availability, as isolated transcripts (http://www.ncbi.nlm.nih.gov/dbEST/dbEST_access.html) (http://image.llnl.gov/). Recently, synthetic oligonucleotides corresponding to each human gene transcript have become available as near-complete sets, providing another representation of the complete range of human transcripts (http://www.operon.com/).

Whole human transcriptomes can be deposited at great density on solid supports using a variety of technologies. DNA microarrays may be constructed using oligonucleotide probes, synthesized *in situ* using the techniques of masked photolithography and solid-phase chemical synthesis (http://www.affymetrix.com/) or by mechanical spotting of cDNA or oligonucleotides onto glass microscope slides[10]. To detect global gene expression in tissues, these arrays are hybridized to fluorescently labelled gene transcripts and detected by the analysis of emission energy after laser excitation. Typically, dynamic intensity ranges in the order of 10^5 are observed, allowing the comprehensive, sensitive and specific evaluation of gene expression.

2.3 The Clinical Classification of Human Tumors by Gene Expression Profiling

Through comprehensive microarray-based gene expression profiles, distinct tumor classifications with novel prognostic relevance have been identified, demonstrating the power of comprehensive tumor bioprofiling using a single technology platform[11]. For instance, human diffuse large cell lymphoma has been fractionated into two important prognostic groups with differing response to therapy based on microarray data[12,13]. Similarly, analysis of human breast and colon cancer samples reveals tumor-specific patterns of gene expression, suggesting the potential for expression-based prognostication and therapy[11,14,15]. Similar approaches have attempted to improve tumor classification in prostate cancer[16]. These approaches will be improved by using higher density arrays and larger patient sample sizes with complete clinical data, including outcomes and therapeutic response. Similar large scale efforts are beginning with other technology platforms, such as protein expression profiling, but the greatest advances will be made when data gathered from multiple genomic and proteomic platforms are comprehensively integrated.

Advances in tumor classification and drug sensitivity prediction will depend on high throughput technological platforms that rapidly and cost effectively produce an entire transcriptome-, genome- or proteome- wide view of tumor biology[17–19]. Integrated gene and protein expression data gathered from these cutting edge technologies and mined using advanced bioinformatics would dramatically transform both our understanding and our approach to human malignancies. These technologies, when harnessed to detailed phenotypic information and investigated in laboratory models, have the power to explain the complex biological phenomenon of tumor progression and direct the development of prognosticators and new therapeutic targets. From the foundation of tumor classification derived from molecular profiles, science is poised to make the next leap into individualized prognostication and treatment based on the unique genetic aspects of individual tumors. As therapeutics are developed to address specific genetic abnormalities, custom therapeutic protocols will become the standard of care. Already, specific aberrantly expressed genes in cancers have been targeted directly, such as Bcl-2, Bcr-Abl and Her2/Neu[20,21]. These efforts are leading the way into specialized and customized therapeutic approaches with lower toxicity based on the tumor's specific aberrations. Genetic and biochemical deviations in cancer cells can not only explain the malignant phenotype but also hold the promise of rational drug design.

2.4 Bioinformatic Analysis of Expression Data

Gene expression profiling of human tumors typically yields tens of thousands of data points for each sample analysed. To extract meaningful information, data sets optimally undergo both a data enrichment phase and a data mining/data analysis phase.

Data enrichment adds layers of external data or prior knowledge to raw bioprofile data. Specifically, it often uses custom web-based crawlers and various bio-analytic tools to assign, derive or predict meta-information (information about the information) associated with microarray data. Identification of clusters of genes which are up-regulated will not necessarily indicate which signalling or metabolic pathways are being affected, which genes work together, or which genes repress one another. The only way this kind of insight could be gained is if one included with the raw microarray data additional protein interaction data (Biomolecular Interaction Database (BIND) http://www.bind.ca) or signalling pathway data (Cancer Genome Anatomy Project (CGAP) database http://cgap.nci.nih.gov/). Dozens of bioinformatics databases are available, including human genome sequence data (GenBank http://www.ncbi.nlm.nih.gov/Genbank/), Federated 2D gel data (Swiss 2D PAGE database http://www.expasy.ch/ch2d/), human mutation data (e.g., P53 mutation database http://p53.genome.ad.jp/), androgen receptor gene database (http://www.mcgill.ca/androgendb) KMDB – Human disease mutation database (http://mutview.dmb.med.keio.ac.jp), human disease information (OMIM http://www3.ncbi.nlm.nih.gov/Omim/), and a wide range of tumor-specific data (Cancer Chromosome Aberration project http://www.ncbi.nlm.nih.gov/CCAP/) Atlas of Genetics and Cytogenetics in Oncology (http://www.infobiogen.fr/services/chromcancer), and Breast Cancer Gene Database (http://condor.bcm.tmc.edu/ermb/bcgd/bcgd.html). Such data adds quantitative or relational information about protein-protein and protein-ligand interactions, homologs, paralogs, functional assignment, gene abundance, tertiary structure, quaternary structure, protein location, disease-causing mutations, protein and RNA turnover rates, chromosomal aberrations, chromosomal location, and karyotypic data. Because genomic data is constantly changing (due to ongoing changes to the databases and improvements to algorithms), self-updating tools are used to automatically update each bioprofile's meta-information on a regular basis.

While new techniques for analyzing array data, such as neural networks, Bayesian belief nets[22], classification and regression trees, discriminate analysis and logistic regression are in development[23], traditional methods, most commonly cluster algorithms, have been successfully adapted for array analysis[24]. These cluster methods group array data in two different ways. Either they group similar genes together, indicating which genes are co-regulated, etc., or they group together similar arrays, indicating which array profiles are similar. For the former, a cluster is a group of genes, while for the latter, a cluster is a group of arrays. The two most commonly used clustering methods are hierarchical clustering and *k*-means clustering.

Hierarchical clustering algorithms may be agglomerative in which data is successively grouped together, or divisive in which data is successively divided. In either case, maximal separation of clusters is sought; the amount of separation can be a good indicator of the quality of the cluster results. Due to the hierarchical nature of the resulting clusters, the number of clusters can be chosen after the algorithm has completed by choosing a level of the hierarchy on which to focus. In contrast, with non-hierarchical clustering, data points are assigned to a predetermined number of groups. *K*-means and self-organized maps (SOM) are frequently used non-hierarchical cluster analysis techniques[25]. The *k*-means method first assigns *k* cluster centers[26]. Pieces of data are then each assigned to a cluster centre in such a way as to minimize the total distance between each piece of data and the cluster centre. The cluster centre is defined as the mean of data assigned to that cluster. This may or may not be an iterative process depending on the flavor of the *k*-means algorithm used. *K*-means clustering has the limitation of needing to specify the total number of clusters ahead of time, which is often done in an *ad hoc* manner. SOM have a similar limitation and determine cluster centers in a slightly different fashion. Data points are mapped within a geometrical configuration. The position of a cluster center migrates iteratively to fit the data points.

All of these algorithms can be said to be either supervised or unsupervised, depending on what information the algorithm requires. Supervised classification schemes depend on prior knowledge of the data set, such as the drug sensitivity phenotype. In some cases, supervised techniques can result in the selection of a small number of genes, which maximally distinguish each group[27,28]. With unsupervised classification schemes, minimal prior knowledge of the data set is necessary. These can be viewed more as class discovery techniques rather than a predictive model builders.

2.5 The Use of DNA Gene Expression Profiling Using Microarrays in the Evaluation of Clinical Anticancer Drug Sensitivity

Cancer researchers have longed for a reliable assay to accurately predict tumor sensitivity to antineoplastic agents. *In vitro* tissue culture-based assays have formed the mainstay of efforts to emulate antibiotic sensitivity testing of bacteria, but they have been limited in their application to cancer by the inability to consistently grow tumor cells in culture and the poor correlation between *in vitro* cell killing and *in vivo* tumor response. While drug response is likely to be a composite between host factors, such as performance status, and tumor factors, such as intrinsic sensitivity, genome-based methodologies have become focused on tumor gene expression as a predictor of clinical outcome. Ultimately, tumor gene expression information will be considered in light of host genomic factors, such as polymorphisms in cytochrome P450 enzymes, drug transporters and repair enzymes to provide custom anticancer drug sensitivity profiles.

As a proof of principle, the drug sensitivity of 60 unstimulated human tumor cell lines has been related to global gene expression[17]. For this study, a bank of cell lines in common use for *in vitro* drug testing by the National Cancer Institute was studied by cDNA expression analysis using microarray techniques. For each cell line, *in vitro* sensitivity data to over 70,000 compounds has long been available, facilitating comparisons between gene expression and drug sensitivity. Of these compounds, 1,400 that had been tested on all lines at least 4 times were included in this study. Of 8000 total gene spots on the microarrays, 1376 were identified that had the most variation among cell lines. While the overall correlation between grouping of cells on the basis of gene expression and that on the basis of drug activity was rather low (r=0.21), interesting correlations between individual compounds and genes were detected. For instance, sensitivity to L-asparaginase and expression of the enzyme that generates this drug's target, asparagine synthetase, were closely inversely correlated. Similarly, gene expression in sub-lines of the breast carcinoma cell line MCF-7 can be related to doxorubicin sensitivity. Acute exposure of MCF-7 cells induces a subset of genes that tends to be over-expressed in sub-lines demonstrating constitutive drug resistance. The conclusion from these studies is that specific gene products, when expressed at the time of drug exposure, may modulate cytotoxic effects and their measurement may predict *in vitro* drug sensitivity.

The use of tumor gene expression profiling to predict clinical response to therapy is a powerful application of this technology. Gene expressions in human prostate cancer cell line xenografts have been analyzed to determine the genetic basis for hormone dependence. Of 5184 genes studied, 37 (0.7%) were elevated more than twofold in a hormone refractory line compared to its hormone sensitive parent, while 135 (2.6%) were reduced by half or more. In this study, over-expression of 2 genes, insulin-like growth factor-binding protein 2 (IGFBP2) and heat shock protein 27 (HSP27), were validated using immunohistochemical analysis of human tissue arrays containing 26 benign prostatic hypertrophy samples, 208 primary prostate carcinomas and 30 hormone refractory local recurrences. IGFBP2 was over-expressed in 100% of hormone-refractory tumors, 36% of primary tumors, and none of the benign samples. Similarly, HSP27 was over-expressed in 31% of hormone-refractory samples, 5% of primary tumors, and in no benign samples.

In an attempt to move gene expression profiling closer to clinical decision making, sensitivity of esophageal tumors to adjuvant chemotherapy was studied in relation to gene expression[29]. An array containing 9216 genes was used to evaluate 20 advanced-stage esophageal cancer tissues from patients who received the same adjuvant chemotherapy containing the drugs cisplatin and 5-fluorouracil (5FU). Expression of 52 genes was incorporated into a drug response score that correlated significantly with individual patients' prognosis. Whether gene expression profiling in this series of esophageal cancers is simply identifying treatment-independent prognostic groups or is predicting response to treatment remains to be determined.

2.6 The Future of Tumor Gene Expression Profiling in Anticancer Drug Sensitivity Testing

The measurement of constitutive and induced gene and protein expression may have clinical usefulness as a measure of intrinsic specific cancer cell drug sensitivity. While powerful, DNA microarray technologies are expensive and difficult to perform, suggesting that widespread clinical studies and application must await robust and readily available techniques. Current statistical methods have the power to identify small numbers of highly predictive gene products. Techniques suited to the analysis of a few gene products in many tumor samples, such as the immunohistochemistry of tumor tissue arrays, may point the way to effective predictive assays. Future medical care of cancer patients will be increasingly guided by the expression of specific cancer genes and by the genetic profile of key drug metabolizing, drug target and repair enzymes. Through these efforts, true custom designed anticancer therapy will be a reality, increasing treatment efficacy and reducing toxicity.

3. GENETIC POLYMORPHISMS

3.1 Single Nucleotide Polymorphism

DNA sequence variations such as variable number of tandem repeats (VNTRs), short tandem repeats (STRs) and single nucleotide polymorphisms (SNPs, pronounced as snips) are the most extensively studied areas of research since the launch of the human genome project[30]. SNPs are simply single base substitutions (point mutations) scattered throughout the genome, and they account for more than 90% of polymorphisms. It is now realized that the vast majority of the human genome is identical (~99.9%) in all individuals. However, the ~0.1% variation in the sequence translates to 3.2 million base changes in the genome, an average of 1 SNP for every 1000 bp or even 350 bp depending on the polymorphisms studied (cSNPs or pSNPs; see below)[31–33]. These variations are fairly stable, are subject to selection pressure, do not exhibit high mutation rates, and are heritable[34]. It is believed that these variations in the genome explain phenotypic differences between individuals and may also serve as a genetic blueprint for susceptibility to disease and response to various drugs[35]. SNPs are defined by their frequency of occurrence (>1%) and are distinct from point mutations which occur at lower frequencies[32].

The international scientific community, and in particular the SNP consortium (TSC), comprised of 13 pharmaceutical companies and the Wellcome trust, have undertaken a detailed and systematic study of SNP discovery and characterization of the entire human genome[36,37]. A total of 1.4 million SNPs are now available in public databases, and rapid progress in SNP genotyping methodologies will soon help to compile the entire chromosomal SNP maps. The availability of SNP maps will greatly influence our understanding of evolution, population genetics (inter- and intra-species variability), association to disease phenotype, correlation to drug therapeutics, and eventually individualized treatments and drug design. Genetic polymorphisms in drug metabolism are now recognized as a critical variable in a patient's response to a drug. Avoiding deaths due to adverse drug reactions, dose optimization for an effective therapy, and identifying patients at increased risk for toxicity, is now possible due to the application of pharmacogenetic screens[37–41]. For instance, the N-acetyltransferase (NAT2) enzyme catalyses the rapid acetylation of the drugs amonafide and caffeine. The polymorphisms observed in genetic screens from Japanese and Egyptian populations showed 90% and 8% rapid acetylation genotypes for NAT2, respectively, and reflect a need to adjust the dose for effective therapeutic levels of the drug to attain a similar response in different populations[31].

Currently, it is estimated that between 240,000 and 400,000 SNPs are present in coding regions of genes (termed cSNPs). An equal number of SNPs are also predicted from 3' or 5' flanking DNA in the immediate vicinity of coding regions (called perigenic SNPs or pSNPs)[31,39,40,42]. These figures are small compared to the total estimated SNPs in the human genome. The remaining SNPs occur randomly in non-coding regions of DNA (rSNPs)[31]. SNP distribution within coding regions varies. Human lipoprotein lipase (*lpc*) and angiotensin converting enzyme (*dcp*1) showed predominantly perigenic SNPs. The non-coding intronic regions of the 10-exon *lpc* gene showed 81 SNPs whereas the coding regions showed nine SNPs. A 24 kb gene containing 26 exons and 25 introns encodes the Dcp1 protein. Of the 78 variable sites in this gene, 63 are in perigenic regions and the remaining SNPs are in the coding region[43]. Several cSNPs and pSNPs in BRCA1, BRCA2 and prohibitin genes are useful markers in predicting breast and ovarian cancer[31,44]. Matrix metalloproteinase-1 protein over-expression due to polymorphism in the promoter region increases risk of lung cancer[45].

Combinations of polymorphisms in cSNPs and/or pSNPs are implicated in the disease outcome in polygenic diseases. Polymorphisms found in several key metabolic pathways such as signal transduction, cell cycle regulation, DNA repair, drug metabolism enzymes, etc., may alter an amino acid, introduce splice site variations or modulate promoters that bind various transcription factors. However, due to redundancy of the genetic code or the conserved nature of amino acid substitutions, most cSNPs lead to synonymous change in the amino acid of the encoded protein. Such mutations do not alter the protein function and are considered harmless, with some exceptions. For example, a SNP (synonymous) in exon 2 of *CYP27*-gene affects sterol 27-hydroxylase activity leading to a sterol metabolism disorder called cerebrotendinous xanthomatosis (CTX). A mutation of G to T at codon 112 (GGG ^{112}Gly to GGT ^{112}Gly) activates a nearby cryptic splice site, giving rise to defective gene transcripts[46]. On the other hand, effects of non-synonymous amino acid substitutions may have a pronounced effect on protein function[42]. Some claim that SNPs in coding or regulatory regions of the human genome that affect gene function are as few as 2000 in number[47].

3.2 Repetitive Genetic Elements are Naturally Polymorphic

Tandem repeats are repeating sequences of nucleotides, also referred to as satellites or VNTRs. Wyman and White in 1980 were the first to describe tandem repeats in human DNA using restriction fragment length polymorphisms (RFLPs)[48]. Work since then shows that the repeating sequences may be as simple as 2 or 3 nucleotides or may be highly complex with sizes ranging up to several thousand base pairs.

Satellites are a common source of genetic variation in the human genome. They are classified as microsatellites, which have repeating base sequences of

10 or fewer, or minisatellites, in which the repetitive element ranges from 11 to 100 base pairs[49]. Satellites may be found in both 5' untranslated regions and in introns, affecting gene expression. Satellites in 5' untranslated regions will affect the spatial orientation of start codons and regulatory elements such as promoters, affecting transcriptional efficiency[50]. They may also affect translational efficiency through unknown mechanisms and splicing of mRNA when found in introns[51,52].

While Wyman and White[48] discovered tandem repeats through identification of RFLP, most studies now use polymerase chain reaction (PCR) amplification of polymorphic regions followed by gel or capillary electrophoresis to measure length[53]. Some investigators have advocated using DNA melting temperature to assign genotypes[54] but others have criticized this as lacking specificity[55].

3.3 Polymorphism and High Density Genetic Maps

Polymorphisms are useful in the construction of high-resolution genetic maps, linkage analysis, positional cloning and loss of heterozygosity (LOH) studies[30,36,56–59]. Most human cancers are characterized by multiple genetic alterations that include deletion or mutations in chromosomal regions. Inactivation of a gene, such as that of a tumor suppressor, may occur due to mutation of one allele (alternative forms of a gene) and loss of the other allele. This kind of allelic imbalance was studied earlier at low resolution using a small number of polymorphic markers (e.g., STRs). With the discovery of SNPs (usually biallelic) and their abundance in the human genome, deletions or copy number changes could be easily detected as LOH by the use of the currently available density of SNPs as markers[33]. Genome sequencing offered the highest resolution map of each chromosome, providing information down to the level of a single nucleotide. Since the coding regions occupy a relatively small fraction of the genome, the functions or the significance of the so-called junk DNA remained elusive. Prior to the human genome project, low-resolution maps were constructed based on known information of genes or other genetic markers on each chromosome. The earliest of the mapping techniques (cytogenetic banding patterns) offered a resolution of 10 million base pairs (Mb). For studies on the inheritance of a particular trait, knowledge on relative locations of specific markers along the chromosome is highly informative. The genetic linkage maps rely on markers that are highly polymorphic and yield information on how frequently two markers are inherited together. These markers need not be in the coding regions as the vast amount of non-coding or junk-DNA is also polymorphic and is of immense value. The closer the markers, the more tightly they are linked and less likely to separate by a recombination event. In inherited diseases, the location of relevant genes can be determined in the individual by following both physical and genetic markers (position of genes) on high resolution genetic maps despite the lack of molecular basis of the disease[60]. In other words, complex diseases can now be traced to a set of genes through association of a group of SNPs or other genetic markers on a linkage map[42,60]. This formed the basis for positional cloning, wherein fine resolution maps help narrow thc region of the responsive genes[59]. Currently, it is estimated that the human genetic map has 1 marker for every 3 Mb. Several hundred genes may lie in between these markers. Many SNPs segregate together and are useful in association studies of polygenic diseases such as cancer, hypertension, diabetes, asthma, susceptibility to infectious diseases, and cardiovascular abnormalities[37,61,62]. In association studies, one looks for the co-occurrence of an allele and disease phenotype in a statistically significant manner[58,63]. Linkage analysis is used to scan the genome with more than one affected individual in the family and often yields information only on strong or high susceptibility factors, and the region defined is usually large. On the other hand, association studies define much narrower regions of the genome, detect weak susceptibility loci, and can be analysed without the need to study multiple individuals in the affected families. While each of these approaches have their inherent strengths, fine mapping of the genome combined with all of the above methods will speed up our understanding of health and disease. The emergence of specialized disciplines of science such as pharmacogenomics, physiological genomics and comparative genomics may have a profound influence on the diagnosis and treatment of patients in the near future[39,40,64].

3.4 Web-based SNP Resources

Many web sites offer current information on human genetic polymorphisms. These include the Human Genome Variation (HGV) database (http://hgvbase.cgb.ki.se/), the SNP Consortium (TSC; http://brie2.cshl.org/genome.shtml), NCBI Genes and Disease (http://www.ncbi.nlm.nih.gov), CDC Genetics and Disease Prevention (http://www.cdc.gov/genetics/info/database.htm), Human Gene Mutation Database (http://archive.uwcm.ac.uk), Human SNP database (http://www-genome.wi.mit.edu/SNP/human/), HUGO Mutation database (http://ariel.unimelb.edu.au/~cotton/mdi.htm) and the University of Utah Genome Center (http://www.genome.utah.edu).

3.5 Genotyping Methodologies

Genomic variability has created interest in genotyping populations to detect genetic factors contributing to diseases or to identify variability in drug metabolism and efficacy. A number of different techniques are currently in use to analyse genetic polymorphisms. Useful techniques for large-scale SNP genotyping studies must be low in cost, permit high throughput, and be accurate. The standard fluorescence based DNA sequencing from a large number of healthy individuals representing diverse ethnic origins is the most robust and reliable method for discovering novel SNPs at a given locus. However, the limited number of fluorophores available prevent multiplex reactions for high throughput analysis of genotypes in fluorescence based technologies. Base excision sequence scanning (BESS, Epicentre Technologies, Madison, WI), RFLP, and real time pyrophosphate DNA sequencing (www.pyrosequencining.com) are used for discovering novel SNPs and/or to study polymorphisms from the well characterized regions of the genome. Several other techniques are also in use today, and we describe here only a select few for reasons of brevity. We encourage the reader to refer to the original articles for their underlying physical principles and for a thorough account of each technique's strengths or limitations.

- **Restriction fragment length polymorphism (RFLP):** This method is based on the premise that polymorphisms in the genome would create or alter restriction enzyme site(s). This method involves digestion of genomic DNA with a panel of restriction enzymes followed by an agarose or polyacrylamide gel analysis for size fractionation. Individual alleles are then identified from Southern blotting profiles. Alternatively, sequences of interest are amplified using PCR followed by restriction enzyme digestion. Gel analysis and DNA staining of the fragments aid in the identification of alleles. This technique, also referred to as PCR-RFLP, is simple, reproducible and scalable for a reasonably large sample size[45,65]. It is estimated that only 50% of polymorphic sites are amenable to analysis using this technique[66]. Lack of restriction enzyme sites at the polymorphic locus precludes analysis in the remaining half, necessitating use of alternative techniques.
- **BESS method:** In this method, regions/loci of interest are amplified by PCR using labelled primer(s) in the presence of dUTP. Cleaving DNA at sites of dUTP incorporation generates sets of nested DNA fragments, which are analysed using high-resolution gel electrophoresis (Epicenter Technologies). This method allows comparison of different DNA samples for mutations (deletions, insertions, frame shifts or SNPs) on a relatively high throughput scale.
- **Pyrosequencing (www.pyrosequencining.com):** The target sequence containing the polymorphic site is amplified using PCR in which one primer is biotinylated. The double stranded template from PCR is immobilized onto a streptavidin-coated matrix and the non-biotinylated strand is washed away by alkali. A primer that anneals to the single stranded template in the proximity of the SNP site is added, along with Klenow polymerase (exonuclease deficient) and dNTPs in a primer extension step. The polymerase catalyzes nucleotide incorporation into a growing DNA chain, resulting in the release of pyrophosphate (PPi). The released PPi is measured in a coupled enzymatic assay after conversion to ATP. Quantitative deoxynucleotide incorporation is measured by coupling ATP synthesis to oxidation of luciferin that results in the generation of light. The light output is measured as peak height from the luminometric assay and is proportional to the number of bases added. The chain extension occurs one nucleotide at a time in a stepwise reaction wherein the deoxynucleotides are added sequentially. Each deoxynucleotide triphosphate (dNTP) is added to the assay and its incorporation is monitored in real time. An enzyme called apyrase degrades the unincorporated nucleotide before the addition of the next dNTP. The rate of dNTP incorporation by polymerase is faster than the rate of degradation by apyrase, favoring the extension reaction. The

nucleotide sequence of the growing complementary strand is determined from the peak heights in the pyrogram. Allele discrimination is achieved by selective addition of dNTPs, the prior knowledge of the sequence near the SNP site and/or separately hybridizing the single stranded template with allele-specific primers. The extension reaction is specific in that the mis-incorporation of a non-complimentary base is almost negligible. The kinetics of incorporation of a matching 3' base is much faster than a mismatched one. Slower reaction kinetics combined with the activity of apyrase prevents chain extension in mismatched primer template configurations. This non-gel electrophoresis technique has the advantage of high throughput, multiplexing, real time sequencing of SNP regions up to 25 consecutive bases, allowing flexibility in primer design and identification of closely located SNPs in a single reaction[67].

- **Conformation sensitive gel electrophoresis (CSGE):** This method is based on PCR amplification of the SNP flanking region and electrophoretic separation of homo- and hetero-duplexes on semi-denaturing polyacrylamide gels. DNA bands are identified by dye staining of the gels. This technique utilizes standard sequencing apparatus and narrower combs that accommodate up to 97 sample loadings. High throughput is achieved by repeatedly loading up to seven samples per well during electrophoresis. Optimum band resolution is achieved by loading samples at defined intervals of time during a run. This technique, though labour intensive, claims a relatively high throughput analysis (672 samples in a single run) in a single workday. The cut off limit for resolution of various bands on a gel is around 450 bp[68].
- **Melting curve analysis:** Melting temperature (Tm) of double stranded DNA depends on DNA length, sequence composition and GC content. Melting curve analysis for SNP genotyping uses a combination of PCR and RFLP without gel separation of restriction digested DNA. Double stranded specific fluorescent dye SYBR green is used to monitor fluorescence in real time as a function of temperature for scoring allele-specific genotyping for up to 96 samples per run. This technique does not require elaborate primer design or the use of biotinylated oligonucleotides that are otherwise required for allele-specific PCR based SNP genotyping methods[70]. This method is somewhat similar to Dynamic Allele-specific Hybridization (DASH) wherein the target sequence is also amplified by PCR and in which one primer is biotinylated. The biotinylated strand is bound to a streptavidin-coated microtiter plate, and the non-biotinylated strand is washed away with alkali. Allele-specific oligonucleotide probes are annealed to the single stranded templates with an intercalating dye that is specific for double stranded DNA, similar to melting curve analysis technique. The sample is gradually heated to its melting point while simultaneously capturing fluorescence intensity. A dramatic lowering of melting temperature is recorded in reactions with single base mismatch between target and probe[69]. Data analysis software is similar for both melting curve analysis and for DASH[71].

- **SNP analysis in a single tube using bi-directional allele-specific amplification:** This method is useful for routine genotyping analysis for known SNPs and involves optimization of magnesium, primer and dNTP concentrations. Two allele-specific primers are designed complementary to non-coding and coding strands of DNA representing the wild type and mutant alleles, respectively. The allele-specific PCR products vary in length, are analysed by standard gel electrophoresis apparatus utilizing a fluorescent DNA stain (SYBR), and are quantitated using standard gel imaging software. This technique is based on the premise that a single mismatched 3'-most nucleotide on the primer would not facilitate extension and amplification of DNA. The reaction conditions are optimized such that only a single band of varying size is expected for each allele, except for heterozygous individuals[72].
- **5' Nuclease assay with TaqMan:** This is a fluorogenic assay that utilizes PCR and Taq polymerase 5' nuclease activity. PCR primers are designed to flank the SNP site and another oligonucleotide (termed probe) is made to anneal at the SNP site, in an allele-specific fashion. The probe has a fluorescent reporter and quencher at the 5' and 3' ends, respectively. During the extension of the DNA strand by PCR, the nuclease activity of Taq polymerase cleaves the probe from its 5' end, releasing the reporter molecule and causing increased fluorescence. When the probe is intact, the fluorescence is quenched due to the proximity of the quencher and reporter dyes. Different reporter dyes are used for various reactions to discriminate alleles. The fluorescence signal accumulates on every round of amplification during the thermal cycling process. A mismatched probe on a target will have a lower melting temperature than a matched probe and is displaced faster by a competing matched probe also present in the same reaction. The 5' nuclease cleaves the reporter end of the probe only when 1-3 nucleotides of the probe are displaced off the template. This process happens much faster with a mismatched probe, leading to un-cleaved reporter and yielding lower fluorescence units than the matched probe and hence the allele discrimination[73].
- **MassArray system (http://www.sequenom.com):** Sequenom's MassArray system is based on measuring the primer's mass (at the 5' end of the SNP site) plus its extension product, which may be 1-4 nucleotides long. This technology uses Matrix Assisted Laser-Desorption/Ionization-Time-of-Flight (MALDI-TOF) mass spectrometry. The target sequence containing the SNP site from the genomic DNA is first amplified using PCR. The unincorporated dNTPs are dephosphorylated using a heat labile phosphatase to prevent incorporation of nucleotides during a primer extension reaction. DNA polymerase is used in the primer extension reaction along with fresh dNTP mix comprised of deoxynucleotides spiked with one allele-specific dideoxynucleotide. The extension reaction is terminated when a dideoxynucleotide is incorporated preventing, synthesis of lengthy extension products. The advantage of this technique is that a single primer (annealing at 1-4 bp upstream of polymorphic site(s)) works for all possible alleles at a given SNP site. Possible variants are identified from the size of the extension product

and the sequence information at which termination occurs. A mass difference of 9 to 24 daltons (depending on the base incorporated in the extension reaction relative to the primer mass) is easily detected by this method. Given the resolution of mass spectrometry at around 3 daltons, the analysis of the extension products and allele discrimination by MassArray system is fairly robust and reproducible. This technique supports high throughput analysis and offers allele calls in real time. The desalted sample is spotted onto a 384-chip array for analysis using a MALDI-TOF mass spectrometry.

- **Masscode system (http://www.qiagengenomics.com):** Cleavable mass spectrometry tags (CMSTs) are incorporated into the allele-specific extension products of PCR DNA. The CMSTs have a photo-labile linker, a mass spectrometry sensitivity enhancer and a variable mass unit, all connected to a lysine moiety. The oligonucleotide is linked to CMST through the 5' amino-hexyl residue. The assay is performed in solution in a two-step PCR format and offers high throughput and multiplexing. Due to the availability of multiple tags (30 in use now) of varying molecular weights which can be detected in a single quadrapole mass spectrometer, 15 simultaneous biallelic measurements are possible in a single run. This method has an advantage over fluorescence-based techniques as the latter are limited by the availability of discrete tags for multiplexing analysis[74].

In addition to the above methods, independent investigators and pharmaceutical companies have reported several genotyping techniques. Some of the more recently published or commercially available methods include SNP-IT process (Orchid Biosciences, http://www.orchid.com), HUSNP mapping assay from Affymetrix (http://www.affymetrix.com), the Acycloprime-FP SNP detection system from Perkin-Elmer (http://lifesciences.perkinelmer.com), Apyrase-mediated allele-specific extension[75], Tetra primer ARMS PCR[76], Ligation-rolling circle amplification[77] and Solid phase invasive cleavage reaction for SNPs [78].

3.6 SNPs and Clinical Drug Resistance

The majority of drug metabolism/detoxification occurs through the cytochrome P450 (CYP) family of hemoproteins (phase I enzymes) and a group of enzymes collectively grouped as phase II enzymes which include N-acetyltransferases (NAT), glutathione transferases (GST), UDP-glucuronosyl-transferases, methyl transferases and sulfotransferases[38,79,80]. These enzymes are predominantly found in organs such as liver, intestine and kidney. Several members of this family of proteins show polymorphism and affect the biosynthesis or degradation of endogenous metabolites or the exogenously administered drugs[38,80,81]. In some instances, these enzymes may also convert an inert compound into intermediates that are very toxic or carcinogenic[80,82] Other phase I enzymes that catalyze oxido-reduction reactions include prostaglandin synthase, alcohol dehydrogenase, and mono- and lipoxygenases. In addition to these enzyme classes, certain transport and receptor protein polymorphisms also affect drug sensitivity and have phenotypic consequences in patients[38,83].

Tuchman *et al.*[84] were the first to report the occurrence of severe 5FU toxicity in a young woman treated with adjuvant CMF (cyclophosphamide, methotrexate, 5FU) chemotherapy. This patient developed severe bone marrow suppression, mucositis and neurological symptoms that progressed to coma. These authors noted that the patient had very high circulating levels of uracil and thymine. Diasio and colleagues[85] reported a second patient with severe neurological toxicity from 5FU and demonstrated a delayed clearance of 5FU, with an increase in the half-life to 189 minutes. They also found low levels of dihyropyrimidine dehydrogenase (DPD) activity in the patient's serum. Meinsma and colleagues[86] first reported a G to A mutation in the GT 5' splice recognition site of intron 14 in a patient with DPD deficiency. This G to A SNP deleted exon 14 and abolished the catalytic activity of DPD[86]. Raida *et al.*[87] subsequently determined frequencies of this SNP in normal controls, colorectal cancer patients and patients with grade 3/4 5FU toxicity. Normal controls had a heterozygote frequency of 0.87% and colorectal cancer patients had a heterozygote frequency of 0.88%. In contrast, patients who had experienced grade 3/4 5FU toxicity had a heterozygote frequency of 20% and had a 4% frequency of homozygous splice mutations.

Methylene tetrahydrofolate reductase (*MTHFR*) has a SNP at position 677 from a C to T mutation. This mutation is found in 5% of the general population and results in a more rapidly degraded protein[88]. This SNP has been associated with an increased pool of reduced folates[89]. Stevenson and colleagues[90] hypothesized that an increased pool of reduced folates would compete with raltitrexed for thymidylate synthase (TS) binding. They confirmed this in a study of irinotecan and 5FU combination chemotherapy; they demonstrated that *MTHFR* TT homozygotes had less elevation of liver transaminases, neutropenia, and asthenia than CT heterozygotes or CC homozygotes[90].

3.7 Cytochrome P450 Enzymes and Drug Metabolism

The *CYP* genes show extensive domains of homology, an indication that gene duplication or transposition events occurred during their evolution. More than 50 human *CYP* genes have been reported and are grouped into families based on sequence conservation[80,90–93]. Some of the well characterized *CYP* gene members and their relevance to drug metabolism are discussed here in brief. The consequences of polymorphism in CYP1 (A1, A2, B1), CYP2B6 and CYP2C8 enzymes are not clear at the moment. These proteins metabolize endogenous substrates as well as exogenous compounds such as benzopyrene (CYP1A1); acetaminophen, amonafide, caffeine and propranolol (CYP1A2); estrogen metabolites (CYP1B1); cyclophosphamide and aflatoxin (CYP2B6) and retinoic acid (CYP2C8). Mutations in *CYP2A6* affect nicotine metabolism leading to cigarette addiction; *CYP2C9* polymorphism affects the anticoagulant action of warfarin; *CYP2C19* variants influence peptic ulcer response to omeprazole and cure rates in *Helicobacter pylori* infections; *CYP2D6* variants affect the metabolism of beta blockers, antidepressants, codeine, dextromethorphan, etc. Variants of *CYP1A2* were shown to rapidly metabolize antipsychotic drugs, leading to treatment resistance[94–96] Polymorphisms in *CYP2E1* affect metabolism of ethanol, linking to the possible effects of alcohol consumption[39,40,97,98]. Polymorphisms in *CYP2C9* were associated with colorectal cancers due to high enzyme activity leading to metabolic activation of the substrates. Enhanced clearance of substrates including non-steroidal anti-inflammatory drugs may further enhance the risk for colorectal cancers[99]. Genetic variants of *CYP19* (aromatase) were implicated in breast cancer risk[100–102]. Aromatase polymorphisms in coding or 3'-non-coding regions may alter the metabolism of endogenous steroids, particularly the conversion of estrogens from androgens. At least 50% of breast cancers respond to hormonal treatment, supporting the role of altered estrogen metabolism in higher incidence of cancers[102]. Adverse drug reaction to fluoxetine was noted in *CYP2D6* polymorphisms with one reported incidence of death due to poor metabolism of drug[103]. Sequence and organization of the *CYP1A* locus revealed the presence of xenobiotic response elements, suggesting a role for upstream regulatory regions in the expression of the *CYP1A1* and *CYP1A2* genes[104]. In addition to the above, modulation (presumably through polymorphisms in related genes) of some non drug-metabolizing proteins such as TNFα, interleukin 6, drug transporters and homologs of p53 were implicated in the drug resistance phenotype in cancer cells[105–108].

The *CYP3A* locus is 231 kb, encodes 4 genes and 3 pseudo genes, and has been studied extensively in recent years. The proteins encoded by these genes are believed to metabolize 50% or more of the known endogenous steroids and various drugs including antidepressants, HIV protease inhibitors, calcium channel blockers, and cholesterol lowering drugs and immunosuppressants[109–111]. The CYP3A proteins may account for up to 30-50% of the P450 content in the liver. The proteins encoded by *CYP3A* locus include CYP3A4, CYP3A5, CYP3A7 and CYP3A43. While CYP3A7 (expressed in fetal liver) and CYP3A43 (low levels in adult liver but highly expressed in prostate) are differentially regulated, CYP3A4 is the major isozyme involved in drug metabolism. Polymorphism in *CYP3A4* determines drug efficacy and accounts for up to 60-90% of the inter-individual responses to a drug. For instance, African Americans and Caucasians express 60% and 33%, respectively, of CYP3A4 activity. The role of CYP3A5 is less certain, but it is interesting to note that this isozyme also shares similar substrate specificity to CYP3A4, with some exceptions[111]. Differential metabolism of aflatoxin B1 and absence of quinidine hydroxylation has been noted for CYP3A5[112].

Polymorphism in the coding or regulatory regions of the genes for *CYP2C9*, *CYP2C19* and *CYP2D6* are well documented and underlie the variations observed in the drug response phenotypes in the population. On the other hand, the coding region SNPs for *CYP3A4* have not shown significant effects on drug metabolism. These observations may implicate polymorphisms in the promoter/regulatory regions of this gene in the drug metabolism phenotypes. It has been recently reported that a novel family of nuclear receptors termed pregnane X receptor (also called PAR or SXR) forms a heterodimer with retinoid X receptor and binds to agents such as rifampicin. These receptor-ligand complexes were shown to bind to regulatory regions of *CYP3A4* and to modulate its expression[93,109,113,114]

Drug metabolism phenotypes due to polymorphisms are designated as PM, EM and UM for poor, efficient and ultra-rapid metabolizers, respectively. These mechanisms are common for both phase I and phase II enzymes, forming the basis for the observed adverse drug reactions or chemo-resistance mechanisms[41]. For instance, variants in CYP2D6 using perphenazine as a substrate showed serum levels of the drug at 10 times the serum concentration in PM individuals compared to the EM, indicating low clearance of the drug. Similarly, the PM phenotype of omeprazole treated patients (in *CYP2C19* variants) showed a larger effect of the treatment when compared at a similar dose with EMs. The UM phenotype arises as a result of gene duplication. Two or more active genes (2-13 copies) on the same allele for *CYP2D6* have been reported. The clearance of drugs such as nortrityline and debrisoquine were shown to be proportional to the gene copy number. Apparent lack of feedback mechanisms for regulation of gene expression may explain this phenotype. The evolutionary significance of gene duplication indicates a beneficial role and is predominantly observed in certain ethnic populations, presumably due to selection pressures imparted by dietary factors[39,40].

3.8 Repetitive Elements and Drug Metabolism

Thymidylate synthase (TS) and uridine glucuronosyltransferase 1A1 (UGT1A1) are enzymes important for chemotherapy sensitivity and they contain satellites within their 5' untranslated regions. TS is the only *de novo* source of thymidylate and is inhibited by several chemotherapeutic classes of drugs such as the fluoropyrimidines 5FU and ftorafur[115] and the antifolates raltitrexed and pemetrexed[116]. UGT1A1 metabolizes irinotecan's active metabolite 7-ethyl-10-hydroxycamptothecin (SN38) to an inactive glucuronide conjugate[117].

Takeishi *et al.*[118] showed that the promoter of TS has a satellite of a tandemly repeated 28 bp sequence. Horie *et al.*[119] demonstrated that this satellite was polymorphic in length due to different numbers of the 28 bp tandemly repeated sequence, with a 19% allele frequency for 2 random repeat (2R) alleles and 81% for 3 tandem repeat (3R) alleles. Kawakami and colleagues[51,118] demonstrated that the number of these repeats affects TS mRNA translation. Colorectal cancer specimens from patients homozygous for 3R alleles have higher TS protein levels than those from 2R/3R heterozygotes. When compared to the 2R-containing TS gene promoter *in vitro*, expression from 3R-containing promoters increased TS protein levels due to increased translational efficiency and not to increased mRNA expression[118]. This observation has relevance to anticancer chemotherapy with the nucleoside analogue capecitabine. Capecitabine is a prodrug that is metabolized to 5FU, which in turn inhibits TS. Park and co-workers[120] showed that among patients with metastatic colorectal cancer the response rate to capecitabine was 14% in 3R TS homozygotes and 80% in 2R homozygotes. The same group showed that response rates in colorectal cancer patients to another thymidine competitor, 5FU, was 57% in those who were 2R TS homozygotes, 14% in 2R/3R heterozygotes and 8% in 3R homozygotes (P=0.02)[121]. Villafranca *et al.*[53] studied the effect of TS polymorphisms in 65 patients with colorectal carcinoma treated with preoperative 5FU and radiation. They found that only 22% of patients with a homozygous 3R TS genotype were downstaged after chemotherapy, in contrast to 60% of 2R/3R heterozygotes and 2R/2R homozygotes (P=0.036). The 2R/2R and 2R/3R genotype patients had a 3 year disease free survival of 81% while 3R/3R genotype patients had a 3 year disease free survival of only 41% although this difference did not reach statistical significance[53].

UDP glucuronyltransferase polymorphic tandem repeats explain phenotypic variability in bilirubin metabolism and drug metabolism. Bosma and co-workers[122] determined that Gilbert's syndrome, a chronic unconjugated hyperbilirubinemia, was caused by variability in the *UGT1A1* promoter. The wild type satellite in the *UGT1A1* promoter region consists of the sequence TATATATATATATAA, sometimes abbreviated to $(TA)_6TAA$. In ten unrelated patients with Gilbert's syndrome, a condition of hyperbilirubinemia, seven repeats of the dinucleotide TA ($(TA)_7TAA$) occur instead of six TA repeats observed in individuals with normal bilirubin levels[122].

Introduction of irinotecan in the late 1980s has made UGT1A1 polymorphisms medically relevant. The active metabolite of irinotecan, SN38, is metabolized by UGT1A1 to an inactive glucuronide[117]. Wasserman *et al.*[123] first reported that patients with Gilbert's syndrome were predisposed to irinotecan toxicity. Iyer *et al.*[124] showed *in vitro* that *UGT1A1* genotypes effected SN38 glucuronidation. In a clinical study, patients homozygous for $(TA)_7TAA$ were less efficient in glucuronidating SN38 to inactive SN38 glucuronide than those having the $(TA)_6$-containing genotype. The ratio of SN38 glucuronide to the unconjugated form was 9.3 in $(TA)_6TAA$ homozygotes, 4.0 in $(TA)_6TAA/(TA)_7TAA$ heterozygotes, and 2.4 in $(TA)_7TAA$ homozygotes. Patients who are homozygous for *UGT1A1* $(TA)_6TAA$ had no grade 3 diarrhea compared to 25% in those having $(TA)_7TAA$ homozygosity[125].

The study of polymorphic satellite sequences in *TS* and *UGT1A1* promoters is yet to become integrated into clinical practice. Since *TS* promoter polymorphisms effect tumor response to TS inhibitors such as 5FU and capecitabine, 3R/3R genotype patients may benefit from avoiding TS inhibitors in favor of different classes of drugs. Similarly, measurement of *UGT1A1* promoter polymorphisms can predict irinotecan toxicity, providing a rationale for custom cancer therapy. The metabolism of other agents will be found related to genetic polymorphisms expanding what is now a small list, permitting greater individualization of care with safer and improved outcomes.

4. METABONOMICS: CLINICAL GENOMICS AND DRUG METABOLISM

Analysis of drug or metabolic by-products in body fluids, referred to as clinical genomics or metabonomics, is now gaining importance as an emerging technology that could complement or augment the strengths of genomics and proteomics in understanding health and disease (<www.ciit.org><www.chenomx.com>)[126,127]. Small molecules in biological fluids may be used as biomarkers for diseases, therapeutic drug efficacy and toxicity. Xenobiotics may exert their effects directly at the pharmacological level without affecting gene expression. Unlike the semi-quantitative genetic or protein analysis, metabolite profiles in body fluids reflect dynamic metabolic responses in living systems to environmental challenges or genetic modifications. Liver and kidney are major organs engaged in metabolism and excretion of xenobiotic compounds. The metabonome approach may also help determine these vital organs' function in health and disease. Areas of immediate application for metabonomics are in the studies on metabolism of drugs/measurement of by-products and secondly to compare the metabolite profiles in body fluids in health and disease. Certain inborn errors of metabolism, as well as diseases that affect energy metabolism, can be readily analysed by a metabonomic approach since the end products of the metabolism under these conditions are well documented[126,128].

Up to 500 metabolites with molecular weights less than 20 kDa could be analysed using high-resolution ^{1}H Nuclear Magnetic Resonance (NMR) spectroscopy in body fluids such as urine, plasma, saliva and cerebrospinal fluids[128]. The technique is amenable to high-throughput analysis, cost effective, non-invasive, and rapid with little or no sample preparation times and yields both qualitative and quantitative information on several metabolic pathways in a single measurement. NMR spectroscopy is widely used in analysis and characterization of small metabolites and proteins. This method separates, identifies and quantitates compounds based on chemical shifts without the need to purify individual components by chromatographic or electrophoretic techniques. Spectral identification is based on pattern recognition and is done automatically by deconvolution software. The concentrations of metabolites are calculated from the peak areas[126].

The metabolism of drugs in humans varies widely among populations due to inherent genetic differences such as polymorphisms, mutations or deletions. Polymorphisms in genes coding for drug metabolizing enzymes may significantly contribute to dynamic changes in metabolite fluxes in body fluids and may be visible as characteristic signatures in the NMR spectrograms[128]. Unlike other diagnostic methods, this technique requires monitoring a number of metabolites and their concentrations to evaluate drug toxicity. This is analogous to predicting disease association (or prediction of drug efficacies/adverse drug reactions) with genetic polymorphisms. The technique is sensitive enough even to detect sub-clinical levels of toxicity/metabolic dysfunction that may go unnoticed by classical clinical diagnostic approaches. Analysis of metabolites in body fluids may become a standard practise in pre-clinical and clinical trials for testing drugs by the pharmaceutical industry in the near future[127,129]

CONCLUSION

Individualized therapies for the treatment of cancers is now increasingly recognized as a viable concept. Implementation of such therapies requires a close collaboration of many disciplines. Interpretation of the vast data collected from diverse classes of experiments involving gene expression, genetic polymorphisms, metabolite fluxes and proteomics is not trivial. The tools available today for data analysis are at best suited for the interpretation of individual classes of experiments described above. Development of comprehensive computational tools would one day help create a virtual clinical laboratory for screening patients prior to initializing therapy. For instance, unequivocal clinical diagnosis of the tumors by gene expression, proteomics and metabolite profiling combined with information on drug metabolizing enzymes will help target therapies to individuals.

ACKNOWLEDGEMENTS

This work was supported by grants from Alberta Cancer Board and Alberta Health and Wellness. We thank Dr. Michael Weinfeld and Jennifer Listgarten for helpful suggestions.

REFERENCES

1. Foulds L. Multiple etiologic factors in neoplastic development. Cancer Res, 25:1339-1347, 1965.
2. Knudson AG Jr. Mutation and cancer: statistical study of retinoblastoma. Proc Natl Acad Sci USA, 68:820-823, 1971.
3. Preisler HD. Resistance to cytotoxic therapy: a speculative overview. Ann Oncol, 6:651-657, 1995.
4. Dalla-Favera R, Bregni M, Erikson J, *et al.* Human c-myc onc gene is located on the region of chromosome 8 that is translocated in Burkitt lymphoma cells. Proc Natl Acad Sci USA, 79:7824-7827, 1982.
5. Ben-Neriah Y, Daley GQ, Mes-Masson AM, *et al.* The chronic myelogenous leukemia-specific P210 protein is the product of the bcr/abl hybrid gene. Science, 233:212-214, 1986.
6. Hollstein M, Sidransky D, Vogelstein B, Harris CC. p53 mutations in human cancers. Science, 253:49-53, 1991.
7. Chan HS, Grogan TM, Haddad G, *et al.* P-glycoprotein expression: critical determinant in the response to osteosarcoma chemotherapy. J Natl Cancer Inst, 89:1706-1715, 1997.
8. Chan HS, Lu Y, Grogan TM, *et al.* Multidrug resistance protein (MRP) expression in retinoblastoma correlates with the rare failure of chemotherapy despite cyclosporine for reversal of P-glycoprotein. Cancer Res, 57:2325-2330, 1997.
9. Subramanian G, Adams MD, Venter JC, Broder S. Implications of the human genome for understanding human biology and medicine. J Amer Med Assoc, 286:2296-2307, 2001.
10. Pollack JR, Perou CM, Alizadeh AA, *et al.* Genome-wide analysis of DNA copy-number changes using cDNA microarrays. Nature Genet, 23:41-46, 1999.
11. West M, Blanchette C, Dressman H, *et al.* Predicting the clinical status of human breast cancer by using gene expression profiles. Proc Natl Acad Sci USA, 98:11462-11467, 2001.
12. Alizadeh AA, Eisen MB, Davis RE, *et al.* Distinct types of diffuse large B-cell lymphoma identified by gene expression profiling. Nature, 403:503-511, 2000.

13. Shipp MA, Ross KN, Tamayo E, *et al.* Diffuse large B-cell lymphoma outcome prediction by gene-expression profiling and supervised machine learning. Nature Med, 8:68-74, 2002.
14. Alon U, Barkai N, Notterman DA, *et al.* Broad patterns of gene expression revealed by clustering analysis of tumor and normal colon tissues probed by oligonucleotide arrays. Proc Natl Acad Sci USA, 96:6745-6750, 1999.
15. Perou CM, Sorlie T, Eisen MB, *et al.* Molecular portraits of human breast tumours. Nature, 406:747-752, 2000.
16. Abate-Shen C, Shen MM. Molecular genetics of prostate cancer. Genes Dev, 14:2410-2434, 2000.
17. Scherf UD, Ross T, Waltham M, *et al.* A gene expression database for the molecular pharmacology of cancer. Nature Genet, 24:236-244, 2000.
18. Hanash S. Mining the cancer proteome. Proteomics, 1:1189-1190, 2000.
19. Martin DB, Nelson PS. From genomics to proteomics: techniques and applications in cancer research. Trends Cell Biol, 11:S60-65, 2000.
20. Banerjee D. Genasense (Genta Inc). Curr Opin Investig Drugs, 2:574-580, 2001.
21. Rudlowski C, Rath W, Becker AJ, *et al.* Trastuzumab and breast cancer. N Engl J Med, 345:997-998, 2001.
22. Greiner R, Grove AJ, Schuurmans D. Learning Bayesian nets that perform well. Thirteenth conference on uncertaininty in artificial intelligence, Providence, RI, 1997.
23. Hooper PM, Zhang H, Wishart DS. Prediction of genetic structure in eukaryotic DNA using reference point logistic regression and sequence alignment. Bioinformatics, 16:425-438, 2000.
24. Celis JE, Kruhoffer M, Gromova I, *et al.* Gene expression profiling: monitoring transcription and translation products using DNA microarrays and proteomics. FEBS Lett, 480:2-16, 2000.
25. Toronen P, Kolehmainen M, Wong G, Castren E. Analysis of gene expression data using self-organizing maps. FEBS Lett, 451:142-146, 1999.
26. Costoya JA, Pandolfi PP. The role of promyelocytic leukemia zinc finger and promyelocytic leukemia in leukemogenesis and development. Curr Opin Hematol, 8:212-217, 2001.
27. Golub TR, Slonim DK, Tamayo P. Molecular classification of cancer: class discovery and class prediction by gene expression monitoring. Science, 286:531-537, 1999.
28. Brown MP, Grundy WN, Lin D, *et al.* Knowledge-based analysis of microarray gene expression data by using support vector machines. Proc Natl Acad Sci USA, 97:262-267, 2000.
29. Kihara C, Tsunoda T, Tanaka T, *et al.* Prediction of sensitivity of esophageal tumors to adjuvant chemotherapy by cDNA microarray analysis of gene-expression profiles. Cancer Res, 61:6474-6479, 2001.
30. Brookes AJ. The essence of SNPs. Gene, 234:177-186, 1999.
31. Nebert DW, Ingelman-Sundberg M, Daly AK. Genetic epidemiology of environmental toxicity and cancer susceptibility: human allelic polymorphisms in drug-metabolizing enzyme genes, their functional importance, and nomenclature issues. Drug Metab Rev, 31:467-487, 1999.
32. Kruglyak L, Nickerson DA. Variation is the spice of life. Nature Genet, 27:234-236, 2001.
33. Stoneking M. Single nucleotide polymorphisms. From the evolutionary past. Nature, 409:821-822, 2001.
34. Fallin D, Schork NJ. Accuracy of haplotype frequency estimation for biallelic loci, via the expectation-maximization algorithm for unphased diploid genotype data. Amer J Human Genet, 67:947-959, 2000.
35. Chakravarti A. To a future of genetic medicine. Nature, 409:822-823, 2001.

36. Lehnert V, Holzwarth J, Ott M, *et al.* A semi-automated system for analysis and storage of SNPs. Human Mutat, 17:243-254, 2001.
37. Sachidanandam R, Weissman D, Schmidt SC, *et al.* A map of human genome sequence variation containing 1.42 million single nucleotide polymorphisms. Nature, 409:928-933, 2001.
38. Evans WE, Johnson JA. Pharmacogenomics: the inherited basis for interindividual differences in drug response. Annu Rev Genomics Human Genet, 2:9-39, 2001.
39. Ingelman-Sundberg M. Genetic susceptibility to adverse effects of drugs and environmental toxicants: The role of CYP family of enzymes. Mutat Res, 482:11-19, 2001.
40. Ingelman-Sundberg M. Pharmacogenetics: an opportunity for a safer and more efficient pharmacotherapy. J Intern Med, 250:186-200, 2001.
41. Phillips KA, Veenstra DL, Oren E, *et al.* Potential role of pharmacogenomics in reducing adverse drug reactions: a systematic review. J Amer Med Assoc, 286:2270-2279, 2001.
42. Cargill M, Altshuler D, Ireland J, *et al.* Characterization of single-nucleotide polymorphisms in coding regions of human genes. Nature Genet, 22:231-238, 1999.
43. Nebert DW. Pharmacogenetics and pharmacogenomics: why is this relevant to the clinical geneticist? Clin Genet, 56:247-258, 1999.
44. Jupe ER, Badgett AA, Beas BR, *et al.* Single nucleotide polymorphism in prohibitin 39 untranslated region and breast-cancer susceptibility. Lancet, 357:1588-1589, 2001.
45. Zhu Y, Spitz MR, Lei L, *et al.* A single nucleotide polymorphism in the matrix metalloproteinase-1 promoter enhances lung cancer susceptibility. Cancer Res, 61:7825-7829, 2001.
46. Chen W, Kubota S, Teramoto T, *et al.* Silent nucleotide substitution in the sterol 27-hydroxylase gene (CYP 27) leads to alternative pre-mRNA splicing by activating a cryptic 5' splice site at the mutant codon in cerebrotendinous xanthomatosis patients. Biochem, 37:4420-4428, 1998.
47. Lewis R. SNPs as windows on evolution. The Scientist, 16:16-18, 2002.
48. Wyman AR, White R. A highly polymorphic locus in human DNA. Proc Natl Acad Sci USA, 77:6754-6758, 1980.
49. Richard GF, Paques F. Mini- and microsatellite expansions: the recombination connection. EMBO Rep, 1:122-126, 2000.
50. Kennedy GC, German MS, Rutter WJ. The minisatellite in the diabetes susceptibility locus IDDM2 regulates insulin transcription. Nature Genet, 9:293-298, 1995.
51. Kawakami K, Salonga D, Park JM, *et al.* Different lengths of a polymorphic repeat sequence in the thymidylate synthase gene affect translational efficiency but not its gene expression. Clin Cancer Res, 7:4096-4101, 2001.
52. Turri MG, Cuin KA, Parker AC. Characterisation of a novel minisatellite that provides multiple splice donor sites in an interferon-induced transcript. Nucleic Acids Res, 23:1854-1861, 1995.
53. Villafranca E, Okruzhnov Y, Dominguez MA, *et al.* Polymorphisms of the repeated sequences in the enhancer region of the thymidylate synthase gene promoter may predict downstaging after preoperative chemoradiation in rectal cancer. J Clin Oncol, 19:1779-1786, 2001.
54. Marziliano N, Pelo E, Minuti B, *et al.* Melting temperature assay for a UGT1A gene variant in Gilbert syndrome. Clin Chem, 46:423-425, 2000.
55. von Ahsen N, Oellerich M, Schutz E. Limitations of genotyping based on amplicon melting temperature. Clin Chem, 47:1331-1332, 2000.
56. Clifford R, Edmonson M, Hu Y, *et al.* Expression-based genetic/physical maps of single-nucleotide polymorphisms identified by the cancer genome anatomy project. Genome Res, 10:1259-1265, 2000.

57. Mei R, Galipeau PC, Prass C, *et al.* Genome-wide detection of allelic imbalance using human SNPs and high- density DNA arrays. Genome Res, 10:1126-1137, 2000.
58. Schork NJ, Fallin D, Lanchbury JS. Single nucleotide polymorphisms and the future of genetic epidemiology. Clin Genet, 58:250-264, 2000.
59. Bader JS. The relative power of SNPs and haplotype as genetic markers for association tests. Pharmacogenomics, 2:11-24, 2001.
60. McCarthy JJ, Hilfiker R. The use of single-nucleotide polymorphism maps in pharmacogenomics. Nature Biotechnol, 18:505-508, 2000.
61. Riley JH, Allan CJ, Lai E. The use of single nucleotide polymorphisms in the isolation of common disease genes. Pharmacogenomics, 1:39-47, 2000.
62. Wang Z, Moult J. SNPs, protein structure, and disease. Human Mutat, 17:263-270, 2001.
63. Schork NJ, Nath SK, Fallin D, Chakravarti, A. Linkage disequilibrium analysis of biallelic DNA markers, human quantitative trait loci, and threshold-defined case and control subjects. Amer J Human Genet, 67:1208-1218, 2000.
64. Sadee W. Genomics and drugs: finding the optimal drug for the right patient. Pharm Res, 15:959-963, 1998.
65. Xie D, Shu XO, Deng Z. Population-based, case-control study of HER2 genetic polymorphism and breast cancer risk. J Natl Cancer Inst, 92:412-417, 2000.
66. Landegren U, Kaiser R, Sanders J, Hood L. A ligase-mediated gene detection technique. Science, 241:1077-1080, 1988.
67. Alderborn A, Kristofferson A, Hammerling U. Determination of single-nucleotide polymorphisms by real-time pyrophosphate DNA sequencing. Genome Res, 10:1249-1258, 2000.
68. Leung YF, Tam PO, Tong WC, *et al.* High-throughput conformation-sensitive gel electrophoresis for discovery of SNPs. Biotechniques, 30:334-335, 338-340, 2001.
69. Akey JM, Sosnoski D, Parra E, *et al.* Melting curve analysis of SNPs (McSNP): a gel-free and inexpensive approach for SNP genotyping. Biotechniques, 30:358-362, 364, 366-367, 2001.
70. Howell WM, Jobs M, Gyllensten U, Brookes AJ. Dynamic allele-specific hybridization. A new method for scoring single nucleotide polymorphisms. Nature Biotechnol, 17:87-88, 1999.
71. Prince JA, Feuk L, Howell WM, *et al.* Robust and accurate single nucleotide polymorphism genotyping by dynamic allele-specific hybridization (DASH): design criteria and assay validation. Genome Res, 11:152-162, 2001.
72. Waterfall CM, Cobb BD. Single tube genotyping of sickle cell anaemia using PCR-based SNP analysis. Nucleic Acids Res, 29:E119, 2001.
73. Livak KJ. Allelic discrimination using fluorogenic probes and the 5' nuclease assay. Genet Anal, 14:143-149, 1999.
74. Kokoris M, Dix K, Moynihan K, *et al.* High-throughput SNP genotyping with the Masscode system. Mol Diagn, 5:329-340, 2000.
75. Ahmadian A, Gharizadeh B, O'Meara D, *et al.* Genotyping by apyrase-mediated allele-specific extension. Nucleic Acids Res, 29:E121, 2001.
76. Ye S, Dhillon S, Ke X, *et al.* An efficient procedure for genotyping single nucleotide polymorphisms. Nucleic Acids Res, 29:E88-98, 2001.
77. Qi X, Bakht S, Devos KM, *et al.* L-RCA (ligation-rolling circle amplification): a general method for genotyping of single nucleotide polymorphisms (SNPs). Nucleic Acids Res, 29:E116, 2001.
78. Stevens PW, Hall JG, Lyamichev V, *et al.* Analysis of single nucleotide polymorphisms with solid phase invasive cleavage reactions. Nucleic Acids Res, 29:E77, 2001.

79. Board P, Blackburn A, Jermiin LS, Chelvanayagam G. Polymorphism of phase II enzymes: identification of new enzymes and polymorphic variants by database analysis. Toxicol Lett, 102-103:149-154. 1998.
80. Taningher M, Malacarne D, Izotti A, *et al.* Drug metabolism polymorphisms as modulators of cancer susceptibility. Mutat Res, 436:227-261, 1999.
81. Nelson DR. Cytochrome P450 and the individuality of species. Arch Biochem Biophys, 369:1-10, 1999.
82. Guengerich FP. Forging the links between metabolism and carcinogenesis. Mutat Res, 488:195-209, 2001.
83. Nebert DW. Drug-metabolizing enzymes in ligand-modulated transcription. Biochem Pharmacol, 47:25-37. 1994.
84. Tuchman M, Stoeckeler JS, Kiang DT, *et al.* Familial pyrimidinemia and pyrimidinuria associated with severe fluorouracil toxicity. N Engl J Med, 313:245-249, 1985.
85. Diasio RB, Beavers TL, Carpenter JT. Familial deficiency of dihydropyrimidine dehydrogenase. Biochemical basis for familial pyrimidinemia and severe 5-fluorouracil-induced toxicity. J Clin Invest, 81:47-51, 1988.
86. Meinsma R, Fernandez-Salguero P, Van Kuilenburg AB, *et al.* Human polymorphism in drug metabolism: mutation in the dihydropyrimidine dehydrogenase gene results in exon skipping and thymine uracilurea. DNA Cell Biol, 14:1-6, 1995.
87. Raida M, Schwabe W, Hausler P, *et al.* Prevalence of a common point mutation in the dihydropyrimidine dehydrogenase (DPD) gene within the 5'-splice donor site of intron 14 in patients with severe 5-fluorouracil (5-FU)-related toxicity compared with controls. Clin Cancer Res, 7:2832-2839, 2001.
88. Kang SS, Wong PW, Jhou JM, *et al.* Thermolabile methylenetetrahydrofolate reductase in patients with coronary artery disease. Metabolism, 37:611-613, 1988.
89. Kawakami K, Omura K, Kanehira E, Watanabe G. Methylene tetrahydrofolate reductase polymorphism is associated with folate pool in gastrointestinal cancer tissue. Anticancer Res, 21:285-289, 2001.
90. Stevenson JP, Redlinger M, Kluijtmans LA, *et al.* Phase I clinical and pharmacogenetic trial of irinotecan and raltitrexed administered every 21 days to patients with cancer. J Clin Oncol, 19:4081-4087, 2001.
91. Lewis DF, Watson E, Lake BG. Evolution of the cytochrome P450 superfamily: sequence alignments and pharmacogenetics. Mutat Res, 410:245-270, 1998.
92. Graham SE, Peterson JA. How similar are P450s and what can their differences teach us? Arch Biochem Biophys, 369:24-29, 1999.
93. Waxman DJ. P450 gene induction by structurally diverse xenochemicals: central role of nuclear receptors CAR, PXR, and PPAR. Arch Biochem Biophys, 369:11-23, 1999.
94. Dojo M, Azuma T, Saito T, *et al.* Effects of CYP2C19 gene polymorphism on cure rates for Helicobacter pylori infection by triple therapy with proton pump inhibitor (omeprazole or rabeprazole), amoxycillin and clarithromycin in Japan. Dig Liver Dis, 33:671-675, 2001.
95. Ozdemir V, Kalow W, Okey A, *et al.* Treatment-resistance to clozapinein association with ultrarapid CYP1A2 activity and the C $\rightarrow$ A polymorphism in intron 1 of the CYP1A2 gene: effect of grapefruit juice and low-dose fluvoxamine. J Clin Psychopharmacol, 21:603-607, 2001.
96. Ozdemir V, Kalow W, Posner P, *et al.* CYP1A2 activity as measured by a caffeine test predicts clozapine and active metabolite steady-state concentration in patients with schizophrenia. J Clin Psychopharmacol, 21:398-407, 2001.
97. Hiratsuka M, Mizugaki M. Genetic polymorphisms in drug-metabolizing enzymes and drug targets. Mol Genet Metab, 73:298-305, 2001.

98. Raunio H, Rautio A, Gullsten H, Pelkonen O. Polymorphisms of CYP2A6 and its practical consequences. Br J Clin Pharmacol, 52:357-363, 2001.
99. Martinez C, Garcia-Martin E, Ladero JM, *et al.* Association of CYP2C9 genotypes leading to high enzyme activity and colorectal cancer risk. Carcinogenesis, 22:1323-1326, 2001.
100. Pike MC, Spicer DV, Dahmoush L, *et al.* Estrogens, progestogens, normal breast cell proliferation, and breast cancer risk. Epidemiol Rev, 15:17-35, 1993.
101. Sourdaine P, Parker MG, Telford J, Miller WR. Analysis of the aromatase cytochrome P450 gene in human breast cancers. J Mol Endocrinol, 13:331-337,1994.
102. Kristensen VN, Harada N, Yoshimura N, *et al.* Genetic variants of CYP19 (aromatase) and breast cancer risk. Oncogene, 19:1329-1333, 2000.
103. Sallee FR, DeVane C, Ferrell RE. Fluoxetine-related death in a child with cytochrome P-450 2D6 genetic deficiency. J Child Adolesc Psychopharmacol, 10:27-34, 2000.
104. Corchero J, Pimprale S, Kimura S, *et al.* Organization of the CYP1A cluster on human chromosome 15: implications for gene regulation. Pharmacogenetics, 11:1-6, 2001.
105. van den Heuvel-Eibrink MM, Sonneveld P, Pieters R. The prognostic significance of membrane transport-associated multidrug resistance (MDR) proteins in leukemia. Int J Clin Pharmacol Ther, 38:94-110, 2000.
106. Conze D, Weiss L, Regen PS, *et al.* Autocrine production of interleukin 6 causes multidrug resistance in breast cancer cells. Cancer Res, 61:8851-8858, 2001.
107. Di Marco S, Hel Z, Lachance C, *et al.* Polymorphism in the 3'-untranslated region of TNFalpha mRNA impairs binding of the post-transcriptional regulatory protein HuR to TNFalpha mRNA. Nucleic Acids Res, 29:863-871, 2001.
108. Vikhanskaya F, Marchini S, Marabese M, *et al.* P73a overexpression is associated with resistance to treatment with DNA-damaging agents in a human ovarian cancer cell line. Cancer Res, 61:935-938, 2001.
109. Eichelbaum M, Burk O. CYP3A genetics in drug metabolism. Nature Med, 7:285-287, 2001.
110. Gellner K, Eiselt R, Hustert E, *et al.* Genomic organization of the human CYP3A locus: identification of a new, inducible CYP3A gene. Pharmacogenetics, 11:111-121, 2001.
111. Kuehl P, Zhang J, Lin Y, *et al.* Sequence diversity in *CYP3A* promoters and characterization of the genetic basis of polymorphic CYP3A5 expression. Nature Genet, 27:383-391, 2001.
112. Hustert E, Haberl M, Burk O, *et al.* The genetic determinants of the CYP3A5 polymorphism. Pharmacogenet, 11:773-779, 2001.
113. Blumberg B, Sabbagh W Jr, Juguilong H, *et al.* SXR, a novel steroid and xenobiotic-sensing nuclear receptor. Genes Dev, 12:3195-3205, 1998.
114. Lehmann JM, McKee DD, Watson MA, *et al.* The human orphan nuclear receptor PXR is activated by compounds that regulate CYP3A4 gene expression and cause drug interactions. J Clin Invest, 102:1016-1023, 1998.
115. Grem J. 5-Fluoropyrimidines. *In*: Cancer Chemotherapy and Biotherapy, B Chabner, D Longo (eds.), Lippincott-Raven, Philadelphia, PA, 1996.
116. Chu E, Allegra CJ. Antifolates. *In*: Cancer Chemotherapy and Biotherapy, B Chabner, D Longo (eds.), Lippincott-Raven, Philadelphia, PA, 1996.
117. Iyer L, King CD, Whitington PF, *et al.* Genetic predisposition to the metabolism of irinotecan (CPT-11). Role of uridine diphosphate glucuronosyltransferase isoform 1A1 in the glucuronidation of its active metabolite (SN-38) in human liver microsomes. J Clin Invest, 101:847-854, 1998.
118. Takeishi K, Kaneda S, Ayusawa D, *et al.* Nucleotide sequence of a functional cDNA for human thymidylate synthase. Nucleic Acids Res, 13:2035-2043, 1985.

119. Horie N, Aiba H, Oguro K, *et al.* Functional analysis and DNA polymorphism of the tandemly repeated sequences in the 5'-terminal regulatory region of the human gene for thymidylate synthase. Cell Struct Funct, 20:191-197, 1995.
120. Park D, Soehlmacher J, Wu Z, *et al.* Human thymidylate synthase gene polymorphism determines response to capecitabine chemotherapy in advanced colorectal cancer. Proc Amer Soc Clin Oncol, 129a, Abstract #514, 2001.
121. Pullarkat S, Ghaderi V, Ingles SA, *et al.* Human thymidylate synthase gene polymorphism determines response to 5-FU chemotherapy. Proc Amer Soc Clin Oncol, 243a, Abstract #942, 2000.
122. Bosma PJ, Chowdhury JR, Bakker C, *et al.* The genetic basis of the reduced expression of bilirubin UDP-glucuronosyltransferase 1 in Gilbert's syndrome. N Engl J Med, 333:1171-1175, 1995.
123. Wasserman E, Myara A, Lokiec F, *et al.* Severe CPT-11 toxicity in patients with Gilbert's syndrome: two case reports. Annu Oncol, 8:1049-1051, 1997.
124. Iyer L, Hall D, Das, S, *et al.* Phenotype-genotype correlation of in vitro SN-38 (active metabolite of irinotecan) and bilirubin glucuronidation in human liver tissue with UGT1A1 promoter polymorphism. Clin Pharmacol Ther, 65:576-582, 1999.
125. Iyer L, Hall D, Das S, *et al.* UGT1A1 promoter genotype correlates with pharmacokinetics of irinotecan (CPT-11). Proc Amer Soc Clin Oncol, 178a, Abstract #690, 2000.
126. Nicholson JK, Lindon JC, Holmes E. 'Metabonomics': understanding the metabolic responses of living systems to pathophysiological stimuli via multivariate statistical analysis of biological NMR spectroscopic data. Xenobiotica, 29:1181-1189, 1999.
127. Holmes E, Nicholls AW, Lindon JC, *et al.* Chemometric models for toxicity classification based on NMR spectra of biofluids. Chem Res Toxicol, 13:471-478, 2000.
128. Holmes E, Nicholson JK, Tranter G. Metabonomic characterization of genetic variations in toxicological and metabolic responses using probabilistic neural networks. Chem Res Toxicol, 14:182-191, 2001.
129. Robertson DG, Reily MD, Sigler RE, *et al.* Metabonomics: evaluation of nuclear magnetic resonance (NMR) and pattern recognition technology for rapid in vivo screening of liver and kidney toxicants. Toxicol Sci, 57:326-337, 2000.

Index